Medicare's Prescription Drug Pricing

Inflation, Challenges and Affordability

New York

Health Care in Transition Series

Tipping the Boundaries: Health and Well-Being of Sustainable Development
Sandeep Poddar, PhD
and Waliza Ansar, PhD (Editors)
ISBN: 979-8-89530-146-3
eBook ISBN: 979-8-89530-378-8

The Future of Universal Health Insurance
Seher Nur Sülkü
and Yağmur Tokatlıoğlu (Editors)
ISBN: 979-8-89530-107-4
eBook ISBN: 979-8-89530-192-0

Nursing Beyond Borders: The Indonesian Diaspora
Ferry Efendi, PhD,
Gading Ekapuja Aurizki, MSc and
Rifky Octavia Pradipta, M.Kep
eBook ISBN: 979-8-89113-859-9

Handbook of Data Analysis of Electronic Health Records (EHR) using SAS Software
Behrouz Ehsani-Moghaddam, PhD
ISBN: 979-8-88697-372-3
eBook ISBN: 979-8-88697-437-9

Mobile Health: Advances in Research and Applications – Volume II
Gaurav Gupta, PhD,
Varun Jaiswal, PhD,
Manju Khari, PhD
and Nagesh Kumar, PhD (Editors)
ISBN: 978-1-68507-988-8
eBook ISBN: 979-8-88697-247-4

Novel Perspectives in Economics of Personalized Medicine and Healthcare Systems
Marinko Škare, PhD,
Romina Pržiklas Družeta, PhD
and Sandra Kraljević Pavelić, PhD
(Editors)
ISBN: 978-1-68507-390-9
eBook ISBN: 978-1-68507-393-0

More information about this series can be found at
https://novapublishers.com/product-category/series/health-care-in-transition/

Lloyd M. Porter
Editor

Medicare's Prescription Drug Pricing

Inflation, Challenges and Affordability

snova
New York

NOTICE TO THE READER

The Publisher has taken reasonable care in the preparation of this book, but makes no expressed or implied warranty of any kind and assumes no responsibility for any errors or omissions. No liability is assumed for incidental or consequential damages in connection with or arising out of information contained in this book. The Publisher shall not be liable for any special, consequential, or exemplary damages resulting, in whole or in part, from the readers' use of, or reliance upon, this material. Any parts of this book based on government reports are so indicated and copyright is claimed for those parts to the extent applicable to compilations of such works.

Independent verification should be sought for any data, advice or recommendations contained in this book. In addition, no responsibility is assumed by the Publisher for any injury and/or damage to persons or property arising from any methods, products, instructions, ideas or otherwise contained in this publication.

The Publisher assumes no responsibility for any statements of fact or opinion expressed in the published contents.

This publication is designed to provide accurate and authoritative information with regard to the subject matter covered herein. It is sold with the clear understanding that the Publisher is not engaged in rendering legal or any other professional services. If legal or any other expert assistance is required, the services of a competent person should be sought. FROM A DECLARATION OF PARTICIPANTS JOINTLY ADOPTED BY A COMMITTEE OF THE AMERICAN BAR ASSOCIATION AND A COMMITTEE OF PUBLISHERS.

Additional color graphics may be available in the e-book version of this book.

Library of Congress Cataloging-in-Publication Data

ISBN: 979-8-89530-728-1 (Hardcover)
ISBN: 979-8-89530-803-5 (eBook)

Published by Nova Science Publishers, Inc. † New York

Contents

Preface

There is nothing in our health-care system as broken as the way Americans pay for their lifesaving medicines. This failed system has forced millions of Americans daily to make gut-wrenching decisions between medicines or other necessities of life. The drug companies have Americans over a barrel, with Medicare barred from negotiating better prices. This program represents tens of millions of seniors, and even more taxpayers, has to take on big pharma with both hands tied behind its back. The consequences are clear when you contrast the prices Americans pay with the prices in other countries.

Chapter 1

Prescription Drug Price Inflation: An Urgent Need to Lower Drug Prices in Medicare*

Committee on Finance

Wednesday, March 16, 2022
U.S. Senate, Committee on Finance,
Washington, DC.

The hearing was convened, pursuant to notice, at 10 a.m., via Webex, in Room SD–215, Dirksen Senate Office Building, Hon. Ron Wyden (chairman of the committee) presiding.

Present: Senators Stabenow, Carper, Cardin, Brown, Bennet, Casey, Whitehouse, Hassan, Cortez Masto, Warren, Crapo, Grassley, Cornyn, Portman, Toomey, Cassidy, Lankford, Daines, and Young.

Also present: Democratic staff: Raghav Aggrawal, Detailee; Shawn Bishop, Chief Health Advisor; Michael Evans, Chief Health Advisor; Anne Kaltenboeck, Senior Health Advisor; and Joshua Sheinkman, Staff Director. Republican staff: Kellie McConnell, Health Policy Director; Connor Sheehey, Health Policy Advisor; Gregg Richard, Staff Director; and Jeffrey Wrase, Deputy Staff Director and Chief Economist.

---

* This is an edited, reformatted and augmented version of Hearing Before the Committee on Finance United States Senate, Publication No. S. HRG. 117–809, dated March 16, 2022.

In: Medicare's Prescription Drug Pricing
Editor: Lloyd M. Porter
ISBN: 979-8-89530-728-1

Opening Statement of Hon. Ron Wyden, A U.S. Senator from Oregon, Chairman, Committee on Finance

The CHAIRMAN. We meet this morning because there is nothing in our health-care system as broken as the way Americans pay for their lifesaving medicines like insulin. This failed system has forced millions of Americans daily to make gut-wrenching decisions between medicines or other necessities of life.

The drug companies have Americans over a barrel, with Medicare barred from negotiating better prices. This program that represents tens of millions of seniors, and even more taxpayers, has to take on big pharma with both hands tied behind its back. The consequences are clear when you contrast the prices Americans pay with the prices in other countries.

In preparation for this hearing, the Finance Committee, our investigators, looked at pricing data for several of the most commonly prescribed brand-name drugs in Medicare. We looked at the prices of top-selling drugs in the United States and comparable Western countries, and we compared the figures from 2015 and 2020.

The list includes medications for conditions such as arthritis, diabetes, and cancer. In every case, colleagues, the U.S. price in 2015 started higher than the international price. In every case from 2015 to 2020, the U.S. price went up, while the international price remained flat.

In 2015, Americans had been paying two, three, even four times as much as international patients paid for these medications. By 2020, that gap has roughly doubled for many of the most expensive drugs.

Here is a specific example. I have a Humira pen. It contains one dose—one dose of a treatment for rheumatoid arthritis, Crohn's disease, and other autoimmune conditions—painful diseases that afflict millions of Americans. Patients typically inject one of these pens every 2 weeks. As of 2020, the price per pen in Quebec, Canada, was $563. List price in the United States was $2,778.

Americans see this infuriating price gouging, and it is clear that big pharma is treating Medicare like they have cracked an ATM. Prescription drugs in Medicare may be the only case across the entire government where negotiating a better price is actually legally prohibited. It is long past time for that to change.

Democrats have a plan that would finally allow Medicare to negotiate for lower prices for brand names and refocus on the costliest products, the ones that monopolize the market. In addition, our plan would cap co-pays for insulin at $35 a prescription. It would set a $2,000 out-of-pocket cap for seniors' medications in Medicare Part D and spread those costs over the year, instead of front-loading them all in January. It also would create tough new price-gouging penalties for drug companies that raise prices faster than inflation, and there are a lot of companies that did that early this year.

A number of these ideas were developed in this committee with bipartisan support, and that remains. However, there is just no substitute, none, for the number one reform, which is allowing Medicare to negotiate like any other payer. Without negotiation, the job is just not done.

For example, setting out-of-pocket caps without negotiation just passes the price on to somebody else, and that is usually taxpayers. That is not sustainable. It just puts more pressure on Medicare's finances in the long run.

Unfortunately for American patients, Mitch McConnell has blocked any changes—even the proposals that had bipartisan support—and repeated big pharma's talking points against real reform.

The drug companies say that allowing negotiation—and you will hear this today—is bad for the market; Western civilization is pretty much going to end; it will not be possible to have pharmaceutical innovation any longer. That claim does not hold up to scrutiny, and we will be looking at it today. First of all, it is true that pharmaceutical companies do develop breakthrough treatments. It is also true that most of the so-called new drugs released at higher and higher prices are actually older drugs, but they have just been re-packaged in new ways. A relatively minor tweak to an old drug, say a different syringe or a change in dosage, just keeps the profits rolling in.

And second, a large and growing percentage of American seniors ration their medications or skip them entirely because they are just too expensive. Almost half the cancer patients, many of them on Medicare, burn through all their savings within 2 years.

If the prescription drug market prices out millions of patients and bankrupts many others, how can anybody say that is healthy or functional for our country? I am here to tell you the scandal is what is legal. Today big pharma has a legal right to set whatever prices they wish and expect Medicare to pay them.

Drug companies can game the system and maintain monopolies and protect their best cash cows. Without fail, the Republican leadership controlling the agenda for their party and Congress is out there protecting the status quo. That is a recipe to stifle innovation, not promote it.

As we meet this morning, there are people all over the country who know that they are going to get mugged every time they show up at the pharmacy counter. High drug prices force people to have to make terrible choices. Far too often, choosing your health also means choosing hunger.

I am going to close with this. The American people have waited too long for action. This has been the longest-running battle since the Trojan War. And the country has heard and told us what this is all about.

So, it is time for action. Democrats have a plan. We need to act quickly.

I want to thank our witnesses, and of course our friend Senator Crapo will be recognized now for his opening remarks.

[The prepared statement of Chairman Wyden appears in the appendix.]

Opening Statement of Hon. Mike Crapo, A U.S. Senator from Idaho

Senator CRAPO. Thank you, Mr. Chairman, and thank you to all of our witnesses for being here today.

Congress plays an important role in ensuring access to affordable prescription drugs for Americans from all walks of life. To that end, last year I reintroduced the Lower Costs, More Cures Act. This comprehensive legislation contains dozens of concrete proposals aimed at lowering out-of-pocket costs at the pharmacy counter, in addition to strengthening supply chain oversight, and combating foreign freeloading.

With inflation at 40-year highs straining family finances for far too many Americans, the Lower Costs, More Cures Act would bring peace of mind to seniors across the Nation by placing a hard cap on out-of-pocket drug spending under Medicare Part D.

Our bill would allow beneficiaries to access additional Part D plan choices, including low-deductible and reduced cost-sharing options, as well as plans that pass more discounts on directly to consumers at the pharmacy counter.

For seniors with diabetes, we would build on the work of the Trump administration, which established a game-changing program that guarantees access to insulin at no more than $35 a month. Our legislation would permanently protect and extend this initiative, which already covers more than two in every five seniors enrolled in Part D.

Nearly 2 decades ago, I joined bipartisan majorities in both chambers in voting to enact Medicare's prescription drug benefit. Since then, Part D has achieved incredible success, coming in at half of its projected cost, with stable premiums, high satisfaction rates, and more than 50 plan options for the average enrollee.

The Lower Costs, More Cures Act would build on these successes, advancing scores of pro-patient solutions for Medicare and the broader prescription drug market. Our legislation would strengthen cost-comparison tools, remove disincentives for prescribing lower-cost medications, enlist a Chief Pharmaceutical Negotiator to drive better trade deals for Americans, and facilitate outcomes-based arrangements for cutting-edge therapies, to name just a few provisions.

Importantly, all of these solutions could pass both chambers of Congress with overwhelming support. Virtually every provision in the Lower Costs, More Cures Act reflects a bipartisan proposal with broad buy-in across the political spectrum.

This bill, if allowed to advance, could head to the President's desk within days, delivering meaningful relief to Americans. Unfortunately, all signs seem to indicate a partisan path forward on drug pricing based on the deeply problematic policies included in the House-passed Build Back Better Act.

These proposals would impose bureaucratic government price controls with a host of bad consequences for consumers, patients, and small businesses. According to a recent study from the University of Chicago researchers, innovative R&D would decline by nearly one-fifth under these proposed price controls, leading to a staggering 135 fewer new drug approvals in the next 2 decades.

Another report found that Medicare payments for physicians and other front-line health-care providers would also fall under the proposed government price-setting program with add-on payments slashed by an average of 40 percent for those targeted.

These policies, which borrow from the failed experiments of the past, would do nothing to tame inflation. In fact, they would trigger a launch price increase for new medications. By enacting these drug price controls, we would hand a competitive edge to our global rivals, including the Chinese Communist Party.

At home, we would see fewer new treatments and cures, higher prices for new drugs, more health-care provider strain and burnout, and an alarming expansion of the Federal bureaucracy, giving Washington, DC more control again over our health-care system.

We have a responsibility to pursue solutions that reduce out-of- pocket drug spending, particularly for seniors. The Lower Costs, More Cures Act provides a practical blueprint for this type of initiative, leveraging targeted policies with bipartisan backing to address the needs of Americans at the pharmacy counter, the hospital, and the doctor's office.

In the weeks ahead, we should move toward consensus-driven legislation with broad buy-in, rather than partisan price controls likely to double down on the most deficient aspects of our health- care system. We also need to identify policies that tackle the root causes and drivers of inflation, which rose to a staggering 7.9 percent year over year last month.

This means reducing our crippling deficit, unleashing American energy, streamlining costly regulations that have strained small businesses, and protecting the tax reforms implemented under the Tax Cuts and Jobs Act of 2017, which led to record-high levels of business investment, historic lows in unemployment and poverty, and record-high incomes during the past administration.

With that, I thank our witnesses again for joining us to testify today, and thank you, Mr. Chairman.

[The prepared statement of Senator Crapo appears in the appendix.]

The CHAIRMAN. I thank my colleague. I am just going to make one quick point and go to the witnesses.

Our colleague talked about Part D of Medicare being the answer. I was one of the Democrats who crossed the aisle and voted for Part D. I took a lot of flak for it too. The problem was, and why we are here, it tied the government's hands behind its back to be able to negotiate better prices. We're glad to get the coverage. Today is about getting price relief to those seniors from sea to shining sea who are getting clobbered with these prices that go through, whether it is Humira, insulin, or a variety of others.

Let's go to our witnesses. Let me introduce them briefly. Professor Rena Conti, Ph.D., is associate professor of markets, public policy, and law in the School of Business at Boston University. She has done extensive research in the economics of the prescription drug market. She is a co-director of the Technology Policy and Research Institute, and between 2006 and 2018, Professor Conti was faculty at the University of Chicago.

The committee's next witness will be Dr. Douglas Holtz-Eakin, president of the American Action Forum. Prior to founding the organization, he was the Chief Economist of the President's Council of Economic Advisors, and he also served there as a senior staff economist. He was also Director of the

Congressional Budget Office and has done extensive research in economic policy in a variety of areas.

Then we have Mr. Stephen Ezell. He is the vice president of global innovation at the Information Technology and Innovation Foundation. He focuses on science and technology policy, and has also studied the practice of innovation in a variety of industries.

Finally, Steffany Stern, MPP, is currently the National Multiple Sclerosis Society vice president of advocacy. She works in this role with volunteers across the country to make sure that folks with MS are heard. The Society is the largest private organization supporting MS research globally, and provides a range of services for people affected by MS. And I know how valuable that is, having just talked with your mother as well about having to navigate the Byzantine system of trying to get help, and we will discuss that.

Let's go right to our witnesses, and we will make your prepared remarks a part of the record in their entirety.

And why don't we begin with you, Dr. Conti?

Statement of Rena Conti, Ph.D., Associate Professor, Department of Markets, Public Policy, and Law, Questrom School of Business, Boston University, Boston, MA

Dr. CONTI. Thank you so much. Chairman Wyden, Ranking Member Crapo, and members of the committee, it is my honor to speak with you today.

I am Rena Conti. I am an economist at Boston University's Questrom School of Business. I have studied and taught the pharmaceutical industries for the better part of 2 decades.

I am here to explain to you why proposals to reduce drug prices will not harm innovation. Prior debates on how to make drugs more affordable have been weighed down by unproven industry claims that reducing drug prices will also reduce the number of new cures. These claims are greatly exaggerated, particularly for negotiation. Our system balances innovation with competition. Negotiation will modestly reduce revenues for companies selling a small number of very high-priced and old drugs. These drugs are targeted for negotiation because their companies took excessive price increases for years, have harmed patients, and have forestalled competition. These behaviors go directly against the fundamentals of our system.

Here is why the industries' claims do not hold.

First, the independent Congressional Budget Office estimates that under reforms currently discussed, the number of drugs that would be introduced into the U.S. market would be reduced by one in the 1st decade, approximately four in the subsequent decades, and approximately five over the decade after that.

In the same time period, under current law approximately 1,300 new drugs will be approved. Thus, proposed reforms will result in a minimal loss of new drugs amounting to less than a tenth of 1 percent under conservative assumptions.

Second, new drugs are not the same as new breakthroughs. Yet CBO's score counts all new drugs the same, without regard for improvements in disease symptoms, quality of life, or survival benefits.

Third, new breakthroughs come from new science. Taxpayers support the type of new science that empirical research demonstrates brings new, transformative drugs to market. These include Gleevec, tezeplumab, and paclitaxel, which have all transformed the lives of persons living with cancer.

Taxpayers also support robust financing to develop new drugs. The pandemic is expected to pump another $80 billion into this industry in excess of pre-pandemic production. Last week's omnibus increased the NIH budget too. Current proposals do not reduce funding to the NIH, basic science carried out by universities, nor will they reduce support for university spinouts or company startups.

Consequently, paying jobs in the world's most successful biotech corridors such as Boston, New Jersey, and Pennsylvania, should remain stable.

Fourth, pharmaceutical companies strongly prefer to launch new drugs in the U.S., where they fetch the highest prices. Yet, inflated prices on existing drugs simply pad corporate balance sheets. They do not relate to the public's better health.

Why should Americans continue to pay more for their prescriptions as a consequence of such bad behavior? The reforms that members of the committee are considering would reestablish the social compacts between the American public and pharmaceutical companies. They are pro-innovation and pro-consumer.

The pharmaceutical industry is the most profitable sector of the U.S. economy. They are staffed with exceptional scientists. Thus, you should feel confident knowing that when these companies are forced to compete by innovating, they rise to the moment. Look at COVID.

Change has come to this industry in the past, and they have thrived. Under the proposed reforms, the U.S. will remain the most highly supportive of innovative activity and the largest market for pharmaceuticals in the world.

Under proposed reforms, it will remain the most profitable sector in our economy. In other words, contemplated reforms are likely to have the opposite effect on innovation.

Finally, detractors of reform minimize that real drug prices have real consequences for real seniors. Without reform, a third of Americans will remain unable to afford the drugs they need to stay alive, locked out of the benefits of existing innovation.

The proposed reforms will also benefit taxpayers, saving approximately $160 billion over the next 10 years. As a consequence, more than 80 percent of voters across the aisle want Congress to act now.

In sum, proposed reforms, including Medicare negotiation, inflation caps, and pricing redesign, represent a modest but decisive step towards limiting the economic burden of inflated drug prices placed on patients. With these reforms, Congress will restore the social compact between pharmaceutical companies and the American public so that we can all benefit from the fruits of innovation without going broke.

Thank you so much for your attention.

[The prepared statement of Dr. Conti appears in the appendix.] The CHAIRMAN. Thank you very much.

Let's go to Dr. Holtz-Eakin.

Statement of Douglas Holtz-Eakin, PhD., President, American Action Forum, Washington, DC

Dr. HOLTZ-EAKIN. Chairman Wyden, Ranking Member Crapo, and members of the committee, thank you for the privilege of being here today.

Let me make a few points at the outset. Number one is that one should not conflate high prescription drug prices, or the pricing of pharmaceuticals in general, with the economy-wide consumer price inflation which we are experiencing right now.

First of all, prescription drugs are not the driver of the economy- wide consumer price inflation. Prescription drugs went up year to year 2.4 percent in the Consumer Price Index. Overall, it was up 7.9 percent year over year. The kinds of policies we are discussing today would have a one-time impact on the level of prescription drug prices, and not impact the overall growth rate over a long period of time. And most of the proposals would be phased in over time and would have no immediate impact in 2022, little impact in 2023, and those are the years that matter for households who are facing a combined 8.4-percent increase in the food, energy, and shelter components of their budgets, and that is over 50 percent of most household spending.

So this hearing is not really about that problem. It is about prescription drugs.

The second point is that the idea of negotiation by the government for Part D, I think, is an important issue. I was the CBO Director during the passage of the Medicare Modernization Act, and I wrote letters, and my successors wrote letters, indicating that in the absence of something else, giving the Secretary of HHS the power to, quote, "negotiate" would have little impact on the overall level of prescription drug prices in Part D.

That something else you needed was a formulary and thus, telling America's seniors they cannot have some drugs, or another instrument of some sort. The instrument in this case is a Draconian tax of up to 95 percent on the domestic revenues of those firms that are somehow not negotiating in good faith, where the Secretary gets to decide when that is. That is not a negotiation, and no one should confuse this with negotiation.

This is a government price-setting mechanism that will reach into every corner of the health-care sector, and government price- setting mechanisms have a long track record of having unintended consequences and being detrimental.

In this case—and this is the third point—I will politely disagree with Dr. Conti. These would be counterproductive proposals. Drug development is an extremely risky business. Only about 80 percent of those drugs that enter trials ever make it to market. It takes 10 years and about $3 billion to develop the drug. And if you cut off the payoff to development of those drugs, you will get less drug development.

The only question is, how much less. But the direction is unmistakable. And the notion of inflation taxes, which would, again in the commercial market as well as in the Medicare and Medicaid spaces, just lead to higher launch prices, and perversely, at the moment—with prescription drug inflation at 2.4 percent, and overall inflation at 8 percent—it is an invitation for drug companies to raise the prices more than they would otherwise. I do not think that is what we want. A classic case of unintended consequences. My final point is that there are things about which there is agreement across the aisle and among those who have studied this area, and which would provide some benefits. And they are Part D redesigns. The redesigns share some key features; number one, for the first time, we would cap the exposure of seniors' out-of-pocket expenses. That is a very desirable thing to do.

Number two, we can protect the taxpayer from picking up the bulk of the cost in the Part D program by shifting responsibility in the reinsurance area to the manufacturers and the prescription drug plans. That has the additional benefit of giving them incentives to keep seniors from getting into that region of the benefit. That means lower prices. That means utilization management. And it gives you an incentive for stronger price negotiations among the private firms, which has been the foundation of Part D's success over the years.

This is a benefit that everyone points out came in cheaper than I thought it would be by 40 percent. That is true. And it has been a tribute to the power of the private negotiations. Strengthening those incentives would be a good thing to do at this time.

So I think the risk of dramatic changes with unintended consequences is real. We could make a Part D redesign and see what we can get from that—it is a big chunk of the national drug spend—and then do further reforms for targeted problems as they arise.

Thank you for the chance to be here, and I look forward to your questions.

[The prepared statement of Dr. Holtz-Eakin appears in the appendix.]

The CHAIRMAN. Thank you.

And just very, very briefly on one point. Dr. Holtz-Eakin says that CBO has indicated negotiation does not save money. Now the old analysis, this outdated analysis, seemed to indicate that there would be modest savings. That study, however, is completely out of date. And what our new effort does—and this is the heart of the case—is we have enforcement in it, and our plan for Medicare negotiation now has real teeth to keep drug companies at the negotiating table. And what is relevant, so that the committee understands it, is not the outdated estimate of savings that Dr. Holtz- Eakin has talked about, but CBO is now estimating very, very substantial savings, billions of dollars in terms of negotiation.

Mr. Ezell?

Statement of Stephen J. Ezell, Vice President, Global Innovation Policy, Information Technology and Innovation Foundation, Washington, DC

Mr. EZELL. Good morning, Chairman Wyden, Ranking Member Crapo, and members of the committee. I appreciate the opportunity to testify this morning.

The United States leads the world in biopharmaceutical innovation. In fact, over the past 2 decades, drug companies in America have delivered just under half of the world's new drugs. It is therefore imperative we preserve the broad policy environment that has been so successful in making America the world leader, especially at a time when we are looking to turn the page on a 3-year pandemic and gear up for a Cancer Moonshot.

To that end, I would like to address three themes this morning: first, the contention that drug prices are rising significantly; second, that drug prices constitute a major contributor to inflation; and third, that drug price controls would not harm new drug development or patients' access to medicines.

First, drug expenditures for retail prescriptions as a share of America's total health expenditures have been roughly stable for the past 2 decades at about 9 percent of total health-care cost. Projections suggest they will remain stable for the rest of this decade. Moreover, U.S. pharmaceutical spending as a share of total health expenditures is right in line with those of OECD nations, and in fact, most others are higher. Nor are prices rising significantly. In fact, the Bureau of Labor Statistics finds that over the past 15 years, American consumer expenditures on health care overall almost doubled, but their expenditures on drugs actually went down by 8 percent. Likewise, drug prices are not driving today's inflation. Over the past year, prescription drug prices have risen only 2.4 percent, just one-third of the increase in the Consumer Price Index. Meanwhile, drug innovation is becoming ever more risky, expensive, difficult, and transformative. Deloitte reports that the average cost of creating a new drug has doubled over the past decade, now surpassing $2.5 billion.

Yet, despite the fact that America's biopharmaceutical sector— the world's single most R&D-intensive industry—plowed 24 percent of its revenues back into R&D every year, the sector's R&D productivity has been steadily declining. That is because these companies are working to tackle still unsolved challenges at the frontiers of biomedical science, such as trying to develop solutions for diseases like Alzheimer's, Parkinson's, and pancreatic cancer.

Life sciences companies depend on revenues earned from one generation of innovation to finance investment towards the next generation of innovation. Yet drug price controls constrain the ability to earn those revenues. This is why virtually all academic studies find that a reduction in drug revenues leads to decreases in future research and new drug discoveries. For instance, one study found that a 1-percent reduction in revenue leads on average to a 1.5-percent decrease in R&D investment. Applying that to the drug price control provisions in the Build Back Better Act, it suggests that America may have as many as 135 fewer new drugs by 2039. Americans consistently enjoy access to innovative drugs earlier and more extensively than citizens of countries employing extensive drug price controls. For instance, of about 350 new medicines launched globally since 2011, 310 are available to American patients. But less than half are available to Canadians. In other words, if you are a Canadian, your medicine cabinet is just half as full as if you are an American.

Now that is similar in Germany, France, and Japan. And speaking of those nations, the extensive drug price controls they implemented in the 1980s and 1990s decimated their biopharmaceutical industries. That is one reason why Japan's share of the global pharmaceutical industry cratered by 70 percent over the past 25 years.

Instead of applying broad price controls, policymakers should focus on promoting affordability, especially through mitigating out- of-pocket costs for individuals, especially seniors. That is why ITIF supports many of the Medicare Part D cost-control proposals, including implementing a $2,000 cap on beneficiaries' annual out-of-pocket costs, as well as monthly caps on patient expenses for drugs treating chronic conditions, like insulin for diabetes.

Further, the Federal Government needs to focus on costs, not just prices. Here it would do well for policymakers to consider how to help increase R&D and production efficiencies, including by launching a significant new effort to assist the private sector in increasing their efficiency in drug discovery, development, and manufacturing.

In conclusion, while there are some issues to address regarding drug pricing, what is needed is reform, not wholesale transformation. Widespread drug price controls would almost certainly reduce America's biopharmaceutical competitiveness against China, and slow the rate of new drug developments.

Thank you.

[The prepared statement of Mr. Ezell appears in the appendix.] The CHAIRMAN. Thank you very much.

Ms. Stern?

Statement of Steffany Stern, MPP, Vice President of Advocacy, National Multiple Sclerosis Society, Minneapolis, MN

Ms. STERN. Chairman Wyden, Ranking Member Crapo, and members of this committee, my name is Steffany Stern, and I am the vice president of advocacy for the National Multiple Sclerosis Society.

I joined the Society as a staff member 7 years ago, but I have been part of the MS community since I was a year old in 1981 when my mom was diagnosed with MS. Until 1993, there were no treatment options for MS. All my mom could do was try to take care of herself and hope that her relapses did not take away too much from her life.

While we now have effective treatments, people with MS and their families, like my parents, struggle with drug prices. My parents moved to a smaller house, replaced their cars with less expensive options, and have cut every possible corner to make ends meet. My dad is 69 years old, and he has his own health challenges. And he has had to get a job driving a city bus in town just to pay the bills. Without the charitable assistance that they receive, they could not pay the $2,400 they owe for her medication month after month.

It just seems wrong to us that people with health-care coverage still need charitable assistance. And my parents are not alone. It is extraordinarily personal to publicly share one's personal financial and health challenges, but person after person has given me permission to do so because they want you to understand and to change the status quo. And I sit here in front of you representing all of them.

The first, most troubling fact that I want to share with you is that 40 percent of people with MS surveyed by the MS Society alter the use of their disease-modifying therapies, which we call DMTs, due to cost, including stopping, skipping, or delaying their treatments.

For example, Laurie Lee from Oregon changed her MS medication twice after joining Medicare because the price would have bankrupted her and her husband. During these changes, Laurie's MS symptoms increased substantially and she transitioned from the relapsing form of MS to the progressive form of the disease.

Therese Humphrey Ball in Indiana was forced to change the DMTs after her costs soared to $6,000 a month. But the next DMT she went on did not work for Therese. Her MS progressed, bringing lingering cognitive issues among other problems.

And Bob Miller in Minnesota made the difficult decision to stop taking his MS drug altogether because he did not want to financially devastate his family, even though he has Medicare.

These kinds of choices are terrifying for people with MS. Any gaps in their medication could mean disease progression, and that could mean a permanent loss of mobility or cognitive function.

A significant percentage of people with MS report stress or emotional impacts, and they make lifestyle sacrifices to afford their DMT. Medicare out-of-pocket medication expenses for Lisa McRipley in Michigan average a debilitating $9,000 a year. She often uses her charge cards to cover the costs and relies on her family to pay for food and other expenses.

Wayne Harven in South Carolina has to take $13,000 out of his 401(k) every year to cover his share of Medicare costs. I could be here all day telling stories.

Early and ongoing treatment with a DMT is the best way to manage MS and prevent the accumulation of disabilities. More than 20 MS DMTs have transformed the treatment of MS over the last 29 years. Or more accurately, they have transformed the treatment for those who can afford it.

We call on this committee to bring forth legislation to enact a Medicare out-of-pocket cap and smoothing mechanism to spread patients' costs throughout the year. But just those policies are not enough.

The first medication my mom took in the mid-1990s was priced at $11,000. Today the price of that same DMT is over $111,000. Her current medication has a list price of nearly $104,000 per year. This medication's price has increased 5.7 percent in the last year, and 35 percent over the last 5 years.

In February 2022, the median annual price of brand MS DMTs was close to $94,000, an increase of nearly $34,000 in less than 10 years. Six of the MS DMTs have increased in price more than 200 percent since they came on the market. Nine are now priced over $100,000. Medications on the market for more than 20 years still have annual price increases. Patients are not only paying out of pocket but more in premiums for their drug coverage due to the costs of their medications.

The current system is not working in the best interests of people with MS and other chronic conditions. It is unconscionable that in 2022 people with MS and other health conditions who cannot pay for their medications would be in the same position my mom was in in 1982 with no treatment options.

We strongly believe that Medicare negotiation and inflationary rebates, along with out-of-pocket caps, strike that right balance between creating affordability and maintaining incentives for manufacturers to innovate.

We look forward to working with this committee as you work to address the high price of medications.

Thank you.

[The prepared statement of Ms. Stern appears in the appendix.]

The CHAIRMAN. Thank you very much, Ms. Stern. I really appreciated talking to your mom as well, because I walked away and said your mom's only sin was to get sick in a country where big pharma has never lost a fight. And we are going to be changing that. We are going to change that.

Let's start with Dr. Conti. Dr. Conti, you said Medicare negotiations and penalties for price inflation would not be harmful to consumers or the economics of the pharmaceutical industry. Your seatmate there, Dr. Holtz-Eakin, obviously feels differently—big difference of opinion.

What evidence do you have, Professor Conti, that Medicare negotiations and stopping price gouging when they are just scoring prices way above inflation, would not be harmful to consumers or the economics of the pharmaceutical sector?

Dr. CONTI. Thank you so much for the question. There are 2 decades of economic research suggesting that taxpayer support for basic science, intellectual property protections, and the financial market drive innovation, including work by Harvard-based economist Scott Stern and Berkeley economist Bronwyn Hall.

Taxpayer support for basic science, university labs, startup companies, et cetera, and the best financial ecosystem for investment in new products also do not change with this legislation.

We know from some of the work of Daniel Lee at MIT and my colleague at BU, Iain Cockburn, that with these types of continuing investments, innovation will follow. In addition, the U.S. supports Americans' access to drugs, the largest market for these products in the world—and the best-paying through insurance provisions. Insurance provisions such as Part B and Part D have clearly benefited consumers. Insurance provisions also drive innovation, according to the work of MIT-based economists Amy Finkelstein and Pierre Azoulay. Indeed, much of CBO's score on the impacts of this reform is based on an economic model of Part D implementation, where they find that expansions in insurance drive new product innovation.

David Dranove at Northwestern and Amy Finkelstein at MIT suggest that most of the new products that came from the expansion of Part D were not breakthroughs, but rather slight modifications of existing products in already-crowded therapeutic classes.

Professor Finkelstein's work, now validated by others, suggests that companies just simply took products off the shelf after the change.

The CHAIRMAN. Thank you, Dr. Conti.

Ms. Stern, let me go to you, because I thought all night—and I have been doing this since my days as director of the Gray Panthers, and I cannot recall a situation more infuriating than hearing your mom basically describe how you all have to beg charities to give you some extra help so she can pay her share of the $111,000 price tag that the manufacturer charges for the drug.

So you say to yourself, it's the company that escalates the prices way beyond what the rest of the world is paying, but then they are going to say to you and your mom, you guys have to beg—and she describes the situation where if she does not get the begging going at the right time, then things go by the boards and her husband is driving a bus. I mean, what in the hell is going on here?

This is not the debate of a technical issue. Something is way out of whack when people like your mom are begging for a little bit of help, which really is a lifeline for us. Tell the committee exactly how this works, and how—I mean, here you are. You are a professional in the field, and you are helping your mom. I ran a legal aid program for the elderly, the Gray Panthers, so I could help people. What are people going to do here, other than just beg and beg and beg to be able to get a lifesaving drug, or at some point I guess people just give up and pass.

Ms. STERN. Yes; so yes, it is a terrible situation. It is very common for people with MS, like my mom, to have to rely on some kind of financial assistance to afford their costs. Our studies show around 70 percent of people rely on financial assistance just so they can pay their out-of-pocket. But a lot of people are shocked when they transition to Medicare and they find they cannot get assistance from the drug companies anymore. They have to rely on these charitable funds. And the charitable funds are so hard to get into. They run out of money all the time. Last year they only opened four times for a total of 25 days. So you can call and call and call and still not get the help you need. And we have a lot of stories from people, like Ms. Dixon in Ohio in my testimony, who cannot navigate the process and go off of their meds.

It is a very draining process, and people with MS have a lot of fatigue and cognitive challenges. It is just unbelievable to have this system where people who have health coverage still have to chase down that financial help to afford their life-changing medication. And just as you said, my mom described it as just begging every year.

The CHAIRMAN. Yes. What is always striking is, members of this committee always hear from the industry that we need certainty and predictability. I certainly share that view. But it is time to give some certainty and predictability to folks like your mom who are going to know that they are not going to have to go through this water torture exercise just to get their medicine.

Thank you. Senator Crapo?

Senator CRAPO. Thank you, Mr. Chairman. It is becoming obvious that the whole focus here of the difference between us on how to proceed with regard to prescription drug pricing is over this notion of government price negotiation. I know that a number of my colleagues and other advocates of this approach call it Medicare negotiation. The reality is, it is government price controls. And we need to understand that.

I do not think that there is any disagreement that we need to strengthen the negotiation process over our drug pricing. There is an impression created by some that there is no negotiation going on with the drug companies, which is just flatly untrue. The negotiations today, though, are occurring in the private sector between the insurance plan providers and the drug producers and drug companies. And those negotiations need to be strengthened and improved so that we can really put true private-sector negotiation power into the development of price in our prescription drug markets, not the imposition of Federal price controls.

What we have seen right now, for those who want to have the government step in and control, is just what we saw when we did, under Obamacare, put so much more Federal control in place over the insurance industry, the plan providers. And what do we have now? We have very limited plan options. We have people with massive deductibles and copays. Their costs are being driven through the roof because there is not a truly functional private-sector approach to developing the best type of plans. And we are going to see the same type of thing in the prescription drug market if we go there.

I would like to direct my question to you, Dr. Holtz-Eakin. You mentioned that we do need to reform our negotiation system and have truly effective and powerful negotiation over drug prices. But that does not mean having government price controls—or that is what I heard you say.

And I referenced my legislation, the Lower Costs, More Cures legislation, which does exactly that. It seeks to try to reform the incentives and develop a pressure point so that we can move back toward having true, powerful, functional negotiations going on in the prescription drug system.

Could you discuss that a bit? And if you would like to, I invite you to respond, if you want to, to the chairman's comments about your reference to CBO's scoring.

Dr. HOLTZ-EAKIN. On the CBO scoring, the scoring was of genuine negotiations, telling the Secretary that he or she could call the manufacturer and start negotiating a price. That is not what I have seen in, for example, the House-passed Build Back Better Act, which begins with a statutory maximum of 40 to 75 percent of the average manufacturing price. A genuine negotiation does not start with a statutory price control. And then it is augmented by the quite Draconian sales tax of up to 95 percent, which just gives the Secretary disproportionate leverage. They are the judge and jury as to whether the negotiation is going well, and they can threaten the domestic markets for that firm. That does not strike me as negotiation. That is price controls.

With Part D, it would be a good idea, I think, to strengthen the private-sector negotiations, which have worked well, but which I think have been undercut a bit with developments over the years. We have seen, over time, that taxpayers are picking up the bulk of the cost, especially for very expensive patients. And so let's put the manufacturers and the prescription drug plans on the hook for those catastrophic costs so they have incentives to keep people out of the catastrophic region through managing the quantity and also the price of those prescription drugs. And certainly, having a maximum out-of-pocket for seniors solves a lot of the price problems we heard about from Ms. Stern.

I mean, this is a situation where you really can do a tremendous amount of good, and genuinely have it operate like an insurance product should. Those with extreme costs are protected, and those costs are distributed across a large population. That is what the Part D reforms, yours included, would do. And I will not pick favorites when I am out in front of you, but yours is great. And any of them, I think, will be a step in the right direction.

Senator CRAPO. Well, thank you for that.

And I will just conclude with a comment rather than another question. Again, I want to focus on the notion—there has been an effort to try to make it look like this is a debate over whether we should have negotiations in prescription drug pricing. That is not the issue.

We have negotiations now. They are not as good as they should be, and we need to provide the appropriate incentives in the private sector for those negotiations to work exactly as an insurance market should work and move those costs not only away from the taxpayer, but away from the seniors with provisions like those that are in the legislation I suggested—which I remind everybody has broad, bipartisan support.

We have got to get past this notion of having the government be put in charge of everything, including insurance policies—and how did that work for us—and pricing of prescription drugs. And it is not going to work for this, either. What will work is when we put the proper market incentives in place for the proper negotiation of drug pricing, and then include some of those caps on seniors out- of-pocket, and protections such as we have seen for the successful insulin drug pricing programs that we are already working on and are already working, as we talked about.

So, I just conclude with that, and thank you very much, Mr. Chairman.

The CHAIRMAN. Before we move to Senator Stabenow—and I will just be very brief—let's make sure we are clear on what is going on here.

Number one, the old analysis at CBO is no longer relevant. We have new estimates that indicate billions of dollars would be saved. Two, all we are talking about is saying that it is wrong for Medicare in this one area to be the only outlier to not be able to negotiate. Everybody else is negotiating. That I what this is about. Senator Stabenow?

Senator STABENOW. Well, thank you very much, Mr. Chairman and Ranking Member. And I have to say, I wish we had hours to debate this, because we are hearing the same old, same old about how we have to pay the highest prices in the world as Americans. And it just does not add up.

And in fact, Americans do pay the highest drug prices in the world. And it is not even close. We pay three times more for brand- name drugs, and every year it gets worse. That is a fact. According to AARP, over the past 15 years the price of the most common brand-name drugs has risen 300 percent. Yes. We are not talking about inflation; we are talking about way beyond what would be considered inflation.

Just since January, drug companies have increased the prices of nearly 800 different drugs. This is devastating for the financial and physical health of American families, especially our seniors. Imagine if other prices rose as fast as prescription drug prices over the last 15 years. Gas would be more than $12 a gallon—it is already too high. A movie ticket would be about $25. A gallon of milk would be more than $13. That is what's happening with prescription drugs. We would not accept that in any other area of the economy. Why in the world do we accept it from the drug companies?

The good news is, it does not have to be this way. You are going to hear a lot today from my Republican colleagues who say there are ways to cut costs, and negotiation is going on. I would suggest, based on the incredibly high prices, they are pretty bad negotiators.

In the end, their proposals are all about one thing: protecting the drug companies' profits at the expense of American consumers.

What we are proposing is very straightforward: allow Medicare to really start negotiating drug prices, like the VA does—and they pay 40 percent less for veterans; put in place a $2,000 out-of-pocket cap for seniors in Medicare Part D, a cap on insulin at $35 a month for everyone; penalize drug companies that raise prices faster than inflation. That is the plan. We will make sure seniors can afford the prescription drugs they need, and we will preserve and even strengthen the great engine of innovation in the country.

So, a simple question, Ms. Stern—and thank you so much for being here and representing people who really need a voice in this discussion. You said the first MS drug your mom used costs $100,000 more today than it did 30 years ago. Does the drug work any better today than it did 30 years ago?

Ms. STERN. No. It is my understanding that it is the same medication. I have heard they have made small tweaks to the injector, making it an auto-pen, but, no, it is the same medication.

Senator STABENOW. Yes, and that is true in so many areas. Insulin was actually discovered and developed 100 years ago—100 years ago.

So, Dr. Conti, let me just say first, thank you for being here, thank you to all of you. American taxpayers provide billions in research funding, as you said, for new treatments and cures every year, with tremendous results. And I support that strongly. In fact, taxpayer-funded research contributed to every single drug approved in the last decade. A House Oversight Committee investigation recently found that the leading 14 drug companies spent $577 billion on stock buy-backs and dividends—$56 billion more than they spent on research and development—between 2016 and 2020. The top 10 companies also paid their executives more than $2.2 billion—billion dollars—over the same period.

Dr. Conti, if we pass the reforms that I outlined, will there be less investment in innovation and treatments and cures?

Dr. CONTI. Thank you——

The CHAIRMAN. I don't think that mic is working. Can you speak right into it?

Dr. CONTI. I can. I am from Brooklyn, so I will just talk loud. The industry tries to separate public investments in research and development from the activities that they perform. However, this is just simply not the case. New drugs come from new science, and nothing about this proposal is going to alter the public support for new science. The transformative drugs that we have seen over the past 2 decades, their source is the NIH. These include, but are not limited to Gleevec, Avastin, paclitaxel, PrEP for HIV, and the new hepatitis C drugs, which are virtual cures.

Conversely, lost drugs do not mean lost therapies, as I stated before. The COVID vaccines and therapeutics are paradigmatic. We spent $39 billion bringing these products to the American consumer and ensuring that anyone who wants them can get them for free. Imagine, just 24 months ago they did not exist. We were locked in our homes.

Public Citizen among others has demonstrated that all of the science behind the MRNA vaccine for COVID–19 was supported by U.S. taxpayers. Much of it dates back to investments in the human genome project and continuing work for the next 20 years.

The reason the infection itself was so swiftly identified is because of the existence of open science pioneered by the U.S. Government. The vaccines have IP protections guaranteed by the U.S. Government, including their base ingredients.

Private money poured in. Why? Because the U.S. Government assures that that investment will get paid back. It is less risky than it otherwise would be.

The CHAIRMAN. Thank you very, very much, professor, for making those important points.

Senator Grassley?

Senator GRASSLEY. I am going to submit my questions for the record, and speak only.

[The questions appear in the appendix.]

Senator GRASSLEY. First of all, I thank you very much for holding this hearing, the first of this Congress. I am disappointed that the entire Senate is not moving on a bipartisan bill that will get 60-plus votes.

Three years ago, I led an effort on this committee to lower drug costs. We brought in pharmacy CEOs, PBMs, and insurance executives and advocates and experts. And we did it to discuss this problem and to seek solutions. We introduced bipartisan legislation. We marked that legislation up and, throughout the last Congress, we continued to make improvements in that legislation. And I suppose we could still say that there are some improvements that can be made.

Our bill contains stuff I liked, and it contains stuff that I didn't like, but that is the way the bipartisan process works. When we first passed the Medicare Modernization Act, we did it in a bipartisan way. Twelve Democrats in the Senate voted for it, including two members currently on this committee. At the time, this was the first major improvement in the Medicare program in nearly 40 years. Today, 49 million seniors have prescription drug coverage.

Eighteen years later, we have a growing problem: prescription drug affordability. AARP says brand-name drugs are going up more than twice the rate of inflation. Estimates suggest 31⁄2 million seniors are having difficulty affording their prescription drugs. The Kaiser report says 50 percent of the Part D drugs and 48 percent of the Part B drugs had price increases greater than inflation.

At our July 2019 Wyden-Grassley markup, Senator Wyden said this, quote: "Who is going to come first, patients and taxpayers or the pharmaceutical giants?", end of quote. That is still a legitimate statement.

If the majority keeps debating partisan ideas, however, on the issue of drug pricing, we will get nowhere. And then what? Pharma will win, and patients and taxpayers will lose.

I urge my colleagues to work with me to pass Wyden-Grassley. It caps out-of-pocket expenses at $3,100. It eliminates the donut hole. It caps rising drug prices in Medicare at the inflation price index, ending uncapped taxpayer-funded subsidies to big pharma. It brings more sunshine and accountability as well.

It saves $72 billion for seniors, $95 billion for taxpayers. Each one of these things is a very big deal. I share my colleague's passion for solving high insulin costs. I have investigated insulin makers, and Wyden was right there with me when we did it together. We also investigated PBMs and worked to hold all of these accountable.

If we want to settle the high drug costs of insulin, we have to pass comprehensive reform like Wyden-Grassley. Let's work to advance a bipartisan drug pricing bill that can pass with 60-plus votes. I continue to meet with Democrats and Republicans to advance Wyden-Grassley. I will work with anyone who wants to pass this bipartisan legislation.

Just to show you that, while the Democrats were trying to pass prescription drug bills as part of Build Back Better—which now obviously, according to Manchin, is dead—I met last year with Pelosi, and I met last year with the House problem solvers group of 50 people. I met with the 10 Democrats who sent Pelosi a letter saying we need a bipartisan bill, not a partisan approach. I met with McCarthy. I met with Peter Welch, a leader in that area. I met with McMorris Rodgers, and I think, in all of these efforts I said to them, you know, Wyden-Grassley is out of business if Democrats can pass a bill with 50 votes. But if you cannot pass the bill, I want you to know what is around that we can get through the United States Senate.

If we can get it through the U.S. Senate, you ought to be able to get it through the House of Representatives.

So we need to be working on it, just on the chance—and I hope this happens—that we have a Republican Congress next time. But I think you suggested the difficulty of passing something like this in a Republican Congress. So you have an opportunity to do it right now, when Democrats and Republicans can work together to accomplish this. If we want to reduce drug prices, then we need to do it now.

Thank you.

The CHAIRMAN. I thank my colleague. And I am going to be very brief on this. There is no question that the committee came together in the last Congress and came up with a number of constructive, bipartisan reforms—period, full stop.

The problem is, if that is all you do—let's say you do not do anything other than the out-of-pocket cap. If you do not have the reform that we are talking about, the key reform, the ability to negotiate, what happens is, with an out-of-pocket cap, everything just gets shifted to everybody else, particularly the taxpayers.

So what we need to do is what everybody else in America does, which is hardball negotiation. And my colleague probably remembers, this country is overwhelmingly in favor of people being able to negotiate. Sometimes when I am home and I ask people, "Anybody here opposed to negotiation?", I walk away and say that anybody who opposes it in my home State must be in a witness protection program, because I cannot find anybody who is against negotiation.

So that is what this debate is about. We have the bipartisan reform from before, but if we do not have negotiation, then we have what we pursued in the last session, and the cost-shifting will be massive and taxpayers and consumers will get hurt.

Senator Cornyn?

Senator CORNYN. One person's negotiation is another person's price controls. Dr. Holtz-Eakin, why shouldn't we have price controls on prescription drugs? Isn't that a way to solve the cost problem?

Dr. HOLTZ-EAKIN. It will solve the cost problem in the near term, but it will have detrimental effects down the road, particularly on the innovation and competition in the pharmaceutical sector.

A great example of this debate is a $35 cap on insulin, which would end the innovation in insulin tomorrow. We would not see any advancements in insulin versus what we are seeing right now with one biosimilar, two authorized generics, and insulin prices down 6.2 percent over the past 3 years.

So create entry, create competition, and lower cost. That is the solution.

Senator CORNYN. Senator Stabenow mentioned the VA, but I note that the Veterans Administration leverages a closed formulary. In other words, they do not have the broad range of drugs that are available to seniors under Medicare Part D. Apparently, the VA would cover just about 52 percent of the top 200 Part D drugs, while Part D plans cover nearly three-quarters of that, on average. And that is the benefit of competition, as opposed to price controls. Is that correct, Doctor?

Dr. HOLTZ-EAKIN. I think that is right. The formulary has a powerful impact on the negotiations. There is no question about that. And people talk a lot about how other countries' prices are lower, but in many cases those countries simply say "no," and the drugs are not available. So you either pay in the form of a financial price or you pay in the form of a lack of access to modern therapies. But there is no cheap way through this.

Senator CORNYN. Well, I am amazed, as I think most Americans are, by American science and the ability of the drug companies to innovate. Operation Warp Speed produced a vaccine in a historically short period of time and helped us start bending the curve on COVID–19. And hopefully, it will ultimately restore us to some semblance of normalcy. So there is no question that we all benefit from the great science and innovation in the drug industry. And of course we grant, under our patent laws, we grant exclusive rights to a drug that somebody comes up with for a period of time. But then of course, that patent expires, and then it is open to generic or other competition.

I think there are things we could do that would enhance the competitive nature of the generic drug market if we could just beat back some of the gamesmanship when it comes to the patent system.

Senator Wyden mentioned Humira, which has, to my knowledge, more than 120 different patents designed to create what has come to be known as a "patent thicket." And that makes it less likely that competitive generic companies can compete with that drug as they do, for example, in Europe today to the benefit of the consumers.

Senator Blumenthal and I had a bill called the Affordable Prescriptions for Patients Act, which addressed the patent thicket issue, and the product hopping, which is another aspect of it where you tweak the formula a little bit and then basically it prevents generic competitors from competing with that drug.

Unfortunately, we tried last year before the general election to get that passed in the Senate several times, since it did have broad bipartisan support, and for some reason unbeknownst to me, Senator Schumer objected to the unanimous consent request in the Senate. Unfortunately, it seems like we end up talking about problems more than we do trying to solve the problems.

But let me ask you, Dr. Holtz-Eakin, one of the other aspects of our drug pricing system that just is mystifying, I think to most of us, is the rebate system and the perverse incentives that can be created. So you have a list price, but then the drug company will actually kick back some money, and so the actual price is lower and presumably will help lower the insurance premium for the plan that covers that drug.

For example, insulin prices have been noted. The list prices have been growing over the years, and the net price has stayed stable or fallen because of higher rebates by PBMs to get on formulary. But for example, Sanofi has noted that in 2021 49 percent of their gross sales were given back in rebates. At the same time, Viatris launched an interchangeable biosimilar to Sanofi's Lantus and needed to have two price points, one to get on formulary and a significantly lower price for the uninsured. But it seems like that is a perverse incentive for manufacturers to continue to raise list prices to continue patient access.

Can you talk briefly—because my time is up, Dr. Holtz-Eakin— about other misaligned incentives in this space that contribute to higher drug prices?

Dr. HOLTZ-EAKIN. Well, I certainly would be happy to give you a longer answer for the record, but I think, briefly, there was a debate about passing those rebates through to consumers, which would have some real advantages. You would be negotiating, not over the list and rebates, but over the net price to the consumer. And that is what the coinsurance and the copays are coming off of. That would be beneficial, but it would have the detrimental effect, in the eyes of some, of raising premiums. But again, you are shifting the cost from a very few seniors with extremely high drug bills to the broad population. That is what insurance is supposed to do. So, directing indirect remunerations the same way, rebates, you can either redesign the insurance contracts—we have seen what it is like for the government to manage the insurance designs—or you could change the nature of the competition between the PBMs and the manufacturers.

Senator CORNYN. It still seems like a shell game, Mr. Chairman. Thank you.

The CHAIRMAN. Again, as I laid out with Senator Grassley, we tried in the last Congress to get sensible bipartisan reforms. Mitch McConnell opposed those. Now we have the chance to end the shell game, to really stop, say, when you limit out-of-pocket expenses, having the cost shifted.

So I am for getting rid of the shell game, and that is what we are doing in our legislation.

I believe our next questioner will be Senator Cardin.

Senator CARDIN. Thank you, Mr. Chairman. I just really want to underscore the point that you have made. We always look to work together to solve problems on this committee, and I appreciate the leadership of our chairman and ranking member, who have worked to try to bring us together on these issues.

I must tell you, on prescription drugs I am baffled, because the United States is an outlier. What we pay for the cost of medicines is just out of step with the industrial world. And it defies common sense, as the chairman has pointed out, that the Federal Government is the largest payer for prescription drugs—we have the largest market share—and Medicare, which is the largest program, cannot negotiate price. That just does not make sense.

If I am a business owner and I have a market share that I can leverage for price, I leverage it for price. That is how the free market works. And we are now restricting the free market from operating the way the free market is supposed to operate by a prohibition from Medicare to be able to use that market share to negotiate price.

It is just counterintuitive and makes no sense whatsoever. And then we hear the argument on innovation. And we take a look at the amount of funds that go into research in this country to develop new drugs, and the Federal Government is one of the largest providers of research dollars, over $40 billion a year. And the pharmaceutical industry—and they make their own judgments—spends more on advertising than they do on research. So I just do not get the argument.

And lastly on this issue, Mr. Chairman, if a consumer cannot get access to a drug because it is high-priced and they cannot afford it, they are not getting the benefits of innovation.

So, for all those reasons, I think it is just common sense that we need to unleash the power of the government to negotiate fair prices, and no longer for the United States' consumers to be outliers as far as the costs of medicines go.

I want to ask a different question, though, on an area that has me baffled also, and that is drug shortages. The pharmaceutical industry makes a lot of money. There is a lot of money spent in America. We manufacture the drugs here. And yet we have drug shortages, and not inconsequential drugs. A lot of the sterile injectables are in short supply. We had shortages in the prescription drops that are put in a newborn baby's eye in order to prevent infection. They were not available for a while. BCG, which is a treatment for bladder cancer, an inexpensive drug, is not available because of various factors. As I understand it, it is mostly single-sourced, and it is not a very profitable drug. That is, it does not cost a lot of money, so therefore they use the manufacturing capacity to make more money, causing a shortage of essential drugs here in America.

And considering that the Federal Government programs are the largest single source of funds going into the pharmaceutical industry, can't we at least guarantee to American consumers that we will have adequate supplies here to leverage the government participation in the programs?

So I welcome any thoughts. Let me start with Dr. Conti; your thoughts on this issue as to how we can reform the way that we deal with prescription drug costs and also make sure that there is adequate supply in this country.

Dr. CONTI. Thank you so much for that question. As you know, I spent a long time studying this issue. Drug shortages are indeed a problem for American consumers, and they are also problems for the other persons in the supply chain, most notably hospitals. They impose costs on people in many different ways.

I think we have an issue related to supply chain resilience in the U.S. for low-cost generic drugs that do not have much supply left. And there is a series of recommendations to support increasing the U.S. drug supply resiliency, which includes reshoring and nearshoring drug supply into the U.S., making sure that these products are made in the U.S. so that the products can be better accessed. We also may have to support more innovative manufacturing for these products. We already have some new companies coming into the market to do so. And then lastly, we simply may have to pay more to ensure that these products are adequately supplied.

Senator CARDIN. Thank you.

Thank you, Mr. Chairman.

The CHAIRMAN. I thank my colleague. I think we are waiting for others to come.

I just want to come back to what constitutes a negotiation and innovation. I think Dr. Conti said it very well. But let me even simplify this.

A negotiation, a Medicare negotiation, is just that. It is a negotiation process, not some sort of price control. It is a market-based approach to come to a price between purchaser, Medicare, and a producer. And it is not setting prices. What we are doing is, we are asking manufacturers to prove their product's value, and to earn their keep. That is what this is about.

So I have seen, particularly some of my colleagues on the other side, go to considerable labors to say that every negotiation is some kind of nefarious price control. My friend has his mic on, so I think probably he wants to say something.

But the point really is, what I have tried to spell out, is a market-based approach to get to a price—purchaser, Medicare, producers, manufacturers. It is a negotiation. Come on in. Prove your product's value. Earn your keep. And let's get this done, and do what everybody else in the Western world is doing.

Senator Crapo wants to talk.

Senator CRAPO. Yes, I would like to respond, Mr. Chairman. You know, the notion that the Federal Government, quote, "negotiating" prices is not a price control is just hard to understand. The fact is, you know, we were told back during the Obamacare debate this very type of thing. You know, we are going to have the Federal Government step in and control the plans the insurance companies can provide for our health care. And that is going to drive down the cost of health-care insurance, and everybody is going to be happier and better off.

Now what do we have? Most Americans can only get a choice between a couple of different types of plans. Those are all really expensive plans. Their costs have gone up through the roof. Not only that, but their deductibles and copayments have skyrocketed as well. And there are other private-sector types of plans that could be put into place, that insurance companies would provide, like low-deductible, high-risk plans, and different things like that, that could fit very well into a marketplace and help reduce the cost of insurance.

My point is simply this. I think that the debate here is not over whether we need to have robust negotiations over prices in the prescription drug industry, in the world; the debate is over how should those negotiations be incentivized and strengthened by this committee and by this Congress? And I think there may be some ways, if we can get past the notion that the Federal Government gets to be the one that sets the price.

Now I know you are not saying that. Although I am hearing you say that, I think the proposal that is in the Build Back Better Act is clearly that. If there is a way we can create some reforms to the negotiations that do exist today—there are negotiations today, but they can be strengthened and reformed and made more open, where the risk and the price of the cost of these drugs is placed in the private sector, where we then have the private sector incentivized to negotiate these prices down—we can enhance and strengthen the negotiation system.

But it is all the question as to whether the Federal Government is going to set the price, or whether a market will set the price. And I think we ought to be able to find a way to get to that.

The CHAIRMAN. Let me just respond briefly, because I think our colleagues are coming back, and we want to give all of them a chance to be heard.

What my colleague is talking about is a different type of negotiation. My view is, you would have to change Federal law to do it, because right now the Federal Government is barred from negotiating. It was barred in a legal process in Part D. I was one of the people who voted for Part D, knowing that it did not do as much as was urgent to hold down costs.

Now we have Ms. Stern's mom begging to get some charity to help her pay for her medicine. So what is being done today is not working. And I say that as somebody who voted for the program that my colleagues on the other side were talking about. And the reality is, there are places where negotiation works. One of them is Canada, which is what Ms. Stern told me about the huge price differential on her insulin.

So, my colleagues on the other side have ideas for negotiations. I am all ears. Right now what we are focused on is, big pharma has won and won and won some more on the notion that in Washington, DC, they are the people who never lose. And, shoot, they even fought what Senator Grassley is talking about. They were relentless in fighting what Senator Grassley is talking about and has been for 2 years.

So today is the time to get the job done right. And apropos of what we did in the last Congress—which I was for—it is not enough. Because, if you put a cap over here and you are not negotiating and doing what everybody else does, and what Medicare does in everything else, we are continuing to have cost shifting that hurts taxpayers, and it hurts seniors.

The discussion will certainly continue.

Senator Brown, I think, is next, and he is with us in cyberspace. Senator Brown?

[No response.]

The CHAIRMAN. Senator Brown? Do we have Brown's staff here?

All right, let's go with—Senator Brown, are you out there? Senator BROWN. I'm trying.

The CHAIRMAN. You're good. You're in.

Senator BROWN. Is it working? Okay.

Thanks, Mr. Chairman, and I throw in with exactly what you said and what Senator Cardin from Maryland said earlier. And it is clear that it is not working. It is clear that big pharma has immense power in this institution. Just yesterday, we saw the power that Senator Whitehouse has talked about of dark money in the oil industry, whether it is killing a nomination or stopping legislation. And we know that Americans are concerned about the cost of living. We know it with oil prices, with drug prices. Dr. Conti noted in her testimony that spending in pharmaceuticals has risen 20 percent over the past 10 years. AARP recently released their study that showed that more than 250 brand-name prescription drugs widely used by older American rose twice as fast as overall inflation. Drug companies, like oil companies, like shipping companies, like meat-packing companies, sense opportunity in times of inflation to inflate and raise their prices, because they can.

I am not going to ask a question. I always do in these hearings, but I wanted instead to share a couple of letters I got from Ohio constituents, because I think they show the issue the chairman was talking about and the inability of Congress to do something because of the power of the drug industry, of big pharma. And I sense the frustration of members on both sides on that. You talked about Chairman Grassley—and certainly Senator Whitehouse and Senator Wyden and all of us, and Senator Cardin, share that frustration.

Two notes I will quickly share, and I will stay within my 5 minutes, Mr. Chairman. Gary from Montgomery County in the Dayton area shared with me that he takes medicine for his blood cancer. When first diagnosed, he had employer-sponsored health insurance coverage that covered most of his out-of-pocket drug costs. So he had to pay about $30 a month for his medicine. Today he relies on Medicare for his health insurance, and because the cost of his drugs increased and Medicare is prohibited—this is a choice, this is Medicare by Federal law, because of drug company lobbying. Medicare is prohibited from negotiating for better prices. The chairman said, "Look at Canada. Look at the VA." Gary faces an annual out-of-pocket cost of $8,500 for a single medication. That makes no sense.

Jeff from Delaware County, just north of Columbus, wrote: "Senator Brown, I retired 4 years ago. My drug prices through my employer's insurance ran $68 per year. On Medicare, they continue to rise. Last year my out-of-pocket cost was $3,500. Is anything being done to help with senior citizens' prescription drug costs?"

We know what is not working. We know what would work. Look at Canada. Look at the VA. It is important we do that. We know how to lower costs for Americans like Gary and Jeff. We need a plan to do this. Let Medicare negotiate this. This is the free market working. It is not Federal price controls.

We penalize companies that price-gouge. We cap out-of-pocket costs. That makes so much sense when the cost of living is hitting retired Americans on fixed incomes particularly hard. Now it is time to get that job done.

So, Mr. Chairman, thanks for this hearing. Thank you to our witnesses, and for speaking out on an issue that is so clear to the public. It is only not so clear to members of Congress who seem interested more in what the drug companies think than what the public needs.

Thanks, Mr. Chairman.

The CHAIRMAN. Thank you, Senator Brown, and for your years of advocacy.

Our next four will be Cantwell, Toomey, Bennet, and Cassidy. Okay; Senator Cantwell?

Senator CANTWELL. Okay; thank you, Mr. Chairman. And thank you for this important hearing. I think really at the heart of it is just how many constituents we have all heard from on the high prices of things like insulin. It is just heartbreaking for seniors, or so many individuals who just cannot afford the price of prescription drugs. And this is really about trying to figure out solutions. And so I appreciate all the witnesses.

Dr. Holtz-Eakin, I would like to focus on a couple of things with you, if I could. You know, I definitely believe in market forces. I definitely understand the problem. I explain to people—I worked in software for a while, and you build and ship a product and it only takes about 18 months, so it is pretty easy to get capital for something like that. To get capital for something that takes 18 years is a lot harder—and having people buy into that. But I still think that you should be able to use market forces once that product is developed, and one of those market forces is, if you buy in bulk, you should get a discount. And that is where I feel like States, or individuals who are part of a larger organization, or plans, just as we do with the VA, should get a discount.

So I am a big believer in getting a discount for buying in bulk. I see in your testimony that PBMs and market concentration are two things that you think we should spend a little more time understanding. To me, it is just a little ironic that if the PBM can negotiate a discount, why can't a State negotiate that?

You mentioned the formularies. My State has had a plan for several years called the basic plan, and that is exactly what the State did. Hey, you want to get access to these 40,000 people? Let's negotiate on the formulary. And yes, there were choices there, but it worked out pretty well; again, for those companies too, because they have access to 40,000 people that they would not have otherwise been able to bundle up. So they were the low end of the market: people who worked for employers who did not provide insurance.

So I want to know what you think about focusing on the PBMs, and particularly you mentioned the Federal Trade Commission. I do worry that this concentration within the market—I care immensely about the pharmacists. I think they are part of the healthcare system. I think they are part of the delivery system. I do not want to see them go away.

I worry that we are going to have a concentration of this market that is so deep that not only is it going to be a few people providing prescription drugs by mail, but it will end up undermining the pharmacy system overall. And I believe that they do provide information to the people right at the window when they are filling prescriptions.

So this point that you made about how we should look to the FTC to prevent what is described as them being anticompetitive or deceptive or unfair, I wholeheartedly believe in that. I would like you to expound on that, and also on PBMs and what oversight that we should have on the PBMs because of their market power.

Dr. HOLTZ-EAKIN. So first off, on the FTC. In general, as in other parts of the economy, we ought to care deeply about the quality of competition and the nature of competitive practices to make sure that there is good monitoring of effective market competition. And the FTC opened a narrow investigation into PBMs and decided not to pursue it. My understanding is that some of the Commissioners would like to restart that process with a broader investigation, and we will see if that goes forward. But I think everyone should welcome a good, solid investigation.

Senator CANTWELL. Great. And just to that point, Senator Grassley and I are trying to work on this together, but I definitely believe that this notion of deceptive or unfair practices should be the issue.

Thank you.

Dr. HOLTZ-EAKIN. More generally with PBMs, PBMs exist because their's is a valuable service. They are essentially managed operations risk: if the insulin costs too much, or the market might not be broad enough, you do not get the penetration you would like. And so, that was their economic function.

You could get that economic function with just the insurers paying them with an incentive contract of some sort. "We need this much to control our drug spend. We need this much for generic substitution. You get rewarded for that." We do not have that now. They get part of their money back in manufacturers' rebates, in this direct and indirect remuneration, in pharmacy negotiations, and so one could easily imagine changing the rules on rebates. We had a discussion about that in past years. We could imagine changing the rules around the DIR.

But we should recognize that if we do that, it is not in a vacuum. We are not going to get it for free. We are going to have to get that service which is managing the drug spend somehow.

Senator CANTWELL. But you do not think that they should be able to negotiate a rebate and then pocket a big portion of it themselves.

Dr. HOLTZ-EAKIN. That was never the intent, no.

Senator CANTWELL. But do you think some of them are doing that? Because it feels like they are. It looks like they are.

Dr. HOLTZ-EAKIN. I honestly do not know, and that is what I am hoping the FTC will tell us.

Senator CANTWELL. Thank you. Thank you, Mr. Chairman.

The CHAIRMAN. I thank my colleague also. Having spent years and years on this, I appreciate her efforts.

Okay, I believe Senator Toomey is next, and then Senator Bennet and Senator Cassidy.

Senator Toomey?

Senator TOOMEY. Thank you, Mr. Chairman. Can you hear me okay?

The CHAIRMAN. Yes.

Senator TOOMEY. Terrific. Well, I think we need to talk about how the Democrats' government price-setting proposals will impact research and development, or what that means for improving treatment options going forward.

We have a very good example of a segment of the market where there is universal coverage and a government set price, and that is dialysis. When someone experiences kidney failure and is diagnosed with end-stage renal disease, they become eligible for Medicare, which provides coverage for dialysis. It has been that way since 1972. By the way, Medicare is set up to pay for dialysis and encourages multiple extended weekly visits. There has historically been very little innovation in this space. Dialysis appointments at a dialysis center, every other day for 2- or 3-hour treatments, that remains the default for patients facing kidney failure.

The former Chief Technology Officer of HHS said, and I quote, "dialysis was a miracle therapy for its time, but it hasn't changed in 60 years," end quote. So contrast that to the innovation that we have seen in a product that does not have price controls, say insulin. I know some of my colleagues want Medicare to negotiate the price of insulin, but what they really mean is they want Medicare to be able to set the price and cap the out-of-pocket expenses at $35.

And it seems as though this is because, in their world view, insulin was invented in the 1920s and a price control could have been implemented back then and would have made it affordable ever thereafter. But this completely ignores how the product has changed over time, and how it has improved because incentives for drug companies enable that improvement.

If you do not care that much about the improvements in insulin, there is an option too. Think about Walmart; just a few years ago it was selling insulin at less than $25 per vial. Now that is a version of insulin that was state-of-the-art in the 1980s. If you are satisfied with that, it is available at $25 a vial.

But because we actually do not control prices, we have had tremendous innovation in the insulin space. Products over the last few decades have changed dramatically, and that innovation is what patients happen to choose: synthetic insulin, longer-lasting products, rapid-acting formulations, accurate doses administered via insulin pens. The list goes on and on. These are not the same insulin products of decades ago. And as I said, patients have shown they prefer the newer, better products, and for good reasons.

Some like to point out the original patent for insulin sold for $1 in 1923. But I know most insulin-dependent diabetes patients do not want to go back to the insulin of the 1980s, much less the insulin of the 1920s.

What astonishes me is the inability of some of our colleagues to appreciate the impact that our actions today could have for the innovation of patients in the next 20, 30, or 40 years in the future; or like the case of Medicare coverage for dialysis, maybe we would be freezing a lack of innovation for 60 years or more.

So my question for Dr. Holtz-Eakin is, could you just reflect briefly on how reimbursement and pricing actually make innovation possible and what we can expect to have happen if government just dictates pricing as a normal routine matter?

Dr. HOLTZ-EAKIN. Well, I think Dr. Conti gave a great description of the ecosystem that goes into the development of new drugs and therapies, and that is an ecosystem that has venture capitalists and other financial market players. It has small firms that are developing a drug which they hope to sell to a larger firm as the way they get a return on their investment and pay off their venture capitalists.

We have the larger manufacturers that everyone has talked so much about. But in the end, that entire system is driven by the ability to recoup the return on a risky investment, if it turns out. And it turns out very rarely—92 percent of them fail and do not get to market.

And so these are very risky bets. They take a long time to develop. And if what you get at the end of the day is the promise that the money will not be there, the money at the beginning will dry up. The small firms will not exist. And the big firms will not have access to new therapies and drugs to sell.

So that is a long process, but it is one that relies on the markets that have served us well, and to intervene dramatically in that is going to be a recipe for problems.

Senator TOOMEY. Thank you.

Let me just take my remaining time with a quick observation here. The most recent 12-month print on inflation overall is 7.9 percent. Food is up 7.9 percent. Gasoline, 38 percent. Electricity, up 9 percent. Natural gas, almost 24 percent. These are hugely problematic for ordinary Americans whose wages are not rising nearly as fast.

What is so ironic is the same CPI data shows that prescription drugs and medical care services have had an increase too. It is 2.4 percent. It is less than a third the overall rate of inflation. And yes, we have Democratic colleagues who are using the general inflation, the inflation in everything other than prescription drugs, as a rationale for imposing price controls where the inflation is not nearly as problematic. It is a misdiagnosis, Mr. Chairman.

The CHAIRMAN. Just to be very brief in a response, Senator Toomey was citing dialysis. Well, dialysis payment is part of a rate-setting process. There is not any negotiating. What we are proposing in our bill is negotiation where the manufacturer has a say in the price Medicare is going to pay. And by that theory, higher-value products get higher prices, and generally Americans think that is fair. And if my friend from Pennsylvania—and he and I can talk about these issues for hours—thinks everything is hunky dory with medicine, tell it to Ms. Stern's mom who is begging charity for a little bit of help with a $111,000 expense for that insulin.

Senator Bennet, you are next.

Senator BENNET. That is the issue, Mr. Chairman, that we are facing and hearing from our constituents. I have had so many calls and so many stories, but the other day there was one of a parent at the pharmacy window at the local grocery store who was there to get drugs for their kid. And they got the prescription, and they looked at the price, and they walked away from those drugs that their kid needed. And you know, parents in other industrialized countries do not have to do that. They do not have to walk away from the pharmacy window.

And seniors in other countries do not have to cut their pills in half, or decide whether they are going to take their medicine or feed themselves, or skip a day. So I think we want to have an aspiration of living in a country where we do not have to do that stuff either. I think that is why we are here today.

Dr. Conti, in Colorado we have a lot of access to data through our All-Payer Claims Database to look at the rising cost of drugs and services in the health sector. According to data analysis funded by the Colorado Health Foundation and the Colorado Trust, health costs rose overall for patients in health plans. But when you break it out by services, you see a few things.

From 2013 to 2019, prescription drugs rose in Colorado by 87 percent. Lots of other things rose, but much less than that. And I mean, I feel strongly—Dr. Holtz-Eakin raised this. I respect him, and I actually agree with him. I think we need to have a lot more transparency of data available to better understand the entire drug supply chain, including pharmacy benefit managers and distributors, on top of what we are talking about today.

But, Dr. Conti, could you talk about the need to focus on prescription costs—as we are sitting here today—to lower costs for Americans, recognizing that there is more to be done in other parts of the health-care system as well?

Dr. CONTI. Yes. Thank you so much for the question. Patients pay the prices that pharmaceutical companies set for their products at the pharmacy counter. It is clear that patients are crippled by the increasing costs of these products and are making decisions about whether they are going to pay for these products or pay for rent, homes, schools, and other things that they absolutely need.

Negotiation and the other proposed reforms will reduce the prices that people pay at the pharmacy counter, providing very substantial relief for people who are insulin-dependent, for people with cancer. The reforms will also reduce the cost of taxpayers currently.

Senator BENNET. Could you also—and when you have finished, I would love to hear Dr. Holtz-Eakin on this as well. When you look at the historic investment in drug development for innovative products, I think there is a lot to be proud of.

In Colorado we have a robust biotechnology sector working on vaccines and cancer drugs and other important therapies. We have more work to do, and we need, for example, novel antibiotics. And I am glad that my colleague, Senator Young, is working with me on the PASTEUR Act to create that, and to put the United States in a place to actually lead on a global problem that we need to find a way to address on the front end, not on the back end—as we learned with the pandemic.

But the question is, are we seeing the kind of innovation that we need? And are the revenues in the industry ones that are generated by truly innovative drugs like the ones that we have all worked on together, the breakthrough therapy-designated drugs for example, that people need? Or is the revenue coming from marginally improved innovation? Could you give us a perspective on that, Dr. Conti?

Dr. CONTI. Sure. So we are very fortunate that we live in a country where innovation happens and we can benefit from it. Clearly there are drugs that come to market, breakthroughs as you say, that have transformed people's lives. And yet there are many other products out there that are really marginal improvements over existing products that do not provide much value, and yet we spend very significant amounts of money on them.

Really, the proposed legislation is intended to address a market failure, and that is, that the companies do not want to compete. They want to forestall competition, and they want to take advantage of our system by continuing to raise prices.

That is what we need to address, and these proposals will help do that.

Senator BENNET. I am out of time. I don't know, do you have anything, Dr. Holtz-Eakin?

Dr. HOLTZ-EAKIN. I guess I would say two things. First, I would be quite cautious about the dangers of sort of "me-too" or similar drugs coming on the market because—think about hepatitis C. The first drug comes on the market, and there is an uproar about what it costs and State Medicaid budgets. Then you get two more drugs that are me-toos, like all they do is cure hep C, but prices come down by 50 percent. There is effective competition. So everyone wants lower prices. The way to get lower prices is to have more supply and greater competition.

And so, finding ways to rule out new therapies that look like things you have is a way for high prices too. I would worry about that.

Senator BENNET. I will say—I know I am out of time—I will say that the PASTEUR Act that I have with Senator Young, that deals with an abject market failure that we have to address. If we do not address it, we are going to be in really bad shape. So, thank you.

The CHAIRMAN. Good work on that legislation with Senator Young.

Senator Cassidy?

Senator CASSIDY. Thank you, Senator Wyden.

First a couple of things. Senator Wyden has said on several occasions, with all due respect, that the Wyden-Grassley bill passed by this committee in 2019 merely shifted costs to taxpayers. That is incorrect. It saved $94 billion, per the CBO. And in a Part D redesign, we shifted the cost away from the consumer, from the taxpayer, to the PBM and the pharmaceutical company. We capped out-of-pocket costs to $3,200. And we allowed an amortization of payments over 12 months.

Senator Cornyn had a bill that, unfortunately, had to go through Judiciary that addressed the patent thicket. But if we addressed the patent thicket, then drugs like Humira would actually encounter competition within 12 years. As best as I can tell, this bill would allow them to maintain their high price for 13 years.

So we can actually work within the existing system if we take back up the bill we passed in 2019 on a bipartisan basis—and achieve $94 billion in savings, et cetera.

With that said, I enjoyed all your testimony, but I will focus upon Dr. Conti—nice to see you, Dr. Conti—and Dr. Holtz-Eakin. It somehow seems like I see you sometimes with facial hair and sometimes without. So now, without.

Dr. Conti, you mentioned that negotiations would not harm innovation. But some drugs are going to be particularly purchased by Medicare, over which Medicare would have monopsony power. And if it is an Alzheimer's drug, or certain cancers that tend to occur in older folks, is it only theoretical that if Bernie Sanders was President he would not kind of use this power to kind of squeeze down upon, you know, just kind of the total distrust of the profit motive, and would squeeze down upon innovation and all the venture capital and major investors required for that? You know where I am going with that: that the capital would dry up in the initial stages of development. Is that not an issue?

Dr. CONTI [off microphone].

Senator CASSIDY. Can you come a little closer to the microphone, please?

Dr. CONTI. The connection to the U.S. market is a privilege. I know that Mr. Ezell and Dr. Holtz-Eakin and the industry would love to call this price controls. It is not.

We pay the highest prices in the world, and we are the largest market in the world. With access to our markets comes requirements, such as the FDA's imposing safety and efficacy requirements on the companies. If the companies do not do that, they face penalties.

Senator CASSIDY. Yes, that is in your testimony. I guess my question is, though, is monopsony power here not going to be operative?

Dr. CONTI. I am getting there. Senator CASSIDY. I have limited time.

Dr. CONTI. No problem. So negotiation as proposed sets up a similar structure. It protects consumers and at the same time sets up a real negotiation. Pharma companies get access to this product, and in exchange, they should set their prices reasonably. All negotiation is doing is setting a process for doing it.

Senator CASSIDY. Is there no possibility of the Federal Government being particularly onerous, depending upon what the administration is, in attempting to squeeze prices in a way that would send a signal to investors not to invest in the early stage?

Dr. CONTI. I do not see that. And that is because, again, pricing is voluntary. And so many pharmaceutical companies price reasonably on their own. What we should expect is that companies will do the same here, and if anything, negotiation will occur in a very few set of products, if at all.

Senator CASSIDY. Dr. Holtz-Eakin, I think Dr. Conti makes an interesting case that our current structure encourages companies not to innovate but rather to tweak in order to squeeze a little bit more juice out of a product which is actually, frankly, mature, setting up patent thickets so as to extend the profitability of something long after patents have expired. Is there validity to that argument?

Dr. HOLTZ-EAKIN. So, well, the key here is exclusivity, and we want to provide exclusivity as an incentive for people to have genuine innovation. It is the job of the Patent and Trademark Office to only provide patents for novel innovations which are genuinely new. And so, if they are doing their job, that should not be a pervasive problem.

Nevertheless, concerns remain, and I know Senator Cornyn had some, and I am sympathetic for looking at specific instances where that practice might be detrimental. The thing I am concerned about is that the innovation we rely on is generic entry to control prices. And under the proposed Build Back Better legislation, if you are thinking of making a generic alternative to a brand-name drug, you do not know if the Secretary is going to designate that drug at some point in the future to suddenly have its price cut down to 40 or 75 percent of ANP at a minimum, perhaps lower. That is in the legislation. That is not a negotiation.

And so, are you going to make the investments so that you can enter that market? We just made actual generic competition harder, not better.

Senator CASSIDY. Can I ask a follow-up? Now, that could happen with the biologic follow-ons. I would say that. But let me ask you this. I had eye surgery. They prescribed a nonsteroidal for my eye pain, and it was going to cost me 50 bucks. I had to take it twice a day, or something like that. It has been a while. It turns out they had discontinued my product. It was the same product, now it is given not twice a day, but once a day, and I had to pay $400 for a vial. Is that innovation? Or is that—technically it is innovation, but the tweak made me pay $350 more, an amount that someone else might not be able to afford. Are there different classes of innovation? And should we treat those different classes differently?

Dr. HOLTZ-EAKIN. The way the market would solve that problem is that we would have both side by side——

Senator CASSIDY. But if the same producer stopped——

Dr. HOLTZ-EAKIN. I hear you. So that is how you decide in a genuine market setting. The consumer gets to pay $50, $400, once, twice—I get to pick. So the issue of these hard product hops, where you withdraw one, is an issue that has come up. There is a related issue, which is, you leave them both on the market and you make it very hard to get the $50 version.

Senator CASSIDY. But if somebody is making both, and they decide to take their machinery and not make the cheap one but make the expensive one——

Dr. HOLTZ-EAKIN. Then that product is not even there for a generic entry, in many cases, and that is an issue.

Senator CASSIDY. But then at that point, it is protected for however many years.

Dr. Conti, really quickly?

Dr. CONTI. Yes, thank you. So the legislation, as proposed, actually protects innovation that is truly innovative, and that includes products that are orphan, products that are for rare disease, products that are made by very small biotech companies.

So I think the thought of the legislation is actually thoughtful about this issue, protecting and making a distinction between things that are real innovation from things that are me-too.

Senator CASSIDY. I yield back. Thank you.

The CHAIRMAN. I thank my colleague. And let's be clear what we are talking about. What Professor Conti is talking about, and what I am talking about is, the bottom line here is, these companies can charge whatever they want—whatever they want—which is why Ms. Stern's mom is paying $111,000 dollars and is out there begging for people to try to give her a hand with medicine. I think it is just disgraceful.

Senator CASSIDY. Mr. Chairman——

The CHAIRMAN. Hang on, if I could just finish. And apropos of the companies being able to charge whatever they want, we are going to have money moving every which way—cost shifting in all kinds of different directions.

And I have to move on with my colleague. I gave my friend extra time. We will continue this discussion.

Our next Senator is, I believe, Senator Casey.

Senator CASEY. Mr. Chairman, thanks very much for this hearing, and I want to thank our witnesses.

I will start with Ms. Stern, and then I will have a question as well for Dr. Conti. But, Ms. Stern, I wanted to start with you and start with gratitude for your willingness to testify and share your mother's story and the stories of so many other MS patients.

I think you spoke for a lot of families across the Nation with your testimony and your appearance today. When you combine so many costs in the lives of families that are very high with the cost of prescription drugs, it is like a bag of rocks on someone's shoulder— every day on that individual and their family. And we have—obviously it is not simply prescription drugs. We have other heavy costs that people carry around.

The cost of care is a big one that we do not talk about enough, the cost of child care, which is just crushing families and literally preventing them from getting back to work. And we have not done nearly enough about the cost for care of an older adult, a family member, or the cost of care for people with disabilities.

So you have all these bags of rocks on the shoulders of so many families, all at the same time, weighing people down every day. And if you have Medicare, it prevents you from making the kind of choices you would like to make about how to spend the dollars you have.

On page 4 of your testimony, Ms. Stern, you list eight areas where people make sacrifices to more easily afford prescription medications, including postponing paying other bills they have, or postponing retirement itself, or spending less on their families.

So if Congress passes reforms to cap out-of-pocket costs, what type of financial relief would that bring for people with Medicare?

Ms. STERN. Thank you so much, Senator. It is such an important question. An out-of-pocket cap would be nothing short of lifechanging for the MS community. I hear day in and day out from people with MS like my mom that they cannot afford their costs. Our most recent study showed people are paying an average of $7,000 a year just for their disease-modifying therapies. Even when they get to the catastrophic phase, they are paying $352 a month. So those numbers are so high, even people working in really good jobs would struggle to pay that kind of burden. And people who are seniors who are on fixed incomes, people with chronic health conditions and disabilities, they find those costs insurmountable.

So we do have people making all kinds of really difficult decisions like not paying their bills, postponing retirement, putting their groceries on their credit cards. You know, I do not believe that our intent was ever for seniors with health conditions to choose between taking their meds and paying other bills. It is just the unfortunate outcome.

So yes, it would be a huge step for the MS community, and so many other patient communities, to address out-of-pocket costs.

Senator CASEY. Thanks very much.

Dr. Conti, I had a question for you, but I wanted to ask, are you a resident of Montgomery County, PA?

Dr. CONTI. I am.

Senator CASEY. That is great. Well, I hope you stay there. We need you in Pennsylvania. But I want to thank you for your testimony, and in particular on the basic question of high costs and what we can do about them.

On page 13 of your testimony you noted, quote, that "29 percent of Americans either can't afford their drugs or are rationing their drugs," unquote. And I have heard this from countless people in Pennsylvania, that they are skipping or rationing their medications, or taking other steps to ease that financial burden.

We had a hearing in the Aging Committee back in 2019, and Barbara Cisek—she is from southwestern Pennsylvania—said she needed to manage her costs every month, and would be paying over $1,500 a month if she was taking all of the medications prescribed. In her testimony, Barbara said that she was not only speaking on behalf of herself, but on behalf of other seniors. She said, quote, "We've had to stand at the pharmacy counter and leave something behind," unquote. And that is a lot to leave behind with what they're paying.

So we all believe, no matter where we stand on this issue, that no one should be rationing or choosing not to take medication rather than putting food on their table.

So my question is, can you discuss how permitting Medicare to negotiate would enable people on Medicare to afford not only the medications, but also the basic bare necessities of their lives?

Dr. CONTI. Yes. People have been dealing with price inflation on the drugs they need to stay alive for years. This hurts their finances and their health. Medicare negotiation will directly improve the access to care. It will likely improve outcomes. The people who will be helped will disproportionately be women, Black and Brown Americans, and consequently, this is also going to improve equity.

Senator CASEY. Thanks very much, Doctor. Thank you, Mr. Chairman.

The CHAIRMAN. Thank you, Senator Casey. Senator Lankford is next.

Senator LANKFORD. Mr. Chairman, thank you. Thanks to all of our witnesses. Obviously, it is an exceptionally important topic today in talking through what we are going to do on drug pricing.

This does affect a lot of people. I am the primary caretaker for my mom, who has Parkinson's and has exceptionally expensive medications, and I will continue to be able to monitor her medications in tracking this process with her.

So all of us have stories of our families and what we are doing, and of individuals who are around us in the process on this.

Dr. Holtz-Eakin, I want to pick up on a conversation you had started a while ago on generics. It is an issue that you and I have talked about before. In 2011, 71 percent of the generics were actually listed on the generic pricing tier. That was in 2011. Now, in 2021, 10 percent of the generics are on the generic tier.

So your comment was, the way to solve some of this is to get more generics out there, more competition that drives the price down significantly. The problem with this is, the drug companies and the pharmacy benefit managers are working together to be able to keep generics off the generic tier. So let me give you just two examples.

The generic of Desogen, the acquisition cost for that generic is $45, but the price set by the PBM is $319. The copayment is $105 because it is not on the generic tier. Though it is a generic, it is not being listed on the generic tier. Another example is the generic Gleevec; acquisition cost: $431 for the generic.

It is very expensive. The PBM price for it is $4,620. The copay then is $1,521 because it is not on the generic tier.

So that should be on the generic tier, but it has been negotiated by the PBMs and the drug companies not to be able to do this. This is an issue that has rapidly accelerated in the last 10 years, that generics do not end up on the generic tier. The consumer pays much more for that.

How do we attack that?

Dr. HOLTZ-EAKIN. So first, just to reiterate the importance of generic competition in the U.S., over 90 percent of scripts that get filled are generics. And U.S. generics are cheaper than generics around the world. So——

Senator LANKFORD. Yes, 90 percent of the scrips that are filled are generics, but only 22 percent of the total cost for prescriptions are generics. So they are overwhelmingly cheaper.

Dr. HOLTZ-EAKIN. I am with you on that. So here's the issue. We all think that this is the result of the rebates from manufacturers to the PBMs for different tiers of placement.

So my position as an economist is that pharmacy managers must provide value. We know that managed care organizations provide value, and we hire them. An insurance plan might want to hire someone to manage the benefit, and they could pay them for that service. So the issue is the reimbursement through the manufacturers' rebates and/or the DIR from the pharmacies.

So we have discussed for years in this town the notion of passing that rebate through to the ultimate purchaser at the point of sale. That means that co-insurance and out-of-pocket costs are driven off net prices, not list prices. That takes away the tier discounts that you are talking about. That would be one way to go.

And my only caution is that, given that there is a value that has to be paid for, it means that insurance probably has to pay the PBMs, and it will show up in premiums.

Senator LANKFORD. Yes, but the challenge is, if the larger drug companies are giving a benefit to the PBM to be able to say they will put the generic competition on the higher-priced tier, then the consumer goes to the counter and says, "Hey, this is my script. Is there a generic for this?" And they say, "Yes, there is. It is the same price as the brands." And they will say, "Okay, well then, just give me the brand," which drives out the generic from the market. Then the generics cannot compete in that space, and eventually they drop out and stop producing, and we lose the benefit of it.

If a generic is not put on the generic tier, they do not get the benefit of the lower price. If they get a benefit on that in their particular prescription plan, the consumer does not get it. The PBM gets the kickback on it coming from the pharmaceutical company saying, "Okay, thank you very much for helping us out on that," but the consumer does not see that.

Dr. HOLTZ-EAKIN. And so, passing it through the PBM to the consumer so that the PBM cannot recoup anything from that rebate is one solution to that problem.

Senator LANKFORD. It would be very, very significant. Dr. Conti, you wanted to say something on that?

Dr. CONTI. I did. The problem with passing the rebate all the way to the consumers is that premiums are going to rise, and therefore disparities are going to grow. While I believe that there is cause for concern, particularly the anticompetitive practices of the PBM, we simply need more information.

The story that you just told, that there are branded pharmaceutical companies that are placing their products on a lower tier than the generics, it may happen, but it appears to be rare. We need more information to understand exactly what is happening in this market—what are the benefits, what are the costs of the current configuration—in order to move forward.

Senator LANKFORD. I would only say that 10 years ago, 71 percent of the generics were on generic tiers. Now 10 percent are. There is definitely something happening in the last 10 years. And when Humira has generic competition starting next year, when there are 7 that are coming out on it, we will all be watching very closely to see if those end up on generic tiers, or if those end up on higher-priced tiers for the consumer.

The CHAIRMAN. The time of the gentleman has expired. Senator Carper?

Senator CARPER. Thanks, Mr. Chairman.

One of the concerns I hear most frequently from the folks I represent in the State of Delaware deals with the high costs—not of all prescription drugs, but too many. I have three or four principals I lean on and am guided by when it comes to drug pricing legislation. They are pretty simple, and I just want to mention them here as I start.

One of those is, I believe we need to lower costs for American families. I believe we need to lower the costs for taxpayers in this country, for the Federal Government, if you will. We need to encourage innovation, and I think we need to improve transparency. And it not just one thing we need to do but a number, and those are foremost in my mind.

We came close to achieving these aims about 3 years ago, in 2019. Frankly, I was deeply disappointed that we were unable to pass legislation that this Finance Committee developed in the last Congress, even though I felt that the current Chairman, Senator Wyden, and our previous chairman, Senator Grassley, did a very masterful job in developing the bill with bipartisan support.

While I would prefer to pass a bipartisan bill, we cannot just wait for that relief for patients to meet the needs that I just outlined. And so I see a clear path forward to deliver drug pricing reform for the American people in a way that is balanced and in a way that is fair, and I am confident that these policies can pass through Congress and be signed into law even today—even today. We can cap the price Americans pay, for example, for insulin at $35 per prescription. We can establish the first-ever out-of-pocket cap for seniors in Medicare Part D. We can institute a price inflation penalty where drug companies would pay a penalty to Medicare for raising their prices faster than inflation. And we can allow Medicare to negotiate for lower drug prices, not for every drug under the sun, but some of the most costly products that monopolize the market and do not have much competition.

We know that scientific innovation is driven by American biotech companies that responsibly invest in R&D, and they develop new treatments to improve the lives of people suffering from any number of debilitating conditions. Yet these products are out of reach for too many people. There are so many factors that contribute to rising drug costs beyond the actions of the industry—among them the opportunistic practices of pharmacy benefit managers—that Congress must take a holistic approach to curb costs.

Dr. Conti, here is my question: in your view, how would policies we are debating today walk the line between curbing costs and encouraging innovation? What further steps can Congress take to ensure that our approach is balanced and fair across the sector? Thank you.

Dr. CONTI. Thank you so much for the question. Negotiation is the [audio interruption]. Negotiations also [audio interruption] expire anyway. I support negotiations with these guard rails in place to preserve these incentives for innovation. Thanks you for your question.

Senator CARPER. Unfortunately, I could not hear your answer. You were cutting in and out. Just repeat your answer, please. Thank you. Hopefully I can hear it.

Dr. CONTI. I am so sorry.

Negotiation is modest and thoughtful. It exempts the most innovative products and the most innovative companies from negotiation. Negotiation is also only an option well after product launch, well after monopoly prices were already supposed to expire anyway. Therefore, this set of proposals walks a line between being pro-innovation and pro-consumer.

Senator CARPER. All right.

Is there any question you were not asked today that you wish you had been asked? What would it be?

Dr. CONTI. Again, I think that this is not price control, and this is not profit control. These are thoughtful proposals that will lower out-of-pocket costs for seniors today and preserve the incentives for innovation that we have currently.

Senator CARPER. That was not a question, but thank you for saying that nonetheless. Thank you.

And thank you, Mr. Chairman.

The CHAIRMAN. Thank you, Senator Carper. [Audio interruption.]

The CHAIRMAN. I have to now go and vote. Here's what we are going to do. We will now have Senator Hassan in the chair, after we have the issues with the microphones eliminated. And, Senator Hassan, the order now will be Senator Daines and then you, and I will go vote and come right back.

Okay; Senator Daines?

Senator DAINES. Chairman Wyden, thank you.

Inflation is the worst we have ever seen now in 40 years. In a State like Montana, it is up a jaw-dropping 9.7 percent. Families cannot keep up.

Americans everywhere are feeling the sting of these higher prices. And those who can afford it the least, sadly, they are truly feeling it the most and hurting the most. The seniors in Montana, its workers, are really hit the hardest.

My colleagues on the Republican side of the aisle and I have been calling for common-sense solutions to address inflation. We look at the big picture here: restoring energy independence, supporting all the energy portfolio. When you look at energy, it is not trading one for the other, it is like an additive. Let's continue to add all of the above in the portfolio. That is the way we continue to drive market forces and drive prices down.

We need to get our fiscal house in order and address the issue of the reckless spending we are seeing—deficit spending creates $3 trillion in debt—as well as supporting our small businesses across the country so American workers can thrive.

Sadly, as we watch what is happening, our friends on the other side of the aisle are attempting to resurrect a dangerous and innovation-stifling set of policies from this Build Back Broke agenda. It is staggering to think that they will still be driving that in a moment when so much is going on in the world, so much going on here in our economy.

This bill would not only make inflation worse, but it would reduce patient access to lifesaving medication. It would also undermine American competitiveness with countries like China and strengthen their own pharma sector. We must do better for all of America. We must do better for the people I serve back in Montana.

Today I would urge my friends across the aisle to publicly ditch the BBB and focus on bipartisan policies like capping seniors' out- of-pocket costs in order to provide real relief to Americans who are struggling. Now is the time to get serious and truly come together in trying to find a way to help lower prescription drug costs for our seniors.

Dr. Holtz-Eakin, Democrats have claimed that tax and spend policies in BBB are fully paid for. According to the Biden administration, and I quote, "It would actually ease inflationary pressures."

As the sixth Director of the CBO, you provided budgetary and policy analysis to Congress. How would you respond to the Biden administration's claims when you estimate the impact that BBB might have on inflation?

Dr. HOLTZ-EAKIN. Well, the version that came out of the House, taken at face value, which is to say believing that all of the spending programs would sunset at the dates in the legislation——

Senator DAINES. Do you believe that?

Dr. HOLTZ-EAKIN. The public statements have been that they want these programs to be permanent, so I think there is good reason to doubt that.

Senator DAINES. Yes.

Dr. HOLTZ-EAKIN. And there has been no comparable public statement about future pay-fors. So the sort of imbalance between 10 years of spending and 10 years of taxes is in the trillions of dollars, a huge structural deficit on top of the one we already have. Senator DAINES. Wouldn't it seem to you, or somebody who understands the details of a policy like this in your past experience, that it is gaming the system and these sunsets are just a way here to try to make it all fit? Frankly, it is smoke and mirrors.

Dr. HOLTZ-EAKIN. And the evolution of the legislation, as it went through the House, they tried to scale down the spending. They essentially cut out the tail years of spending, and they front-loaded the spending and added 10 years of pay-fors. So it is front-loaded spending, back-loaded pay-fors; that is a stimulus bill. And so that is not what the U.S. economy needs at this moment. It has already developed a very bad inflation problem in part due to the $1.9 trillion in the American Rescue Plan, which was a major policy error. So another round of that is not a good idea. As it came out of the House, it would be $150 billion in the first year. So that is not nearly the scale of the American Rescue Plan, but it is directionally the wrong way to go.

Senator DAINES. I remember having spirited debates, pushing back on that $1.9-trillion stimulus bill when we had nearly a trillion dollars unspent in COVID dollars at the end of 2020. These numbers here are numbing. And we said, if you launch a $2-trillion spending bill in the midst of additional supply chain constraints, you have stimulated demand in a constrained type of environment as relates to supply, and this is a recipe for inflation fire. We said that. You go back and look at the transcripts; we have warned the American people and our colleagues that this was a bad idea.

And then, furthermore, when you talk about the dollars—I think there was one reputable analysis that said it was $5 trillion of spending, and would add approximately $3 trillion of debt.

Lastly, Mr. Ezell, in your testimony you mentioned how the prescription drug policies in BBB would curtail future innovation—I should say could curtail—and undermine American competitiveness. Can you explain how BBB would advantage countries like China that are seeking to bolster their own biopharma industries?

Senator HASSAN [presiding]. And I will just ask the witness to be relatively brief, because you are over time, Senator.

Mr. EZELL. Mr. Daines, in 1995, European-headquartered drug companies invented twice as many new-to-the-world drugs as American ones. Today, it is reversed. We innovate the vast majority of the world's new medicines. That is because we have created an environment that supports innovation, but we have squared the circle better than any country in the world in terms of being able to innovate new drugs, get them to the patients first, support a competitive biomedical industry, and create pathways for companies to have more time to manage drug costs.

So that is what is at stake in the international competition for leadership in this industry. China certainly is the country that has, for the past 2 decades, seen its share of the global pharmaceutical industry value-added grow by threefold, while ours has shrunk by a third. Competition from China is real.

And if we do not maintain the conditions needed to sustain innovation in the United States, China is ready to nip our heels. And if you look at solar panels, for instance, in the year 2008, China produced 2 percent of the world's solar panels. Today, they produce over 70 percent. China brings every resource to bear to wrest industrial leadership from other countries, and that is why we have to take the challenge seriously.

Senator DAINES. Thank you. Senator Hassan, thank you.

Senator HASSAN. Thank you. I want to thank the chair and ranking member for this hearing, and I want to thank all of the witnesses for being here today. And I really want to get back to the topic at hand. Because while Americans struggle to afford lifesaving medications, pharmaceutical companies continue to raise the prices.

Allowing Medicare to negotiate drug prices is a common-sense solution that will strengthen Medicare and bring relief to Granite State families, and families all across the country. We also need to penalize the companies that arbitrarily make large price increases. And Congress needs to act quickly to pass drug pricing reforms. Patients and families cannot wait any longer, and this is an immediate way to lower costs for families all across this country.

So, Dr. Conti, I want to start with a question to you. The pharmaceutical industry has burdened Americans with one arbitrary price increase after another. These increases fall especially hard on patients using specialty drugs which treat their complex chronic conditions. A Medicare beneficiary from Wilmot, NH with stage one Parkinson's disease contacted me last week. She spent $2,100 last year on copayments for just one of the drugs that she takes.

Dr. Conti, how would allowing Medicare to negotiate prices make specialty drugs more affordable for patients like her?

Dr. CONTI. Thank you so much for the question. Negotiation and inflation caps will directly benefit consumers at the pharmacy counter. They will find immediate price relief for the drugs that they need to stay alive. This will help them afford their medicines, and hopefully it leads to better outcomes.

Senator HASSAN. Thank you. I agree, and that is why it is so essential that we allow Medicare to negotiate prices and pass a drug pricing reform package.

Another question to you, Dr. Conti. As prices skyrocket, Granite Staters have also shared their struggle to pay for insulin. While New Hampshire has taken steps as a State to cap the cost share for insulin products, the State law leaves unprotected the estimated 300,000 Medicare beneficiaries in New Hampshire. The law also does not encompass many individuals who are covered by employer-sponsored insurance, since that insurance is regulated by the Federal Government.

To ease their burden, my colleagues and I introduced the Affordable Insulin Now Act, which would cap out-of-pocket costs for insulin at $35 per month.

Dr. Conti, why are Federal reforms like this one needed?

Dr. CONTI. Thank you. There are 2.3 million seniors who use insulin daily, and these reforms will result in measurable savings immediately at the pharmacy counters. American workers and others who are non-Medicare-insured will also benefit from this change.

Senator HASSAN. Thank you very much.

Ms. Stern, first of all, I just want to thank you for your very moving testimony, and thank you for being here.

Several Granite Staters who have multiple sclerosis recently visited my office to share the financial toll of high drug prices on their families. According to the National Multiple Sclerosis Society, the median price of certain medications for MS is close to $94,000 per year, an increase of almost $25,000 since 2015. These Granite Staters also discussed the strain of worrying about how they will afford to fill their next prescription.

So, Ms. Stern, how do high drug prices exacerbate the stress of managing a chronic condition like yours?

Ms. STERN. That is a great question. First of all, I should point out that these high prices really do translate to real-life impacts for people with MS, and people who are relying on Medicare payment co-insurance for their MS disease-modifying therapy. So they are paying 25 percent, or whatever percent of the cost of that drug, and that can be a huge amount of money.

MS is a condition that is exacerbated by stress, like so many other conditions. Having to navigate the system through MS symptoms such as chronic fatigue and sometimes cognitive issues—it represents a huge burden for the person with MS, for their family, for their support system.

Senator HASSAN. Thank you very much. And again, thank you for being here. It is not always easy sharing your personal experiences in a hearing, but it is really important.

The chair is back, so I will turn it back to him.

The CHAIRMAN. I thank my colleague. It is a busy day. Let's go to Senator Cortez Masto.

Senator CORTEZ MASTO. Thank you, Mr. Chairman. I want to thank you for this important hearing today, and thank you to the panelists for the discussion.

What I have heard this morning is, we all know that there are major market failings in the health-care sector right now. We can see that in really the huge profits that we are talking about today that the pharmaceutical industry rakes in. And that is why Medicare does need tools to negotiate for fair prices from pharmaceutical companies, prices that will let drug companies continue to innovate without gouging seniors or Federal taxpayers.

That is not a popular opinion, unfortunately, among some drug manufacturers. What I have heard today is that it will somehow— they have said it is government price control, and that it will stifle innovation. There is a lot of fear-mongering going on out to the general public, and you have to kind of question why that is happening.

And so let me just put a couple of things on the record here, because I think it is important. This is not price control. And, Dr. Conti, I am going to have you touch on that. What is price control—and you touched on this—is when pharmaceutical companies set the prices and we cannot negotiate lower prices for taxpayers, for Americans across the country. That is price control.

"Government price control" really is a tactic, from what I am hearing from some of my colleagues, to scare people. Because, quite honestly, if we want to talk about what the government does to lower costs, we have a perfect example in the GSA, which literally—the U.S. Government GSA awards contracts to vendors who want to do business with Federal agencies, because there are a lot of Federal agencies, and they are allowed to do that business based upon pricing that is fair and reasonable and would provide the best value at the lowest overall cost.

So the Federal Government is already doing this to get the best price, and in this instance we are looking at negotiation under Medicare to get the best price for people who are in the program. It just astounds me that there is so much fear-mongering going on around here.

So really what I hear on government price controls, what I am hearing is that pharmaceutical companies are afraid for the free market to take place, and negotiations to take place to lower the costs. That is one.

Two, there was conversation about a bill that we passed on July 25, 2019, out of this committee, the Prescription Drug Pricing Reduction Act of 2019. Not only did it pass out of this committee in a bipartisan way—and unfortunately at the time, there were nine Republicans who did not support it—but it passed under a Republican administration and Republican leadership. It went nowhere. It was not passed on the floor of the Senate, but it should have been.

And I agree, not only should that piece of legislation, which we passed out of this committee, get passed on the floor of the Senate and get to the President's desk for signature, but we should also be passing drug price negotiation in Medicare so that we can lower costs for so many people across this country.

It is not working. I mean, just listen to the general public. It is not working right now. It is the number one issue I hear when I am at home. Something is going on.

So, Dr. Conti, can you once again talk about how false this is that somehow if we allow prescription drug negotiation that it is going to inhibit innovation?

And by the way, let me just add, if you are concerned that somehow it is going to inhibit it because it is going to reduce profit for the pharmaceutical companies, then let me add to their profit line. Stop doing those commercials on TV. Let our doctors decide the drugs and prescriptions that patients need and not advertise all over the television with all of these commercials. That could save dollars for the pharmaceutical companies that they could put back into R&D and innovation.

But, Dr. Conti, please tell me. Is it true that it is going to stifle innovation?

Dr. CONTI. It is not true. Nothing about our current ecosystem, which is the envy of the world where we bring the most drugs to market and the most innovative drugs to market, will change after this legislation is passed.

And at the same time, consumers will be able to pay for the products that they need to stay alive, stay well, stay working, and stay to take care of their families.

Senator CORTEZ MASTO. Thank you.

And let me say, Ms. Stern, thank you for being here. Thank you. I have a cousin, a year younger than I am, with MS. And he is in a wheelchair. And the worst thing that I can see is not only how my aunt and he have to manage the costs for their drugs with everything else that they have to do—food on the table, and pay their bills, and a roof over their head—but here is the other thing.

Can you talk about the anxiety that comes with worrying about prescription drug costs, and what toll that takes on a patient who is really having challenges already with their health? What kind of impact does it have on their mental health?

Ms. STERN. Yes. So I would say these are excruciating decisions, right? These are impossible. And I said in my testimony I think it is one of the most compelling findings we have had in the last decade. Forty percent of the people with MS are altering the use of their medications. And they are making those choices, you know, depending on what they are being charged for their meds and what money they have.

So, they might be skipping doses. They might be going off their meds altogether. And with that, you worry about what is going to happen to my disease. Is my MS going to progress? Am I going to lose mobility or cognition or something like that? And will it ever come back?

So I mean, it is anxiety that really compounds the difficulty, as you said, of living with a disease that is already a challenge.

Senator CORTEZ MASTO. Thank you. I know my time is up. Thank you, Mr. Chairman.

The CHAIRMAN. I thank my colleague, and she has been such an advocate—Attorney General, in so many sectors—we really appreciate her leadership.

Next is Senator Young.

Senator YOUNG. Thank you, Mr. Chairman. I welcome the witnesses.

My State of Indiana has a robust life sciences industry. We are very proud of that. The pipeline for new drugs and cures is growing because of alignment between innovators and regulators that recognizes the benefit of innovative therapies.

I am concerned that policies included in the partisan Build Back Better Act will have significant long-term impacts on investment and discoveries to improve, save, and extend lives that are currently being made in this country.

So my question is for Dr. Holtz-Eakin. Doctor, you led the Congressional Budget Office years ago, and there are some differing analyses of the impact BBBA policies will have on new drugs.

Now the Congressional Budget Office and the University of Chicago, for example, are widely differing in their assessments. Can you explain how the CBO has a perception that the Build Back Better Act proposals are more modest and less threatening to drug development compared to other studies?

Dr. HOLTZ-EAKIN. Well, I cannot speak for the CBO any better than they can speak for themselves, so I would direct you to the publications they have. They have a publication on their modeling of the drug industry and the development process.

As with most issues in economics, there is often a range of findings in the research literature. And I think the message to those making policy is, you should move slowly and cautiously in those circumstances where there are such large and divergent differences in the estimates of the impacts on innovation.

I will just point out that there is no one who believes that this is going to put more money into the drug development ecosystem. And so, at best it is zero. And most people conclude that it is negative, and the only question is, how negative?

Senator YOUNG. Yes. And in light of the very serious implications that one might expect through passage of the Build Back Better Act, one would think that we would move slowly and cautiously towards, first adoption of the legislation, and then implementation. And this committee, the Committee on Finance, did not even hold a hearing on the Build Back Better Act. So I think that is troubling.

I am glad we are holding this hearing today, as it relates to some of the facets that we can touch on. The research and development tax credit is something I would like to turn to next.

Senator Hassan and I have introduced the bipartisan American Innovation and Jobs Act to support R&D investments by companies large and small. This bill will restore full and immediate deduction of R&D investments. It will expand the refundable R&D tax credit for our startups by raising outdated credit caps.

I know there is a lot of bipartisan support for this effort, and I think people recognize that, now more than ever, we have to find bipartisan solutions to stimulate our economy, get Americans back to work, and ensure we maintain our global competitiveness on the economic stage.

I recently led a letter, relatedly, with Senator Hassan to Senate leadership to prioritize R&D in any upcoming legislation. And so, Dr. Holtz-Eakin, I ask you: can tax incentives like section 174 and the R&D refundable tax credit for small businesses help in the development of innovative prescription drugs and keep costs down in the long term?

Dr. HOLTZ-EAKIN. I think the evidence is very clear that this is something that has been beneficial for R&D in the U.S. I think it is poorly understood that most R&D is done in the private sector. Our support for that R&D, where there is a clear economic case that not every firm gets the full benefit of the R&D—there are spillovers to the rest of the economy. Our credits are low by international standards and could be more generous. I think it is a big mistake to move to amortizing the R&D. We should be fully expensing it. And the quicker we can reverse that, the better.

Senator YOUNG. Yes.

Mr. Ezell?

Mr. EZELL. Thank you for the leadership on that issue, Senator Young. And to Dr. Holtz-Eakin's point, the United States really invented this instrument as a motivator of innovation in 1981, and for decades America had the world's most generous R&D tax credit. Today we have fallen to 24th out of 32 OECD countries in R&D tax credits. In countries like Brazil and India, you have a tax credit three times more generous than ours.

Brazil and India have a tax credit three times more generous. That is instructive and a powerful example. Where is communist China in terms of their incentives they offer? Well, of course that is an opaque system, but at least what is on paper is actually more generous than ours. It is more generous than ours.

Senator YOUNG. Okay.

Thank you so much, Mr. Chairman.

The CHAIRMAN. I thank my colleague. And just to be clear, I think my colleague said there had not been any hearings and markups on matters relating to Build Back Better. I think my colleagues know that with respect to the centerpiece, which is the Clean Energy for America legislation, we had hearings. We had a long, long markup, and it was actually reported out.

So I just want the record to be clear on that. Senator Warren?

Senator WARREN. Thank you, Mr. Chairman.

Earlier this month you and several others on this committee joined me in sending a letter to PhRMA about two studies that reveal troubling increases in drug prices. The studies showed that in January alone, 1 month, manufacturers raised prices for 16 of the 20 top-selling Medicare Part D drugs, and increased prices for brand-name drugs by an average of over 5 percent.

Now, in their response to our letter, PhRMA revealed that there is no rationale other than industry price gouging for raising prices. And I would like to share some of what we have learned in evaluating PhRMA's weak attempt to justify these price increases.

First, PhRMA claimed that drug manufacturers were not increasing prices at all, that back-door rebates and discounts have caused the average prices of medicine to actually decline. But they very carefully cherry-picked the data on this. In fact, according to the Congressional Budget Office, quote, "Brand-name drugs have experienced substantial growth in average prices."

Dr. Conti, what do you think about PhRMA's claim that prices are secretly declining?

Dr. CONTI. Thank you. It is fiction. PhRMA sets the prices of their products, and we are seeing over and over again that the prices of, particularly specialty drugs have increased both overall, but also for specific consumers at the pharmacy counter.

Senator WARREN. Thank you, Dr. Conti.

You know, I think the data are clear on this. Brand-name drug prices are rising, not falling. And it is absurd to claim otherwise. So let's go to their second argument.

Next, PhRMA claimed that their price increases were not really hurting consumers at the pharmacy counter. Ms. Stern, you represent patients who are forced to pay high drug prices. What do you make of PhRMA's argument that increases in list prices do not actually hurt consumers?

Ms. STERN. You know, I would say right off the bat that that does not reflect the lived experiences of people with MS, and seniors, and people with chronic health conditions across the country who are telling us that they cannot afford their drugs, that they are going off of their drugs, that they are skipping doses. And we do hear, you know—I think I have shown that the MS medications have gone up exponentially and that the patients are paying a percentage of that cost in their co-insurance.

But it is not just our medication. A lot of medications are going up dramatically. And it is like you said, you can kind of cherry-pick those statistics, but that does not mean that people are not faced with the choice of buying their groceries or taking their medication.

Senator WARREN. Okay, so prices are going up. And people are feeling it when they go to fill a prescription.

Let's take a look at PhRMA's third argument. PhRMA blamed everyone but themselves for higher prices. They claimed that middlemen like pharmacy benefit managers, pharmacies, insurance companies, were more to blame than the manufacturers.

And do not get me wrong. I know there are some serious problems with the middlemen, but none of those problems absolve big pharma for their part in the price increases.

So, Dr. Conti, when you think about brand-name drugs, especially the very expensive ones, is it fair to say that brand-name drug manufacturers collect more revenue from drug sales and have higher profit margins than the middlemen that PhRMA is trying to blame for the price increases?

Dr. CONTI. Yes, absolutely. Research shows that the industry itself is benefiting off of the high list prices they are setting and the year-over-year price inflation they are experiencing on these products.

The only way that the PBMs are enriched by that is if there is competition in these markets. There is no competition in these markets, and therefore there is no rebate, and therefore the PBMs are not benefiting.

It is the companies themselves that are benefiting from the high prices and price increases that they are setting. The companies own documents support this claim.

Senator WARREN. Thank you. And I appreciate your analysis of the data here.

You know, what we have happening in the drug industry is exactly what is happening throughout the economy. Big drug manufacturers have outsized market power, and they face little or no competition for their brand-name drugs. So basically, they are free to increase prices exactly as much as they want to.

That hurts patients. It drives up inflation. And it needs to stop. And that is why we need to pass legislation that lets Medicare negotiate for lower prices and cut costs for beneficiaries. And it is why the administration also needs to use its existing authorities such as compulsory licensing and march-in rights to rein in drug prices immediately.

We know what the solutions are. We just need to put them in place and get it done. Thank you.

Thank you, Mr. Chairman.

The CHAIRMAN. Thank you, Senator Warren. And we have been at it for 3 hours at this point, and I think we know what the bottom line here is. Pharma can charge whatever it wants, period, full stop. And we now have watched over the last 3 hours the bookends, where Ms. Stern describes how her mom, with her help, is out there begging for a good chunk of the year to be able to cover a bit of the $111,000 that her mom has to pay for medicine.

So what is the response from some of my colleagues sitting over here? They say, "Oh, my goodness. We care about prices too, but if you do anything to really negotiate, oh, it is going to be horrible. We will not get innovation. We are not going to be able to make progress with the cures we all want."

So along comes Dr. Conti, who is a professor, a distinguished professor, and she lays out very clearly how when you negotiate in the right ways—and she described our bill as doing that—it is not price control, and it is not going to destroy innovation.

So that is where we are, folks. And to me, it is a serious problem right now. And the staff went out and found that the problem is getting worse. The differential between the international and domestic prices is getting worse.

So my message is—I am heading home this weekend for four town meetings. I have one in every one of my counties open to everybody. I had 1,000 of them. I am going to tell them what I said pretty much today. I am going to do everything in my power to make sure this Congress does not wrap up until the patients whom we have been talking about today get a fair shake, and pharma has not been able once again to derail real reform.

Everybody always bets on pharma because they are so powerful, and they have always been able to hold off change, to stiff-arm it, saying it is going to hurt innovation, and it is this, and it is that. Well, as I said earlier, this has been the longest-running battle since the Trojan War. This is the time now for the people of this country who have said overwhelmingly, we think it is just common sense for Medicare to be able to negotiate the price of medicine, because everybody negotiates everything else. It is just common sense to get that done.

And I want to say "thank you" to all of you. There are differences of opinion on this panel, and it has been a good debate. But I just want to make sure that the word to everybody in this country who is following this issue is, we are the committee that is in charge of it, and I am determined that this is going to be the time when there is real change, and finally the consumer gets a fair shake and is in a position to afford medicine and does not have to beg, and we follow Dr. Conti's counsel that we do it in a way that does not discourage innovation.

With that, the Finance Committee is adjourned. [Whereupon, at 12:49 p.m., the hearing was concluded.]

Appendix

Additional Material Submitted for the Record:

Prepared Statement of Rena Conti, Ph.D., Associate Professor, Department of Markets, Public Policy, and Law, Questrom School of Business, Boston University

Summary of Remarks

There is an urgent need for Congress to reform how Medicare pays for prescription drugs. Proposals to reduce drug prices, such as proposed in the recently passed House bill (H.R. 5376), will not harm pharmaceutical innovation and will improve affordability for the American public. I review the strong empirical evidence base supporting these claims.

My Background and Expertise

I am Rena M. Conti, Ph.D., associate professor of markets, public policy, and law in the Questrom School of Business, and co-director of the Technology Policy and Research Institute, a joint program of Boston University's Business and Law Schools. Between 2006 and 2018, I was faculty at the University of

Chicago. I am a graduate of Harvard University's Interfaculty Initiative in Health Policy, concentration economics.

My research interests are in the economics of the pharmaceutical industry. I have published over 100 peer reviewed articles, many in top economics, policy and medical journals. I have taught health economics and strategy in the pharmaceutical industry for 2 decades.

My research work is supported by grants, including from the National Cancer Institute, the Leukemia and Lymphoma Society, the American Cancer Society and Arnold Ventures.

Overview of Proposed Reforms and Likely Savings

There is a social compact between the American public and pharmaceutical companies: the industry is supported by taxpayer investments to benefit their health at an affordable price.[1] It does so by supporting all aspects of innovation and competition. Yet, some pharmaceutical companies are breaking the social compact. Pharmaceutical companies set prices of prescription drug which are so high they impose financial toxicity on the American public. Twenty-nine percent of Americans either can't afford their drugs or are rationing their drugs.[2] Instead of seeking the next breakthrough, companies delay competition to maintain exceptional revenue.

Reform Provisions Address These Challenges in Several Ways[3]

First, by imposing penalties on pharmaceutical companies to ensure that prices do not increase greater than inflation. These changes will reduce the number of prescriptions Americans don't fill or currently ration due to their expense.

Second, by extending new authority for the Federal Government to negotiate Medicare prices for selected drugs.[4] Negotiation will only target of drugs that have frequently manipulated the FDA rules and patent policy to extend exclusivity far beyond the intent of the legislation that created our patent system.

---

[1] Gruber J., Johnson S., "Jump-starting America: How breakthrough science can revive economic growth and the American dream." NY: Public Affairs, 2019.

[2] Kirzinger A., Lopes L., Wu Bryan, Brodie M., "KFF Health Tracking Poll—February 2019: Prescription Drugs." March 2019.

[3] Conti R.M., Frank R.G., Gruber J., "Regulating Drug Prices while Increasing Innovation." New England Journal of Medicine. 385(21): 1921–1923. November 2021.

[4] U.S. House of Representatives. "Drug Price Investigation. Lost Savings: How Prohibiting Medicare Negotiation Has Cost Taxpayers." Staff Report, Committee on Oversight and Reform. September 2021.

Third, by redesigning seniors' pharmacy coverage to cap out of pocket costs.

Reforms Will Generate Significant Savings for the American Public Over the Next Decade[5]

For example, reform proposals aim to cap seniors' out of pocket costs for insulin at $35 dollars per prescription. For the 2.27 million seniors who use insulin daily, this will result in measurable savings.[6] American workers will also benefit from this change.

With access improvements, better health will likely follow.[7]

Reform will benefit the American public in other ways. Reform will benefit tax-payers. One government estimate suggests reform will generate $160 billion in savings over the next decade.

Reform Will Not Harm Innovation

What These Proposals Will Not Do Is Harm Pharmaceutical Innovation

Prior debates on how to make drugs more affordable have been weighed down by concerns about how reducing any drug prices will reduce the number of new "cures." A particularly colorful version of this claim include the head of PhRMA, the industry lobby group, threatening reform would cause a "nuclear winter" for innovation.[8]

Those claims are not empirically based.

First, CBO Reports That the Proposed Legislation Would Have Very Little Impact on the Number of New Drugs Produced

The non-partisan Congressional Budget Office's report suggests that an earlier version of the latest House proposal would not result in material reductions in

---

[5] Congressional Budget Office. "CBO's Simulation Model of New Drug Development." Working Paper Series 2021–09. August 2021.

[6] Turner A., Conti R.M., Hughes-Cromwick P., "Strategies to Advance Insulin Affordability in the United States." Altarum's Center for Value in Health Care. September 2020.

[7] Chandra A., Flack E., Obermeyer Z., "The Health Costs of Cost Sharing." National Bureau of Economic Research Working Paper 28439. February 2021.

[8] U.S. House of Representatives, Committee on Oversight and Reform. "Drug Pricing Investigation: Majority Staff Report." December 2021.

innovation in the next decade and would have small effects over 30 years—1 less drug over the next decade and 4 less drugs over the subsequent decade.

Even then, the CBO report may have overstated reform's impact on innovation. CBO's estimate does not account for the coincident increases in profits the pharmaceutical industry has realized in the past 2 years and is expected to increase in the next 5 years.[9] CBO assumes pre-COVID–19 growth in revenues derived from pharmaceutical sales. It does not account for the expected effects of pharmaceutical company revenue increases from COVID–19 therapeutics and vaccine sales, and outsized revenues from new product launches in oncology and immunology.

Second, New Drugs Are Not the Same as New "Cures"

In the context of reform, the key policy question for assessing the trade-off is not how many new drugs maybe lost (i.e., absolute quantity of new drugs), but what is the likely impact on breakthrough treatments by reducing prices for a limited number of older high-cost drugs (i.e., quality of new drugs)?

Most of the evidence on which all sides base their claims come from the same "natural experiment", the expansion of Medicare to include the drug benefit or Medicare Part D implemented in 2006.[10] The research consistently showed that the number of new drugs grows as the market increased.

Yet, on the question of quality, the story is different. Research by Dranove and colleagues shows that the new launches following Part D implementation were almost entirely in areas where there were already existing therapies (5 or more, rather than 2 or fewer).[11] They also found that few were truly innovative. Figure 1 from the paper highlights this point clearly.

---

[9] IQVIA. "Global Medicine Spending and Usage Trends: Outlook to 2025." April 2021.

[10] Blume-Kohout M.E., Sood N., "Market Size and Innovation: Effects of Medicare Part D on Pharmaceutical Research and Development." *Journal of Public Economics.* 97: 327–336. January 2013.

[11] Dranove D., Garthwaite C., Hermosilla M., "Pharmaceutical Profits and the Social Value of Innovation." NBER Working Paper 20212. June 2014.

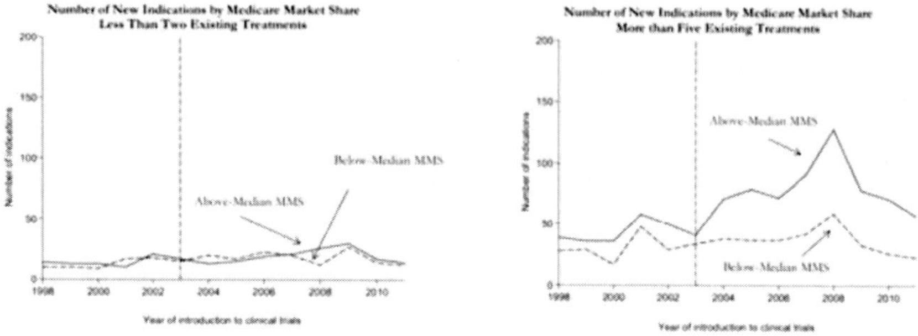

Figure 1. Number of New Indications by Medicare Market Share Less Than or More Than Five Existing Treatments.

Research by Amy Finkelstein[12] provides some insight into the possible mechanisms behind this. Her work argues that the companies took existing products that were "on the shelf" but not sufficiently profitable with the smaller market and launched them as the market grew.

Research by Byrski and colleagues extends this line of analysis.[13] They examine the same data on the impact of the creation of Part D and then looked at the impact of the market expansion on new drugs, new patents, and new published science. What they found was that they could replicate the increase in new drugs found by prior studies and there was no overall evidence of increases in patenting or new published science.

In addition, most of the new pharmaceutical products (excluding generics) approved by the U.S. FDA are not new drugs at all. Data on FDA approvals from 2011 through 2021 show that of all brand name drug products approved only 32 percent were new molecular entities. The rest represent new version of old drugs. This is reflected in industry SEC filings and public testimony showing large R&D investments in new formulations for existing blockbuster drugs.

- Bristol-Myers spent a large part of its 2018–2019 R&D dollars for line extensions for Opdivo and Yervoy existing blockbusters.
- Sanofi testified in the Senate that only 33 of its 81 R&D projects were for new chemical entities.

---

[12] Finkelstein A., "Static and Dynamic Effects of Health Policy: Evidence From The Vaccine Industry." *The Quarterly Journal of Economics.* 119(2): 527–564. May 2004.

[13] Byrski D., Gaessler F., Higgins M.J., "Market Size and Research: Evidence from the Pharmaceutical Industry." National Bureau of Economics Research Working Paper 28858. May 2021.

Third, New Breakthrough Treatments Come From New Science

Drug innovation that is truly transformative for human health often emerges in large part from taxpayer supported research and development, even though this is rarely reflected in the pricing of the resulting drugs, nor in commensurate "payback" to the funding agencies that made them possible.

While the industry often plays an important role in bringing new drugs to market, all drugs brought to market in the U.S. can trace their discovery back to NIH- supported basic and translational science.[14]

Current reforms will not alter the American public's support for these investments.

Therefore, as long as Congress continues funding the National Institutes of Health and university-based scientists, then we can be assured that the next generation of important new treatments will be in the pipeline.

Fourth, Additional Drivers of Innovation Will Not Be Altered by Reform

The pharmaceutical industry wouldn't exist without the support of the American public in many additional ways. These include:

- Patents and other types of intellectual property protections offer the potential for economic rewards to invention of new treatments.[15]
- Public support is also linked to the later-stage development of many transformative drugs at university labs or spin-off small companies before being acquired by large manufacturers.[16] For example, the public supports private sector investments into orphan diseases, antibiotics, COVID–19 therapeutics and vaccines.[17]
- Robust financial markets which affect both the existence and pace of innovation.[18]

---

[14] Kesselheim A.S., Tan Y.T., Avorn J., "The Roles of Academia, Rare Diseases, and Repurposing in the Development of the Most Transformative Drugs." Health Affairs (Millwood).

[15] Lerner J., "150 Years of Patent Protection." *American Economic Review.* 92(2): 221–225. May 2002.

[16] Nayak R.K., Avorn J., Kesselheim A.S., "Public sector financial support for late stage discovery of new drugs in the United States: Cohort study, *BMJ.* 367(l5766). September 2019.

[17] Congressional Research Service. "Operation Warp Speed Contracts for COVID–19 Vaccines and Ancillary Vaccination Materials." March 2021.

[18] Hall B., Lerner J., "The Financing of R&D and Innovation." Chapter 14 in *Handbook of the Economics of Innovation,* vol. 1: pp. 609–639. 2010.

The American public also supports policies that protect consumers from companies taking advantage of this support. For example, the U.S. Food and Drug Administration establishes the level of testing for safety and efficacy that pharmaceutical companies must conduct to avoid patient harm. Policies such as The Drug Price Competition and Patent Term Restoration Act of 1984, commonly known as the Hatch-Waxman Act, support innovation and competition.

Finally, Proposed Reforms Are Further Targeted to Mitigate Potential Harms to Innovation

Empirical evidence suggests even many of the most expensive drugs make in revenue the full costs of research and development within 5 years post-launch.[19] Under currently discussed reforms, drugs are only eligible for Medicare price negotiation after being on the U.S. market for more than a decade. Therefore, the proposed reforms give manufacturers plenty of time to make profits on new drugs while reducing the incentives companies currently face to forestall competition. Reform's focus on older drugs a decade or more post-launch for negotiation obviates another extreme argument the industry propounded earlier in the debate, that companies will refrain from launching their products in the U.S. if they are subject to negotiation.

There Is a Strong Evidence Base for the Reforms Currently Proposed

U.S. Pharmaceutical Spending Levels and Trends

There were 6.3 billion prescription dispensed in the U.S. market in 2020. Older Americans use most dispensed prescription drugs and polypharmacy is common. Nearly 7 in 10 adults aged 40–79 used at least 1 prescription drug in the past 30 days in the United States (69.0 percent) and around 1 in 5 used at least 5 prescription drugs (22.4 percent).[20]

---

[19] United States Government Accountability Office. "Drug Industry: Profits, Research and Development Spending, and Merger and Acquisition Deals." GAO–18–40. November 2017.

[20] Hales C.M., Servais J., Martin C.B., Kohen D., "Prescription drug use among adults aged 40–79 in the United States and Canada." NCHS (National Center for Health Statistics) Data Brief. 347. August 2019.

U.S. pharmaceutical spending currently represents approximately 14 percent of overall health-care spending,[21] including 4 percent of spending in non-retail outpatient clinics and hospital settings. Spending on pharmaceuticals has risen by 20 percent over the past 10 years; an average of 2 percent per year.[22]

U.S. spending on pharmaceuticals is forecast to grow 0–3 percent CAGR over the next 5 years. To put these figures in broader context, industry reports expect global medicine spending through 2025 to amount to about $1.6 trillion. Projected global spending on pharmaceuticals by IQVIA, the industry gold standard, is $88 billion higher than their pre-COVID outlook.

Two types of on patent "branded" pharmaceuticals contribute substantively to drug spending growth: new drugs and the expanded use of existing drugs. Also notable is that specialty drugs, including those in the protected Part D categories of oncology and immunology, have been increasing as a share of spending. In 2020, specialty drugs comprised 47 percent of spending, up from 24 percent 10 years earlier. Specialty drug spending is expected to increase to 60 percent of total pharmaceutical spending in the U.S. by 2025.

According to a recent analysis by the Kaiser Family Foundation, half of all Part D covered drugs (50 percent of 3,343 drugs) and nearly half of all Part B covered drugs (48 percent of 568 drugs) had price increases greater than inflation between July 2019 and July 2020, which was 1.0.[23] Moreover, 23 of the top 25 Part D drugs and 16 of the top 25 Part B drugs had price increases above inflation between 2019 and 2020.[24] See Figure 2 for details.

---

[21] Conti R.M., Turner A., Hughes-Cromwick P., "Projections of US Prescription Drug Spending and Key Policy Implications." *JAMA Health Forum.* 2(1): e201613. January 2021.

[22] IQVIA Institute. "The Use of Medicines in the United States." May 2021.

[23] Cubanski J., Neumann T., "Prices Increased Faster Than Inflation for Half of all Drugs Covered by Medicare in 2020." KFF Issue Brief. February 2022.

[24] Annual price increases are also inconsistent with the notion that prices are optimized for profit maximization at launch and appear unrelated to approval of supplemental indications, additional information about the benefits associated with treatment, and potential increases in manufacturing costs. *See* Bennette C.S., Richards C., Sullivan S.D., Ramsey S.D., "Steady In- crease in Prices for Oral Anticancer Drugs after Market Launch Suggests a Lack of Competitive Pressure." *Health Affairs* (Millwood). 35(5):805–12. May 2016.

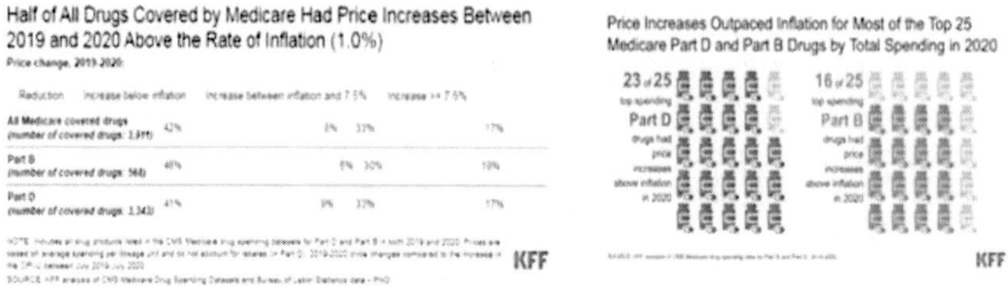

Figure 2. Price Trends Paid by Medicare Beneficiaries Outpace Inflation.

High Pharmaceutical Prices and Price Inflation Are a Result of Pharmaceutical Companies Breaking the Social Compact with the American Public

Paying high prices for new pharmaceuticals is one way among many the American public encourages innovation. The counterweight to paying high prices is competition. Our system relies on competition after patents and other exclusivities expire on pharmaceuticals to bring down prices and reduce spending. We expect companies to move onto innovate the next opportunities.

Yet, there is mounting empirical evidence that this social contract has been violated by some pharmaceutical companies.[25] New reports released by the U.S. House of Representatives' Oversight Committee details drug companies egregious and widespread manipulation of our system to delay competition from lower-priced generics and biosimilars of such drugs a decade or more after launch.

Price inflation is the direct result of pharmaceutical companies ensuring their profitability in drugs by delaying competition.[26] The House Oversight's recent report on Copaxone, an MS drug, suggests Teva played many games to forestall competition, while raising prices.[27] Celgene and Bristol Myers

---

[25] For an explanation and summary of activities, *see* Statement by Michael A. Carrier to House Judiciary Committee (Subcommittee on Antitrust, Commercial, and Administrative Law). House Subcommittee of House Judiciary Committee hearing. April 27, 2021.

[26] *See* for example, U.S. House of Representatives. "Drug Pricing Investigation AbbVie—Humira and Imbruvica." Staff Report, Committee on Oversight and Reform. May 2021. The report states "New documents show that these settlements allowed AbbVie to delay com- petition far beyond what its own internal assessments of the strength of its patent portfolio predicted. In 2014, AbbVie's executives estimated that three to five biosimilar competitors would enter the market by the first quarter of 2017. AbbVie ultimately entered into settlement agreements with four of these competitors, delaying their entry into the market until 2023."

[27] U.S. House of Representatives. "Drug Pricing Investigation Teva—Copaxone." Staff Report, Committee on Oversight and Reform. September 2020.

Squibb's Revlimid,[28] a drug that treats blood cancers launched in the U.S. in 2005, and Abbvie's Humira, a drug that treats arthritis and other inflammatory diseases launched into the U.S. market in 2002 has only recently faced competition. The pricing of these drugs in the U.S. has also increased since launch. A 1-month supply of Revlimid pills now costs approximately $23,000 and a 1-month supply of Humira injections costs approximately $10,000.

Moreover, the significant revenues reaped from these activities by the pharmaceutical companies are not primarily directed into research and development efforts. Instead, high prices, price increases and significant profits lead to higher executive compensation, dividend payments to stockholders and stock buybacks.[29]

Why Should Americans Always Have to Pay the Highest Prices for Pharmaceuticals?

The U.S. is the largest market for prescription drugs in the world.[30] Approximately 40 percent of all prescription drug sales is in the U.S. market.[31] Corporate profits off the sale of prescription drugs are expected to reach over $1.3 trillion in 2021 and the top pharmaceutical companies are more profitable than those in non- pharmaceutical industries, including the technology giants Apple and Amazon.[32]

Pharmaceutical companies strongly prefer to launch new drugs in the U.S. where they fetch the highest prices.[33] Unlike other OECD countries, U.S. payers place no limits on the prices pharmaceutical companies can charge for drugs while they are protected from competition by patents and market exclusivities. These features lead drug companies to set high prices well above standard measures of clinical and economic benefit and pursue price increases

---

[28] U.S. House of Representatives. "Drug Pricing Investigation Celgene and Bristol Myers Squibb—Revlimid." Staff Report, Committee on Oversight and Reform. September 2020.

[29] U.S. House of Representatives. "Industry Spending on Buybacks, Dividends, and Executive Compensation." Staff Report, Committee on Oversight and Reform. July 2021.

[30] nternational Federation of Pharmaceutical Manufacturers and Associations. "The Pharmaceutical Industry and Global Health. Facts and Figures 2021." April 2021.

[31] United States Government Accountability Office. "Drug Industry: Profits, Research and Development Spending, and Merger and Acquisition Deals." GAO–18–40. November 2017.

[32] Ledley F.D., McCoy S.S., Vaughan G., Cleary E.G., "Profitability of Large Pharmaceutical Companies Compared With Other Large Public Companies." *JAMA.* 323(9): 834–843. March 2020.

[33] National Academies of Sciences, Engineering, and Medicine. "Making Medicines Affordable: a National Imperative." Washington, DC: National Academies Press. 2018.

that greatly exceed the general rate of inflation.[34] In fact, evidence suggests pharmaceutical companies target U.S. payers for drug price increases, while at the same time decreasing prices in other countries. Celgene's Revlimid and Teva's Copaxone took significant price increases to increase revenue in the U.S. at the same time as cutting prices in other countries. In a new study of cancer drugs, pharmaceutical companies are observed to increase prices in the U.S. that exceed inflation, while at the same time prices stayed stable or declined in Germany and Switzerland.[35] When Abbvie pursued price increases on Humira, it claimed it did so because it was being "forced" to reduce prices in other countries. While it may make common sense for firm to offset "losses" with gains, this pricing behavior by pharmaceutical companies controverts the companies' own statements to Congress suggesting the prices of prescription drugs in the U.S. are untethered to those in other countries.[36]

While many expensive biologics remain without competition in the U.S., inexpensive biosimilars have been available since 2006 within Europe. In 2021, biologics represented 34 percent of spending in Europe on pharmaceuticals.[37] Despite 2020 being impacted by the COVID–19 pandemic, the volume of biosimilar prescribing in the EU is estimated to have generated a record high in savings from biosimilar competition, of Ö5.7 billion (about $6.8 billion USD) in savings versus the pre-biosimilar cost of the originator by 2020.

When reforms reduce the option for companies to pursue such behavior, pharmaceutical companies will move onto seek revenue by investing in innovative treatments. When the Supreme Court ruled that companies could no longer pay to delay generic entry, the companies that were doing that instead started to pour money into research and development.[38]

---

[34] Schondelmeyer S.W., Purvis L., "Rx Price Watch: Brand Name Drug Prices Increase More than Twice as Fast as Inflation in 2019." AARP Public Policy Institute. November 2019.

[35] Vokinger K.N., Hwang T.J., Carl D.L., Laube Y., Ludwig W.-D., Naci H., Kesselheim A.S., "Price changes and within-class competition of cancer drugs in the USA and Europe: A comparative analysis." *The Lancet Oncology*. March 2022.

[36] Pharmaceutical company executives have dismissed this as a possibility, stating repeatedly that there is no direct relationship between U.S. drug prices and foreign prices. *See* U.S. House of Representatives. "Drug Pricing Investigation AbbVie—Humira and Imbruvica." Staff Report, Committee on Oversight and Reform. May 2021; and PhRMA. Complaint, in Litigation Challenging Legality of the Administration's Most Favored Nation Rule. December 4, 2020.

[37] IQVIA. "The Impact of Biosimilar Competition in Europe." December 2021.

[38] Li X., Lo A.W., Thakor R.T., "Paying Off the Competition: Market Power and Innovation Incentives." NBER Working Paper 28964. June 2021.

American Public "Financial Toxicity" Related to High and Growing Pharmaceutical Prices

Expanded pharmaceutical insurance coverage has benefited many. Yet, too many seniors are locked out of the promise of pharmaceuticals currently available. The prices of some drugs seniors need to stay alive—such as Tysabri and Rebif for MS and Revlimid and Imbruvica for cancer—are now so high that they exceed the costs of a private university education. A recent survey suggests 18 million Americans can't pay for the drugs they need.[39] The substantial costs of cancer care on patients are now so common they are termed "financial toxicity," a play on the commonly encountered medical toxicities patients experience with chemotherapy.[40]

My own work on this topic focuses on the blood cancers, multiple myeloma (MM) and chronic lymphocytic leukemia (CLL), which represent a small percentage of all cancers, but for which treatment costs are among the highest. Treatment advances in both cancer types have resulted in greater survivorship and improved quality of life for patients. Nevertheless, my research group has found that close to half of the blood cancer patients we surveyed report financial difficulties associated with cancer treatment. Reports of financial burden commonly include an inability to pay for basic necessities such as food and utility bills, the presence of medical debt and high out of pocket burdens relative to income.

There is also underuse. In my study, reports of financial burden are associated with worrisome deficits in care—medication non-adherence including skipping medication, taking less medication or not filling recommended prescriptions at all. In other work, while new drugs have transformed calls for the elimination of HIV[41] and the hepatitis C virus by 2030[42] into tangible goals, these drugs remain under- used.

The status quo also imposes costs on taxpayers. Finally, these behaviors harm workers in the form of higher health insurance premiums and lower wages.

---

[39] Witters D., "In U.S., an Estimated 18 Million Can't Pay for Needed Drugs." Gallup. September 21, 2021.

[40] National Institutes of Health, National Cancer Institute. "Financial Toxicity Associated with Cancer Care—Background and Prevalence."

[41] U.S. Department of Health and Human Services. "HIV National Strategic Plan: A Roadmap to End the Epidemic for the United States 2021–2025." 2021.

[42] Hofmeister M.G., et al. "Estimating Prevalence of Hepatitis C Virus Infection in the United States, 2013–2016." *Hepatology*. 69: 1020–1031. November 2018; Centers for Disease Control and Prevention. "CDC Estimates Nearly 2.4 Million Americans Living with Hepatitis C." Press Release. November 2018.

Conclusion

In summary, the consequences of continued congressional inaction on pharmaceutical prices are simply untenable. Currently, 29 percent of Americans either can't afford their drugs or are rationing their drugs. Proposed reforms will not harm innovation. Proposed reforms will not alter the American public's substantial support for basic science, product development, strong universities, nor a highly favorable funding environment. Proposed reforms will not alter patents or market exclusivities pharmaceutical companies selling their products to American consumers currently enjoy nor reduce insurance coverage for these products.

After reform, the U.S. will remain the largest market for pharmaceuticals in the world. After reform, the U.S. pharmaceutical industry will remain the most profitable sector in our economy. After reform, the U.S. economy will remain the most highly supportive of innovation activity globally. Consequently, pharmaceutical companies will continue to invest in innovative products and investors will remain invested in this sector.

What these reforms do represent is a modest step towards limiting the economic burden placed on Americans from pharmaceutical companies' manipulations of our system. In doing so, they help restore the social compact between pharmaceutical companies and the American public.

Prepared Statement of Hon. Mike Crapo, U.S. Senator from Idaho

Thank you, Mr. Chairman, and thank you to all of our witnesses for being here today.

Congress plays an important role in ensuring access to affordable prescription drugs for Americans from all walks of life. To that end, last year, I reintroduced the Lower Costs, More Cures Act.

This comprehensive legislation contains dozens of concrete proposals aimed at lowering out-of-pocket costs at the pharmacy counter, in addition to strengthening supply chain oversight and combating foreign freeloading. With inflation at 40-year highs, straining family finances for far too many Americans, the Lower Costs, More Cures Act would bring peace of mind to seniors across the Nation by placing a hard cap on out-of-pocket drug spending under Medicare Part D.

Our bill would allow beneficiaries to access additional Part D plan choices, includiing low-deductible and reduced cost-sharing options, as well as plans that pass more discounts directly to consumers at the pharmacy counter. For seniors with diabetes, we would build on the work of the Trump administration, which established a game- changing program that guarantees access to insulin at no more than $35 a month. Our legislation would permanently protect and extend this initiative, which already covers more than two in every five seniors enrolled in Part D.

Nearly 2 decades ago, I joined bipartisan majorities in both chambers in voting to enact Medicare' prescription drug benefit. Since then, Part D has achieved incredible success, coming in at half of its projected cost, with stable premiums, high satisfaction rates, and more than 50 plan options for the average enrollee.

The Lower Costs, More Cures Act would build on these successes, advancing scores of pro-patient solutions for Medicare and the broader prescription drug market. Our legislation would strengthen cost-comparison tools, remove disincentives for prescribing lower-cost medications, enlist a Chief Pharmaceutical Negotiator to drive better trade deals for Americans, and facilitate outcomes-based arrangements for cutting-edge therapies, to name just a few key provisions.

Importantly, all of these solutions could pass both chambers of Congress with overwhelming support. Virtually every provision in the Lower Costs, More Cures Act reflects a bipartisan proposal with broad buy-in across the political spectrum. This bill, if allowed to advance, could head to the President' desk within days, delivering meaningful relief to Americans.

Unfortunately, all signs seem to indicate a partisan path forward on drug pricing, based on the deeply problematic policies included in the House-passed Build Back Better Act. These proposals would impose bureaucratic government price controls with a host of bad consequences for consumers, patients, and small businesses.

According to a recent study from University of Chicago researchers, innovative R&D would decline by nearly one-fifth under these proposed price controls, leading to a staggering 135 fewer new drug approvals in the next 2 decades.

Another report found that Medicare payments for physicians and other front-line health-care providers would also fall under the proposed government price-setting program, with add-on payments slashed by an average of 40 percent for those targeted. These policies, which borrow from the failed experiments of the past, would do nothing to tame inflation. In fact, they would trigger higher launch prices for new medications.

By enacting these drug price controls, we would hand a competitive edge to our global rivals, including the Chinese Communist Party. At home, we would see fewer new treatments and cures, higher prices for new drugs, more health-care provider strain and burnout, and an alarming expansion of the Federal bureaucracy, giving Washington, DC more control over our health-care system.

We have a responsibility to pursue solutions that reduce out-of-pocket drug spending, particularly for seniors. The Lower Costs, More Cures Act provides a practical blueprint for this type of initiative, leveraging targeted policies with bipartisan backing to address the needs of Americans at the pharmacy counter, the hospital, and the doctor' office.

In the weeks ahead, we should move toward consensus-driven legislation with broad buy-in, rather than partisan price controls likely to double down on the most deficient aspects of our health-care system.

We also need to identify policies that tackle the root causes and drivers of inflation, which rose to a staggering 7.9-percent rate, year over year, last month. This means reducing our crippling deficit; unleashing American energy; streamlining costly regulations that have strained small businesses; and protecting the tax reforms implemented under the Tax Cuts and Jobs Act of 2017, which led to record- high levels of business investment, historic lows in unemployment and poverty, and record-high incomes during the past administration.

With that, I thank our witnesses again for joining us and testifying today. Thank you, Mr. Chairman.

Prepared Statement of Stephen J. Ezell, Vice President, Global Innovation Policy, Information Technology and Innovation Foundation

Introduction

Chairman Wyden, Ranking Member Crapo, and members of the Senate Finance Committee, thank you for inviting me to share the views of the Information Technology and Innovation Foundation (ITIF) on the issue of the

U.S. life-sciences innovation ecosystem and the relationship between drug prices and patient costs in the U.S. Medicare and broader health-care system.

ITIF is an independent, nonpartisan research and educational institute focusing on the intersection of technological innovation and public policy. As the world's leading science and technology policy think tank, ITIF's mission is to formulate and promote policy solutions that accelerate innovation and boost productivity to spur growth, opportunity, and progress.

While there is a need to reform the Medicare Part D program—notably by capping out-of-pocket patient costs and reforming rebate policies—the reconstructive surgery of drug price controls envisioned in the Build Back Better Act (BBBA), the H.R. 3 legislation before it, or the prior administration's International Price Index (IPI) is not the ideal way to manage America's drug prices.

This testimony begins by contending that U.S. prescription drug expenditures have been broadly stable and consistent over time—and expected to continue to be so in the future—while broadly in line with those of international peers. It will show that prescription drug prices are, in fact, not a contributor to increased U.S. inflation rates and that, overall, consumer prescription drug expenditures have risen at a much lower rate than the increase in total health-care expenditures since 2005.[43] It will contend that to the extent policymakers wish to reform drug pricing challenges, they need to consider the costs that are introduced by all actors across the pharmaceutical supply chain and compare profits in all relevant sectors, where the drug industry has lower profits than most other health-care subsectors. It will then examine the impact America's biopharmaceutical sector has on the U.S. economy and examine the significant value of the medicines and therapies the sector produces on Americans' quality, longevity, productivity, and the economic impacts thereof. It will contend that stringent drug price controls are not only unnecessary and unwarranted but actually quite damaging in a number of ways, including by inhibiting drug research and development (R&D), actually impeding patients' access to innovative medicines, and potentially undermining nations' biopharmaceutical competitiveness, as drug price controls have in other nations. It concludes with policy recommendations to better manage drug prices, including policy actions that could increase the

[43] Gabriel Rubin, "Inflation Reached 7.9 percent in February; Consumer Prices Are the Highest in 40 Years," Wall Street Journal, March 10, 2022, https:// www.wsj.com/articles/us-inflation-consumer-price-index-february-2022- 11646857681.

R&D efficiency of America's biopharmaceutical innovation system and reforms to assist seniors at the pharmacy counter.

America is fortunate to be home to the world's leading biopharmaceutical indus- try—one that leads the world in R&D spending and the introduction of innovative, often breakthrough drugs that improve, extend, and save lives. That America has become the leader as a result in part of intentional and conscientious public policy choices over the past 4 decades to make it so: robust public and private R&D investments, investment incentives like the R&D tax credit, and strong technology transfer and commercialization systems. American policymakers should be proud of this industry and have as their foremost consideration policies that could further enhance its innovation and productivity potential, such as increased National Institutes of Health (NIH) R&D funding, expansion of public-private industrial R&D programs such as the National Institute for Innovation in Manufacturing Biopharmaceuticals (NIIMBL) that seek to enhance the cost-effectiveness of drug discovery and manufacturing practices, and building up America's biomedical STEM (science, technology, engineering, and mathematics) talent pipeline.

On February 2, 2022, President Biden announced an aggressive, revitalized cancer moonshot that seeks to reduce the death rate from cancer by at least 50 percent over the next 25 years while improving the experience of people and their families living with and surviving cancer, thus trying to "end cancer as we know it today."[44] While these are certainly laudable and needed aspirational goals, the last thing policymakers should be doing is introducing stringent drug price controls that would hinder investments needed to meet the challenge.[45] Moreover, this is at a time when competitors, especially China, are seeking to overtake America's lead in the bio- pharmaceutical industry.[46]

Policymakers should proceed very cautiously before drastically reforming a successful system that has enabled America to lead the world in biomedical innovation, to get innovative drugs to patients first, to support a vibrant and

---

[44] The White House, "Fact Sheet: President Biden Reignites Cancer Moonshot to End Cancer as We Know It," February 2, 2022, https://www.white house.gov/briefing-room/statements-releases/2022/02/02/fact-sheet-president- biden-reignites-cancer-moonshot-to-end-cancer-as-we-know-it/.

[45] Robert D. Atkinson, "Op-Art: Drug Price Controls vs. the NIH 'Cancer Moonshot' Initiative," February 21, 2022, *https://itif.org/publications/2022/02/ 21/op-art-drug-price-controls-vs-nih-cancer-moonshot-initiative.*

[46] Robert D. Atkinson, "The Impact of China's Policies on Global Biopharma- ceutical Industry Innovation" (ITIF, September 2020), *https://itif.org/publi- cations/2020/09/08/ impact-chinas-policies-global-biopharmaceutical-indus-try-innovation.*

competitive domestic biopharmaceutical industry, and to do so while maintaining stable prescription drug expenditures (as a share of total health-care expenditures) over time through a system that marries incentives for innovation and conditions for competition with pathways to introduce cheaper generic and biosimilar drugs.

Drug Expenditures Have Been Stable Over Time

Critics contend that drugs have experienced "skyrocketing costs," are rapidly rising, and are a major contributor to U.S. inflation.[47] However, the data suggests that, broadly, U.S. drug expenditures have been roughly stable over time.[48] For instance, according to the Peterson Center on Healthcare and Kaiser Family Foundation, the percentage of total U.S. health-care spending going toward retail prescription drugs was consistent from 2000 to 2017, at mostly under 10 percent, and even dipped slightly to 8 percent in 2020.[49] (See Figure 1.)

Figure 1. Percentage of total health spending going to retail prescription drugs, 2000-2020.[50]

[47] Office of Congresswoman Katie Porter, "Killer Profits: How Big Pharma Take- overs Destroy Innovation and Harm Patients" (January 2021), 15, *https:// porter.house.gov/ uploadedfiles/final_pharma_ma_and_innovation_report_ january_2021.pdf.*

[48] Robert D. Atkinson and Stephen Ezell, "Five Fatal Flaws in Rep. Katie Por- ter's Indictment of the U.S. Drug Industry" (ITIF, May 20, 2021), *https:// itif.org/publications/2021/05/20/ five-fatal-flaws-rep-katie-porters-indictment- us-drug-industry.*

[49] Peterson-Kff Health Systems Tracker, Peterson Center on Healthcare and Kaiser Family Foundation (National Health Spending, accessed March 12, 2022), *https://www.healthsystemtracker.org/health-spending-explorer/.*

[50] Rabah Kamal, Cynthia Cox Twitter, and Daniel McDermott, "What are the recent and forecasted trends in prescription drug spending?" (Peterson Center on Healthcare and

Moreover, the prescription drug share of national health expenditures is expected to remain stable and consistent going forward—just as it has over the past 2 decades. In fact, in a 2020 report, research firm Altarum found that the share should remain roughly stable in the 9 percent range through most of this decade, with non-retail expenditures also roughly stable in the 4.5- to 4.9-percent range over that period. (See Figure 2.) Prescription medicines account for approximately 14 percent (as of 2018, 13.7 percent) of total U.S. health-care spending, with that overall share also looking to remain consistent throughout this decade.[51]

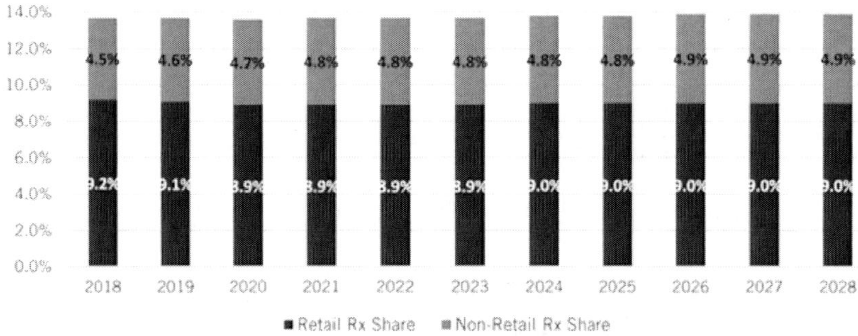

Figure 2. Rojected Prescription drug share of national health ependiture, 2018-2028.[52]

It should also be noted that America's expenditures on pharmaceuticals are well in-line with those of international peers. The Organisation for Economic Co-operation and Development (OECD) provides internationally comparable data on OECD members' expenditures on pharmaceutical drugs as a percentage of their total health spending. For 2020, the United States stood right in line with peer nations, with its 12.6 percent of expenditures (as calculated by the OECD's methodology) just slightly more than Austria, France, Ireland, and Switzerland's 11.9 percent and below Australia and Germany's 13.8 and 14.3 respectively.[53] Sweden's substantially lower share at 9.7 percent and Japan's reportedly higher share at 17.8 percent may well

Kaiser Family Foundation, February 20, 2019), *https:// www.healthsystemtracker.org/ chart-collection/recent-forecasted-trends-pre-scription-drug-spending.*

[51] *Ibid.*

[52] Altarum, "Projections of the Non-Retail Prescription Drug Share of National Health Expenditures," September 2020, 3, *https://altarum.org/publications/ projections-non-retail-prescription-drug-share-national-health-expenditures.*

[53] Note, the OECD uses a slightly different accounting methodology to equiva- lently compare countries' prescription drug health expenditures; the point is meant to be illustrative.

reflect population health peculiarities: Sweden having one of the world's more physically fit populations, Japan a more elderly one that requires more prescriptions. But the broader point stands: on this indicator, as with many others, U.S. pharmaceutical spending as a share of national health spending is quite in line with peer nations and far from out of balance. Moreover, for a roughly equivalent level of national investment, America's life-sciences system gives it so much more, including the ability to field the world's most competitive biopharma industry and lead the world producing innovative medicines and getting them to citizens first.

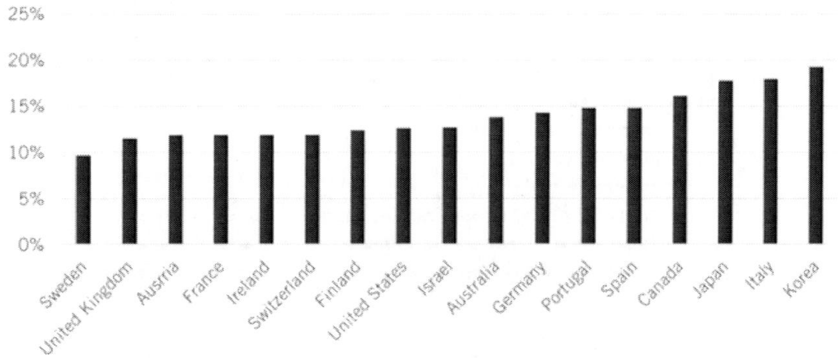

Figure 3. Pharmaceutical spending as % total health spending, 2020 (latest available year)[54]

Thus, both historical and international expenditure trends demonstrate that U.S. prescription drug spending cannot be termed "skyrocketing" or abnormally high. Drug expenditures have largely been stable, suggesting that the historical rate of increase in drug prices has not been excessive compared to other health-care costs.

Moreover, prescription drugs are in no way a significant contributor to the in- creased inflation the United States is presently experiencing. In fact, over the past 12 months, prescription drug prices increased just 2.4 percent, well below the average consumer price index (CPI) increase of 8 percent and less than other parts of the U.S. health-care system, such as health insurance, which experienced a 4.1- percent increase. (See Figure 4.)

[54] Organisation for Economic Co-operation and Development, "Pharmaceutical spending as percent total health spending, 2020 (or latest available year)," *https://data.oecd.org/healthres/pharmaceutical-spending.htm.*

Nor is this recent trend unique. In fact, as calculated by the U.S. Bureau of Labor Statistics, from 2005 to 2020, Americans' reported expenditures on health insurance increased by over 160 percent, and total health-care expenditures increased 94 percent, while consumer expenditures on drugs actually fell by almost 9 percent. (See Figure 5.) Of course, this does not necessarily mean overall drug expenditures fell because health insurance and hospitals also purchase drugs, but it does address consumers' out-of-pocket costs.

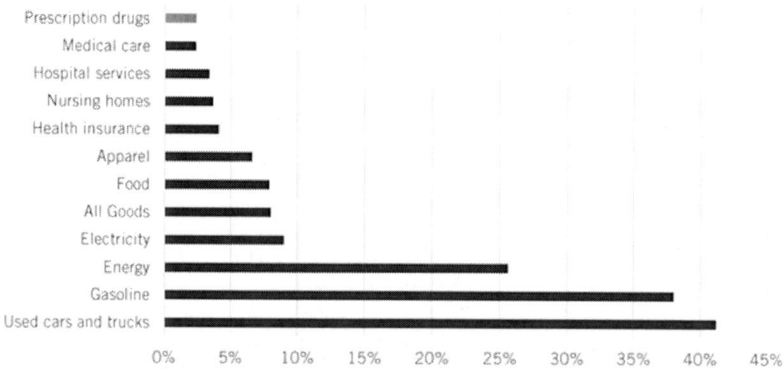

Figure 4. Concumer price index by sector, 12-month change ending in February 2022.[55]

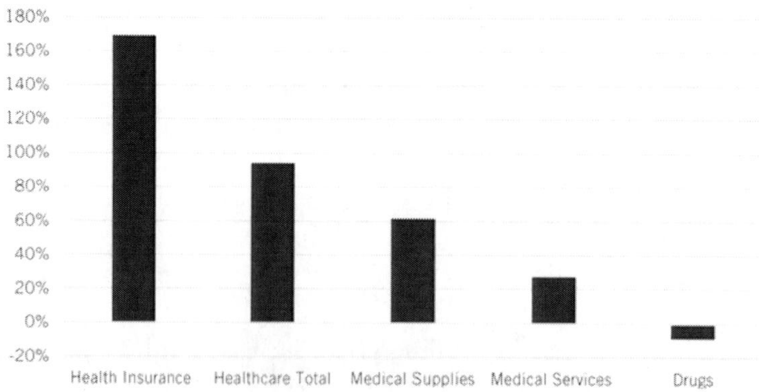

Figure 5. Percent change in consumers' reported healthcare expenditures, 2005-2020.[56]

[55] Bureau of Labor Statistics, Consumer Price Index (accessed March 10, 2022), *https://www.bls.gov/cpi/*.

[56] Bureau of Labor Statistics, Consumer Expenditure Survey (Health care expenditures, 2005–2020), *https://www.bls.gov/cex/*.

While drug expenditures have grown at moderate rates in recent years, an increasing share of those expenditures goes not to the manufacturer but to other actors in the supply chain. When payment is made for a prescription drug at the point of sale, only a portion of that payment accrues to the drug manufacturer. The rest accrues to non-manufacturer stakeholders in the supply chain—pharmacy benefit managers (PBMs), health plans, hospitals, the government, and pharmacies in the form of rebates, discounts, fees, and other payments.[57]

Over time, drug manufacturers have lost a growing share of drug expenditures to other members of the drug supply chain, such as PBMs, health plans, hospitals, the government, and pharmacies. Since 2013, the share of drug expenditures going to manufacturers has decreased by 13 percent. Thus, while total expenditures on brand drugs grew by $268 billion between 2013 and 2020, only 31 percent of the increase accrued to the manufacturers, while 69 percent accrued to other stake- holders. By 2020—for the first time ever—over half of drug expenditures accrued to non-manufacturers. (See Figure 6.)

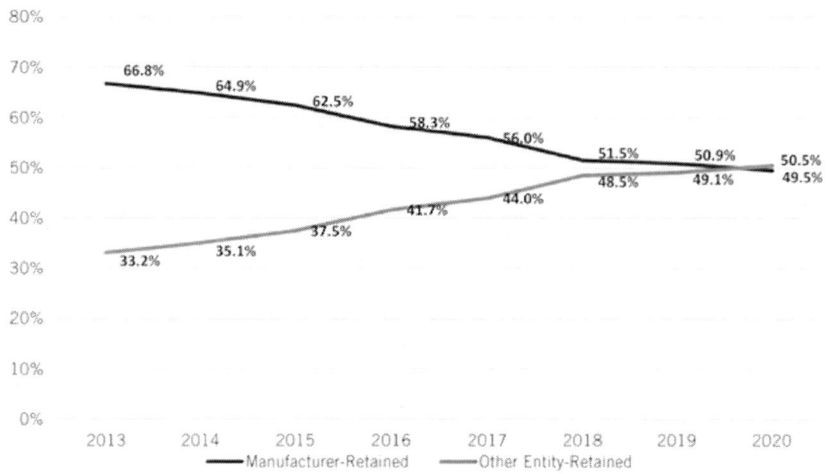

Figure 6. Total gross expenditures for brand medicines received by manufacturers and other stakeholders (2013-2020).[58]

[57] Andrew Brownlee and Joran Watson, "The Pharmaceutical Supply Chain, 2013–2020" (Berkeley Research Group, 2022), 3, *https://www.thinkbrg.com/ insights/publications/ pharmaceutical-supply-chain-2013-2020/.*

[58] *Ibid.*

Indeed, particular attention must be paid to the role played by rebates and discounts. Discussion of drug prices tends to focus on the annually announced increase in the list prices for prescription drugs. However, sales of prescription drugs are subject to substantial manufacturer rebates and discounts, leading to a considerable reduction in manufacturer earnings. Researchers at the University of Pittsburgh School of Pharmacy and Medicine estimate that while the average annual increase in the list price for prescription drugs between 2007 and 2018 was 9.1 percent, the net increase in drug prices after rebates was only 4.5 percent.[59]

In recent years, as list prices have been growing at a slower pace, the volume of discounts and rebates has increased. For example, in 2020, list prices grew at an average rate of 4.4 percent, but net prices decreased by 2.9 percent.[60] As The Wall Street Journal, citing data from the SSR Health Report, notes, "[A]verage U.S. list prices for prescription medicines rose in the past decade, but net prices—after rebates and discounts—rose less sharply and have recently declined."[61] (See Figure 7.) In fact, one study found that more than one-third of drug list prices were rebated back to pharmacy benefit managers and other entities in the supply chain. As that report describes, "Pharmaceutical spending estimates that omit rebates and discounts do not fully reflect the underlying competitive dynamics of the pharmaceutical sector and provide a misleading impression of drug spending."[62]

Fees charged by intermediaries also subtract from drug manufacturer revenues. PBMs nearly quadrupled the fees they charge biopharmaceutical companies—such as administrative and service fees—between 2014 and 2016. Total fees charged to biopharmaceutical companies by these middlemen increased from $1.5 billion in 2014 to $2.6 billion in 2015, and then doubled to nearly $5.6 billion in 2016. Along with rebates, these fees—which are typically based on the list price of a medicine— contribute to a system of

---

[59] Inmaculada Hernandez et al., "Changes in List Prices, Net Prices, and Discounts for Branded Drugs in the US, 2007–2018," *Journal of the American Medical Association,* Vol. 323, No. 9 (2020): 856, *https://pubmed.ncbi. nlm.nih.gov/32125403/.*

[60] Ibid., 27.

[61] Jared S. Hopkins and Peter Loftus, "Flip the Script: Drugmakers Blame Mid- dlemen for Price Increases," The Wall Street Journal, February 5, 2019, https://www.wsj.com/articles/flip-the-script-drugmakers-blame-middlemen-for-price-hikes-11549364401.

[62] Aaron Vandervelde and Eleanor Blalock, "The Pharmaceutical Supply Chain: Gross Drug Expenditures Realized by Stakeholders" (Berkeley Research Group, 2017), *https://www.thinkbrg.com/media/publication/863_Vandervelde_PhRMA-January-2017_WEB-FINAL.pdf.*

misaligned incentives where middlemen make more money when the list prices of medicines increase.[63]

Despite an increase in the share of negotiated rebates shared with health plan and employer clients, total PBM revenue increased between 2014 and 2016. That's in part due to the increasing administrative fees they charged bio-pharmaceutical companies. But PBMs aren't just charging biopharmaceutical companies more than ever before—they also brought in a record total of $22.4 billion in revenue in 2016 by charging more to others in the supply chain, such as health plans and phar- macies.[64]

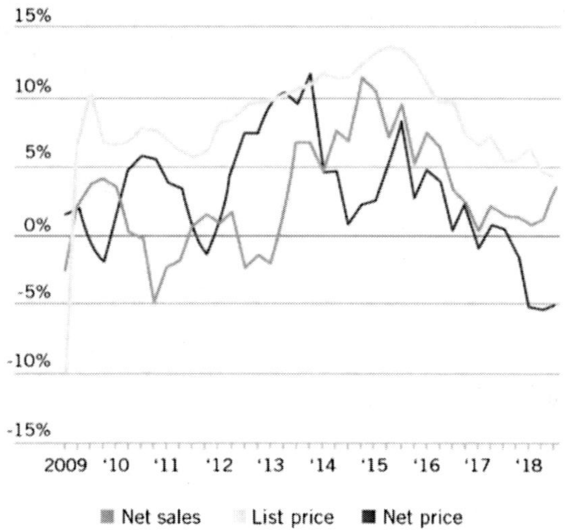

Figure 7. Change from a year earlier in U.S. prespcription brand prices, 2009-2019.[65]

Profitability

America's life-sciences innovation sectors are not enjoying consistently outsized returns, particularly when compared to other actors in America's health-care system. For example, Deloitte's "2020 Global Life-sciences Outlook" report finds that drug intermediaries and retailers—notably

[63] Robert Zirkelbach, "The PBM story you haven't heard: Hidden fees quad- rupled in 2 years," *The Catalyst,* March 20, 2019, *https://catalyst.phrma.org/ the-pbm-story-you-havent-heard-hidden-fees-quadrupled-in-two-years.*

[64] Ibid.

[65] Hopkins and Lotus, "Flip the Script: Drugmakers Blame Middlemen for Price Increases."

pharmacies, wholesalers, and PBMs—generally earned higher returns on investment over the years 2011 to 2017 than the biopharmaceutical and medical device manufacturers who are actually innovating new-to-the-world, life-saving or life-improving drugs and medical devices.[66] By 2017, pharmacies and wholesalers continued to enjoy substantially higher returns on cap- ital (RoC), while PBMs and health plans realized slightly larger returns than pharmaceuticals. (See Figure 8.)

In fact, the report found that of the U.S. health-care sectors it studied (as shown below), life-sciences manufacturers (pharmaceuticals and medical technology) actually experienced the largest drop in returns on capital (ROC), from 17 percent in 2011 to 11 percent in 2017.[67] In other words, the often-made claim that drug prices are too high because of limited competition and excess profits does not hold up to the evidence.

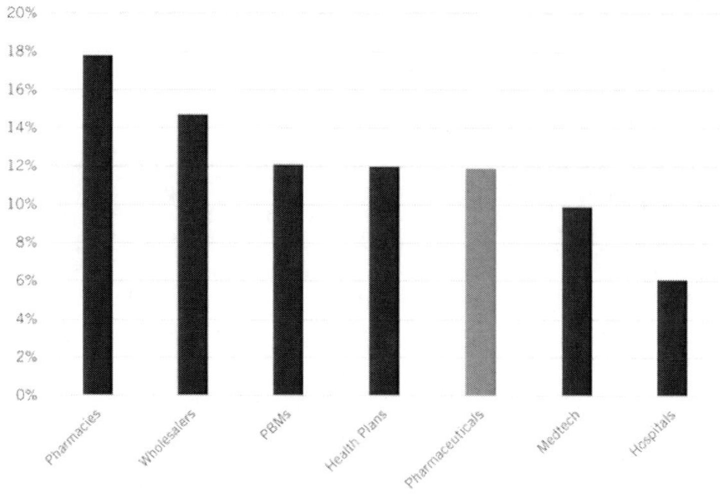

Figure 8. Return on capital performance in health care sectors, 2017.[68]

Researchers at the University of Southern California have sought to estimate excess returns (the extent to which a firm's profits are higher than expected given the risk associated with their investments) for manufacturers and middlemen in the pharmaceutical supply chain. They found that the rate

[66] Greg Reh, "2020 Global Life-sciences Outlook: Creating new value, building blocks for the future" (Deloitte, 2020), 17, *https://www.economist.com/search?q=pharmaceutical + industry+returns.*

[67] *Ibid.*

[68] *Ibid.*

of return on investments of large firms in the pharmaceutical industry between 2013 and 2018 was just 1.7 percent once adjusted for the risk premium paid for capital and the more logical treatment of R&D expenditures as long-term investments rather than current costs.[69] For comparison, the overall S&P 500 had an excess rate of return of more than dou- ble—3.6 percent—over this period.

In an article in the International Journal of Health Economics and Management, Sood et al. found that other players in the pharmaceutical supply chain realized higher excess returns. Specifically, for the period 2003 to 2018, they found that wholesalers earned excess returns of 8.1 percent and that insurers, PBMs, and retailers collectively earned excess returns of 5.9 percent. The authors did find that the cohort of biotechnology firms in their study realized the highest excess returns of any group, at 9.6 percent, though they note this was in part driven by several blockbuster drugs introduced from 2013–2015, notably new hepatitis C drugs, and that by 2018 the sector's excess rate of return had fallen to under 9 percent. More importantly, however, the authors note that, "In contrast with middlemen, monopoly power in the pharmaceutical and biotech sectors—derived through the U.S. patent system—provides [an] incentive for innovation that might not happen otherwise."[70] In other words, as the subsequent section elaborates, society enjoys high-value impacts in terms of quality, productivity, and longevity of life from the latter sector's returns. Sood et al. conclude by fairly noting that "policies that promote competition in all areas of the pharmaceutical supply chain are important avenues" for managing drug spending.

That said, even modestly higher returns for America's biotechnology or pharmaceutical sectors should not be cause for significant concern. As a former Congressional Office of Technology Assessment (OTA) study pointed out, "Pharmaceutical R&D is a risky investment; therefore, high financial returns are necessary to induce companies to invest in researching new chemical entities."[71] Or, as Harvard University industrial organization economist Scherer writes, "Had the returns to pharmaceutical R&D

---

[69] Neeraj Sood, et al., "Do companies in the pharmaceutical supply chain earn excess returns?", *International Journal of Health Economics and Management* (January 4, 2021): 99–114, *https://doi.org/10.1007/s10754-020-09291-1.* The researchers calculated the "risk adjusted rate of return" by subtracting capital costs, which vary with the level of risk across industries.

[70] *Ibid.,* 110.

[71] U.S. Congress, Office of Technology Assessment (OTA), "Pharmaceutical R&D: Costs, Risks and Rewards," OTA–H–522 (Washington, DC: U.S. Government Printing Office, February 1993), 2, *http://ota.fas.org/reports/9336.pdf.*

investment not been attractive, it seems implausible that drugmakers would have expanded their R&D so much more rapidly than their industrial peers."[72]

This is why price controls would be so damaging to the industry. As the OTA study found, "excess returns over R&D costs would be eliminated if the annual revenue per compound was reduced by 4.3 percent over the product's life." This is a similar finding to the OTA's finding that U.S. drug firms had an average profit rate of just 2 to 3 percentage points higher per year than the internal rate of return in control-group industries.[73] In other words, efforts to drive down profits may yield only small price declines, as compared to generating significant R&D reductions, as a subsequent section further elaborates.[74]

Value Created by Innovative Drugs

The reality is that America derives tremendous value from the 14 cents on every health-care dollar it spends on prescription drugs. First, pharmaceutical innovation boosts longevity, productivity, and standards of living. Second, pharmaceutical treatments and therapies that can intervene earlier to prevent, effectively treat, or even cure diseases can save America's health-care system from incurring considerable costs by helping keep patients out of hospitals and physicians' offices. For this reason, far from being viewed solely or even principally as a cost, medicines (and their prices) should be viewed as a key component of the solution to burgeoning overall health-care system costs. For example, if the cost of medicines were to increase by 10 percent, but this could yield 15- or 20-percent savings to the broader health-care system, then surely this would be a tradeoff worth making.

To the first point above, Columbia University professor Frank Lichtenberg finds that pharmaceutical innovation accounted for 73 percent (or 1.27 years of the 1.73- year increase in life expectancy) of the increase between 2000 and 2009 in life expectancy at birth across 30 countries,

---

[72] F.M. Scherer, "Pricing, Profits, and Technological Progress in Pharmaceutical Industry," *Journal of Economic Perspectives,* Vol. 7, No. 3 (Summer 1993): 97–115, *http://pubs.aeaweb.org/doi/pdfplus/10.1257/jep.7.3.97.*

[73] U.S. Congress, Office of Technology Assessment, "Pharmaceutical R&D: Costs, Risks and Rewards," 24.

[74] Robert D. Atkinson, "Why Life-Sciences Innovation Is Politically 'Purple'— And How Partisans Get It Wrong" (ITIF, February 2016), *https://itif.org/ publications/2016/02/22/ why-life-sciences-innovation-politically-purple.*

including the United States.[75] Another study by Lichtenberg found that drugs launched since 1982 have added 150 million life- years to the lifespans of citizens of the 22 countries analyzed, with the average pharmaceutical expenditure per life-year saved being $2,837.[76] In other words, it would cost just $2,837 to extend life 1 year. A related study found that if no new drugs had been launched after 1981, the number of years of life lost would have been more than twice as high as it actually was.[77]

Consider cancer. Since peaking in the 1990s, U.S. cancer fatality rates have fallen by 32 percent.[78] Approximately 73 percent of survival gains in cancer are attributable to new treatments, including medicines.[79] For instance, the development of breakthrough drugs such as Imatinib for chronic myeloid leukemia (CML) has increased the 5-year survival rate for CML patients to 89 percent, with many CML patients now living close-to-normal lifespans.[80] Such innovations explain why American citizens enjoy the highest cancer-survival rates in the world, with over 90 percent of U.S. women suffering from breast cancer still living 5 years later, something which matters greatly when 1 in 2 American women, and 1 in 3 men, are likely to receive a cancer diagnosis in their lifetime.[81]

To the second point, drugs further produce health system value well above their cost. For instance, Lichtenberg finds that from 1997 to 2010, "the value of reductions in work loss days and hospital admissions attributable to

---

[75] Frank Lichtenberg, "Pharmaceutical Innovation and Longevity Growth in 30 Developing and High-income Countries, 2000–2009," *Health Policy and Tech- nology,* Vol. 3, Issue 1 (March 2014): 36–58, *https://www.sciencedirect.com/science/article/abs/pii/S221188371 3000646.*

[76] Stephen Kurczy, "Calculating the Benefit of Drugs," Columbia Business School Ideas and Insights, February 12, 2019, *https://www8.gsb. columbia.edu/articles/ideas-work/calculating-benefits-drugs.*

[77] Stephen Chupaska, "The Value of a Vaccine," *Columbia Business School Ideas and Insights,* March 23, 2020, *https://www8.gsb.columbia.edu/articles/ideas- work/value-vaccine.*

[78] Rebecca L. Siegel et al., "Cancer Statistics, 2021," *CA: A Cancer Journal for Physicians,* (Volume 7, Issue 1): 7–33, *https://acsjournals.onlinelibrary. wiley.com/doi/full/ 10.3322/caac.21654.*

[79] Seth A. Seabury et al., "Quantifying Gains in the War on Cancer Due to Im- proved Treatment and Earlier Detection," *Forum for Health Economics and Policy,* Vol. 19, Issue 1 (November 2015), *https://www.degruyter.com/view/ journals/fhep/19/1/article-p141.xml.*

[80] C. Gambacorti-Passerini et al., "Multicenter independent assessment of out- comes in chronic myeloid leukemia patients treated with imatinib," *Journal of the National Cancer Institute,* Vol. 103, Issue 7 (April 2011): 553–561, *https://pubmed.ncbi.nlm.nih.gov/ 21422402/.*

[81] Stephen Ezell, "Seizing the Transformative Opportunity of Multi-cancer Early Detection" (ITIF, April 2021), *https://itif.org/publications/2021/04/19/seizing-transformative-opportunity-multi-cancer-early-detection.*

pharmaceutical innovation was three times larger than the cost of new drugs consumed."[82] Elsewhere, Lichtenberg found that the mean number of lost workdays, lost school days, and hospital admissions declined more rapidly among medical conditions with larger in- creases in the mean number of new (post-1990) prescription drugs consumed.[83] He further found that "the use of newer prescription drugs also reduced the ratio of the number of workers receiving Social Security Disability Insurance benefits to the working-age population, and has had a positive effect on nursing home residents' ability to perform activities of daily living."[84] Updating this work in October 2021, Lichtenberg estimated the value in 2015 of the reductions in disability, Social Security recipiency, and use of medical care attributable to previous biopharmaceutical innovation. That value, estimated at $115 billion annually, stood fairly close to 2015 expenditures, $127 billion, on drug classes that were first approved by the U.S. Food and Drug Administration (FDA) during the period 1989 to 2006.[85]

Thus, far from being the leading cause of rising U.S. health-care system costs, greater levels of life-sciences innovation will be key to limiting the growth of those costs. Indeed, significant economic benefits could be achieved if innovative medicines could make progress toward addressing some of the most intractable diseases.[86] For instance, even just a 1-percent reduction in mortality from cancer would deliver roughly $500 billion in net present benefits, while a cure could deliver $50 trillion in present and future benefits.[87] Likewise, the financial impact of Alzheimer's disease is expected to soar to $1 trillion per year by 2050, with much of the cost borne by the Federal Government, according to the Alzheimer's Association report "Changing the

---

[82] Frank R. Lichtenberg, "The Impact of Pharmaceutical Innovation on Dis- ability Days and the Use of Medical Services in the United States, 1997– 2010," *Journal of Human Capital*, Vol. 8, No. 4 (Winter 2014): 432–480, *https://www.jstor.org/stable/10.1086/679110.*

[83] Frank R. Lichtenberg, "The Benefits of Pharmaceutical Innovation: Health, Longevity, and Savings" (Montreal Economic Institute, 2016), 5, *https:// www.iedm.org/files/ cahier 0216_en_0.pdf.*

[84] *Ibid.*

[85] Frank R. Lichtenberg, "The impact of biopharmaceutical innovation on dis- ability, Social Security recipiency, and use of medical care of U.S. community residents, 1988–2015," National Bureau of Economic Research, NB21–02 (October 2021), *https://www.nber.org/programs-projects/projects-and-centers/retirement-and-disability-research-center/center-papers/nb21-02.*

[86] Stephen Ezell, "The Imperative of Protecting Life-Sciences Innovation in the TPP" (ITIF, March 2015), *http://www2.itif.org/2015-life-science-tpp.pdf.*

[87] Joe Kennedy and Robert D. Atkinson, "Healthy Funding: Ensuring a Predict- able and Growing Budget for the National Institutes of Health" (ITIF and United for Medical Research, February 2015), 2, *http://www2.itif.org/2015-healthy-funding.pdf.*

Trajectory of Alzheimer's Disease."[88] However, the United States could save $220 billion within the first 5 years and a projected $367 billion in the year 2050 alone if a cure or effective treatment for Alzheimer's disease were found. Overall, the potential economic opportunity associated with curing brain diseases and related disorders could be more than $1.5 trillion per year—equivalent to 8.8 percent of U.S. gross domestic product (GDP).[89] Of course, these kinds of returns aren't limited to the life-sciences industry; they're indicative of the economic value returned by America's innovation industries in general, which is why Yale economist William Nordhaus found that, "Inventors capture just 4 percent of the total social gains from their innovations," while the other 96 percent spills over to other companies and society as a whole.[90]

Economic Impact of America's Biopharmaceutical Industry

America is fortunate to host the world's leading biopharmaceutical industry. In 2017, America's biopharmaceutical industry produced $560 billion in direct economic output, with the ripple effect of this production throughout the economy generating an additional $589 billion in output from suppliers and other economic sectors, bringing the sector's total economic output to over $1.1 trillion. Also, in 2021, the U.S. pharmaceutical industry accounted for $78 billion of exports.[91]

In 2017, the U.S. biopharmaceutical industry employed 811,000 workers directly, with this employment further supporting approximately 3.2 million additional U.S. jobs through the supplier base and from the additional economic impacts stemming from industry and worker spending.[92] In total, the sector supports over 4 million well-paying U.S. jobs. On average, wages for biopharmaceutical workers topped just over $140,000 in 2019, compared

---

88 The Alzheimer's Association, "Changing the Trajectory of Alzheimer's Disease" (2015), *http://www.alz.org/documents_custom/trajectory.pdf.*

89 Adams Nager, "A Trillion-Dollar Opportunity: How Brain Research Can Drive Health and Prosperity" (ITIF, July 2016), *http://www2.itif.org/2016-trillion- dollar-opportunity.pdf.*

90 William Nordhaus, "Schumpeterian Profits and the Alchemist Fallacy" (work- ing paper, Department of Economics, Yale University, 2005), *http://www. econ.yale.edu/ddp/ddp00/ddp0006.pdf.*

91 Trading Economics, "United States Exports of Pharmaceutical Products,"*https://tradingeconomics.com/united-states/exports/pharmaceutical-products.*

92 TEConomy Partners, LLC and PhRMA, "Economic Impact of the U.S. Bio- pharma ceutical Industry," 5.

with $58,200 for all U.S. workers.[93] The industry also supports a number of high-wage manufacturing and construction jobs; in fact, analysis by the Pharmaceutical Industry Labor-Management Association and the Institute for Construction Economic Research (ICERES) shows the biopharma and biotech industry contributed to more than $774 million in union wages for construction workers between 2015 and 2020.[94]

R&D and Innovation Intensity of America's Biopharmaceutical Industry

America's biopharmaceutical industry leads the world in innovation, thanks largely to its world-leading investments in R&D and risk capital (supported by robust intellectual property rights, investment incentives, and effective technology transfer and commercialization mechanisms) as the following sections articulate.

Innovation

While the economic impact of America's biopharmaceutical industry is vitally important, its most important contribution comes in that America's biopharmaceutical industry leads the world in creating new drugs and therapies that are improving, saving, and extending human lives. This was nowhere more on display than during the COVID–19 pandemic, when the industry was able to bring novel vaccines and therapeutics to U.S. and global citizens within just over a year of the virus's discovery. The tremendous bench strength of American talent, scientific research and knowledge base, and biomedical infrastructure—the product of decades of robust private and public investment alike—explains how Gilead Sciences could provide an effective COVID–19 therapeutic, remdesivir, a mere 123 days after the virus was first detected in a patient sample and how the Pfizer-BioNTech vaccine could

[93] U.S. Bureau of Labor Statistics, "Quarterly Census of Employment and Wages" (Employment for NAICS 3254, 541714, 541711).

[94] Russell Ormiston, "An Analysis of Construction Spending in the Pharma- ceutical and Biotech Industry, 2015–2020" (Pharmaceutical Industry Labor- Management Association and the Institute for Construction Economic Re-search (ICERES), June 2021), *https://unionjobs.pilma.org/wp-content/uploads/2021/06/PIL-D-2106-Full-Jobs-Report_FINAL.pdf.*

arrive 347 days after the virus's first detection.[95] Moderna delivered the first doses of its COVID–19 vaccine to the National Institutes of Health for testing on February 24, 2020, a mere 6 weeks after Chinese scientists put the genetic sequence of the novel coronavirus online on January 11, 2020.[96] To put the incredibly rapid COVID–19 vaccine development timeline in context, a GlaxoSmithKline representative had ex- plained in 2017 how, "It can take up to $1 billion and 20–50 years to create and fully distribute a vaccine at scale."[97]

But that's just one example. In the 2000s, U.S.-headquartered biopharmaceutical enterprises generated more new-to-the-world drugs than companies from the next five nations combined.[98] Indeed, in every 5-year period since 1997, the United States has produced newer chemical or biological entities than any other country or region. And from 1997 to 2016, U.S.-headquartered enterprises accounted for 42 per- cent of new chemical or biological entities introduced throughout the world, far out- pacing relative contributions from European Union (EU) member countries, Japan, China, or other nations.[99] Put simply, over the past 2 decades, U.S.-headquartered biopharmaceutical enterprises accounted for almost half of the world's new drugs. Among others, these have included effective breakthrough oncological treatments or therapies for breast, lung, cervical, colorectal, and skin cancer; childhood leukemia; cystic fibrosis; lupus; and even a cure for hepatitis C. Captopril (1981), Prozac (1987), trastuzumab (1998), sirolimus (1999), adalimumab (2002), pembrolizumab (2014), Kymriah (2017), and Luxturna

---

[95] Stephen Ezell, "Ten Reasons Why a COVID–19 TRIPS IP Waiver Is Unwar- ranted," Innovation Files, April 9, 2021, https://itif.org/publications/2021/ 04/09/ten-reasons-why-covid-19-trips-ip-waiver-unwarranted.

[96] Catherine Clifford, "How the Moderna COVID–19 mRNA vaccine was made so quickly," CNBC, July 9, 2011, *https://www.cnbc.com/2021/07/03/how- moderna-made-its-mrna-covid-vaccine-so-quickly-noubar-afeyan.html.*

[97] Peter Wilderford, "How long does it take to research and develop a new vac- cine?", Effective Altruism Forum, June 28, 2017, *https://forum.effective altruism.org/posts/8q MDseJTE3vCFiYec/how-long-does-it-take-to-research- and-develop-a-new-vaccine.*

[98] Ross C. DeVol, Armen Bedroussian, and Benjamin Yeo, "The Global Bio- medical Industry: Preserving U.S. Leadership" (Milken Institute, September 2011, 5), *https://www.life changinginnovation.org/sites/default/files/files/ Global%20Bio_Full%20Report_WEB.pdf.*

[99] Joe Kennedy, "How to Ensure That America's Life-sciences Sector Remains Globally Competitive" (ITIF, March 2018), 37, *https://itif.org/publications/ 2018/03/26/how-ensure-americas-life-sciences-sector-remains-globally-com- petitive;* European Federation of Pharmaceutical Industries and Associations, "The Pharmaceutical Industry in Figures, Key Data 2017," 8, *https:// www.efpia.eu/media/219735/efpia-pharmafigures 2017_statisticbroch_v04-final.pdf.*

(2017) are just some of the headline bio- pharma breakthroughs developed by American life-sciences companies over the past 50 years.[100]

Moreover, amidst the COVID–19 pandemic, several impressive biotech and biopharma breakthroughs went unnoticed. In 2021, the FDA advanced several disease-modifying drugs used to treat the underlying biology of Alzheimer's rather than the symptoms, including by awarding a breakthrough therapy designation to donanemab developed by Eli Lilly.[101] Gingko Bioworks' groundbreaking research on synthetic biology and the Brigham and Women's Hospital's CRISPR research are on the frontlines alongside mRNA for potential designer treatments.[102] Harvard University's research into identifying brain biomarkers is also a game-changer for potentially predicting and treating neurodegenerative diseases.[103]

R&D

The United States leads the world in biomedical innovation in no small part because it invests more in biomedical R&D than any other nation. According to Research America, total U.S. medical and health research and development investment reached $245 billion in 2020, an 11-percent increase since 2019, which included $162 billion (roughly two-thirds) invested by industry and $62 billion by Federal departments and agencies.[104] Indeed, the United States has clearly been the world's largest global funder of biomedical R&D investment over the past 2 decades, a share that some analyses suggested reached as high as 70 to 80 percent over that time period.[105]

Moreover, the U.S. biopharmaceutical industry is both America's and the world's most R&D-intensive industry of any kind. As the U.S. Congressional

---

[100] Cello Health, "15 Breakthrough drug innovations (infographic)," https:// cellohealth.com/ us/views/15-breakthrough-drug-innovations-infographic/.

[101] Matt Fuchs, "6 Biotech Breakthroughs of 2021 That Missed the Attention They Deserved," Leaps.org, January 3, 2022, https://leaps.org/6-biotech-breakthroughs-of-2021-that-missed-the-attention-they-deserved/new-alzheimer-s-therapies.

[102] *Ibid.*

[103] *Ibid.*

[104] Research America and TEConomy Partners, "U.S. Investments in Medical and Health Research and Development, 2016–2020" (Research America and TEConomy Partners, January 2022), 1, https://www.researchamerica.org/ sites/default/files/Publications/Research%21America-Investment%20Report. Final.January%202022.pdf.

[105] Justin Chakma et al., "Asia's Ascent—Global Trends in Biomedical R&D Ex- penditures," *New England Journal of Medicine,* 370 No. 1 (January 2014); ER Dorsey et al., "Funding of US Biomedical Research, 2003–2008," *New England Journal of Medicine* 303 (2010): 137–43, *http://www.ncbi.nlm.nih.gov/ pubmed/20068207.*

Budget Office (CBO) explains, "Over the decade from 2005 to 2014, the industry's R&D intensity averaged 18 to 20 percent per year. That ratio has been trending upward since 2012, and it exceeded 25 percent in 2018 and 2019."[106] This level of R&D investment is substantially more than any other U.S. industry. As the CBO observes, "By comparison, average R&D intensity across all [U.S.] industries typically ranges between 2 and 3 percent" and even "R&D intensity in the software and semiconductor industries, which are generally comparable to the drug industry in their reliance on R&D, has remained below 18 percent."[107] (See Figure 9.) America's biopharmaceutical sector accounts for 18 percent of total U.S. business R&D investment.[108] Importantly, the CBO notes that while "Consumer spending on brand-name prescription drugs has risen, [the industry's] R&D has risen more quickly."[109]

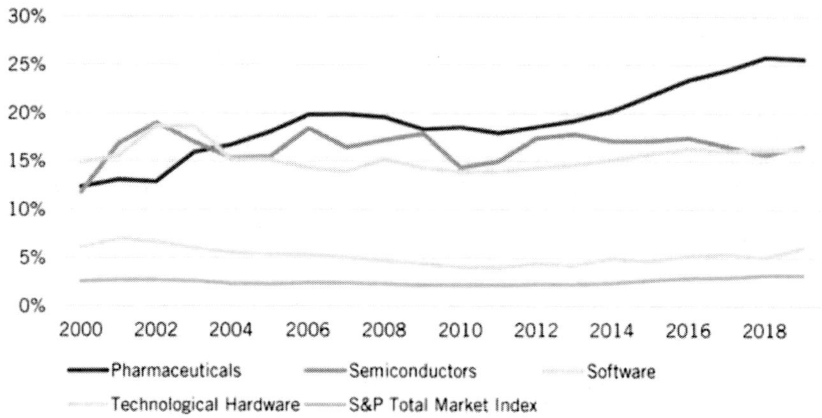

Figure 9. Average R&D intensity for publicity traded U.S. companies, by industry.[110]

Lastly, it's important to note that 23 percent of the American biopharmaceutical industry's workforce can be found at the lab bench in R&D jobs seeking to create new cures, giving the industry a share of employment

---

[106] Congressional Budget Office (CBO), "Research and Development in the Phar- maceutical Industry" (CBO, April 2021), 4–5, *https://www.cbo.gov/publica- tion/57025.*

[107] *Ibid.*

[108] TEConomy Partners, LLC and PhRMA, "Economic Impact of the U.S. Biopharma ceutical Industry," 7.

[109] Congressional Budget Office, "Research and Development in the Pharmaceutical Industry."

[110] Ibid., 5.

dedicated to R&D three times higher than the national average.[111] Moreover, the sector alone employs over one- quarter of America's total R&D workforce. Many of these R&D workers will invest their careers searching for innovative new drugs that never see the light of day. The point is that America's biopharmaceutical industry is fundamentally research-driven and innovation-focused, dedicated to the discovery and development of innovative drugs for the betterment of human society.

As ITIF has written extensively elsewhere, it should be briefly noted here that America's life-sciences innovation ecosystem is also ably supported by an effective set of policies that facilitate the transfer and commercialization of technology (in the life sciences, often molecular compounds) originally developed in private research institutions, universities, or national labs to the private sector for development into innovative drugs to be tested through clinical trials and brought to market.[112] Indeed, academic technology transfer enabled by the Bayh-Dole Act has facilitated the development of approximately 300 new drugs and vaccines that are now protecting public health worldwide.[113]

Another key strength of America's life-sciences innovation system has been creating a financial-markets environment capable of both valuing and marshaling the tremendous amount of capital necessary to finance investment in risky biopharmaceutical innovation.[114] Indeed, nearly three-quarters of worldwide venture capital investments in biopharmaceutical companies are made in the United States.[115] Over the past 2 years, the U.S. biopharmaceutical sector has attracted over $50 billion of risk capital investment.[116] While certainly most of these investments will fail, venture capital investors undertake these risky investments in the hope that successes will yield

---

[111] TEConomy Partners, LLC and PhRMA, "Economic Impact of the U.S. Bio- pharmaceutical Industry," 7.

[112] Stephen Ezell, "The Bayh-Dole Act's Vital Importance to the U.S. Life- Sciences Innovation System" (ITIF, March 2019), 20, *https://itif.org/sites/de fault/files/2019-bayh-dole-act.pdf.*

[113] Association of University Technology Managers (AUTM), "AUTM 2020 Licens- ing Activity Survey" (AUTM, 2020), 3, *https://autm.net/AUTM/media/ SurveyReportsPDF/ FY20-US-Licensing-Survey-FNL.pdf.*

[114] Stephen Ezell, "Ensuring U.S. Biopharmaceutical Competitiveness" (ITIF, July 2020), 34–35, *https://itif.org/publications/2020/07/16/ensuring-us-bio-pharmaceutical-competitive ness.*

[115] TEConomy Partners, LLC and PhRMA, "The Economic Impact of the U.S. Biopharmaceutical Industry"; April 2019 analysis of Pitchbook data, https:// pitchbook.com.

[116] Jacob Pileth, "In 2021 it paid to stay private when the chips were down," *Evaluate Vantage,* January 5, 2022, *https://www.evaluate.com/vantage/arti- cles/insights/venture-financing/2021-it-paid-stay-private-when-chips-were- down.*

commensurate returns, a bet that would be undermined if stringent drug price controls were applied to the relatively few successful drugs that result.

Dynamics of Biopharmaceutical Innovation

As drug innovation becomes more difficult and expensive, companies increasingly depend upon the profits from one generation of biomedical innovation to fund investment in the next, a dynamic that would be undermined if policymakers choose to implement stringent drug price controls, as the following section explains.

Drug Innovation Becoming More Difficult, Risky, and Expensive

As companies try to solve aheretofore intractable and unsolved challenges at the frontiers of biomedical science, the challenge gets ever-more difficult. Indeed, the biopharmaceutical industry must be so R&D-intensive precisely because bringing innovative new drugs to market represents a risky, time-consuming, and expensive process. On average, as many as 5,000 to 10,000 compounds may be screened to get to approximately 250 promising molecular compounds that can enter preclinical testing, with 5 entering actual clinical testing.[117] And that's just getting to the clinical trial stage, as less than 12 percent of candidate medicines that even make it into Phase I clinical trials are ultimately approved by the FDA.[118]

Overall, it takes 11.5 to 15 years of R&D and clinical trials to develop an innova- tive new drug, with the average cost of doing so almost doubling during the prior decade, increasing from $1.19 billion in 2010 to $2.17 billion by 2018, according to the Deloitte Center for Health Solutions. (Other estimates place the figure as high as $2.87 billion). As a Deloitte report notes, "The average cost to develop an asset, including the cost of failure, has increased in 6 out of 8 years."[119] The 2019 version of the report concludes that

---

[117] Pacific BioLabs, "Stages of Drug Development," https://pacificbiolabs.com/ stages-of-drug-development.

[118] PhRMA, "Chart Pack: Biopharmaceuticals in Perspective, Summer 2019" (PhRMA, 2019), https://www.phrma.org/-/media/Project/PhRMA/PhRMA-Org/PhRMA-Org/PDF/P-R/PhRMA_2019_ChartPack_Final.pdf.

[119] Deloitte Center for Health Solutions, "Unlocking R&D Productivity: Meas- uring the Return from Pharmaceutical Innovation 2018" (Deloitte Center for Health Solutions,

the average cost of bringing a new biopharmaceutical drug to market has increased by 67 percent since 2010 alone.[120] At the same time, Deloitte finds that forecast peak sales per asset have already more than halved since 2010. Perhaps most significantly, the biopharma industry has experienced a downward trend in returns to pharmaceutical R&D: Deloitte found that the rate of return to R&D in 12 large-cap pharmaceutical companies declined from 10.1 percent in 2010, to 4.2 percent in 2015, and then to 1.8 percent in 2019.[121] This is evidence that genuinely new biopharmaceutical innovation is becoming more difficult as com- panies try to tackle more difficult maladies previously unsuccessfully solved by bio- medical science: challenges such as pancreatic cancer, Alzheimer's, rare diseases, etc.

Companies Depend Upon Profits to Sustain Biopharmaceutical Investments

That's why there exists a direct link between the expensive and risky process of drug development and the need to earn commensurate returns on successful drugs to sustain the process. This explains why the CBO estimates that, because of the high failure rates, biopharmaceutical companies need to earn a 61.8-percent rate of return on their successful new drug R&D projects in order to match a 4.8-percent after-tax rate of return on their investments (i.e., a risk-free rate they could readily attain in public markets).[122]

Indeed, the claim that any individual drug generates very high profits cannot be viewed in isolation. All the drugs that did not make it through clinical trials to the marketplace by definition generated no profits, only losses. But even many drugs that make it to the market do not cover their costs. In a

2018), https://www2.deloitte.com/global/en/pages/life-sciences-and-healthcare/articles/measuring-return-from-pharmaceutical-inno- vation.html.

[120] Deloitte Center for Health Solutions, "Unlocking R&D Productivity: Meas- uring the Return From Pharmaceutical Innovation 2019" (Deloitte Center for Health Solutions, 2019), 2, *https://www2.deloitte.com/content/dam/Deloitte/uk/Documents/life-sciences-health-care/deloitte-uk-ten-years-on-measuring-re-turn-on-pharma-innovation-report-2019.pdf.*

[121] Deloitte Center for Health Solutions, "Ten years on: Measuring the return from pharmaceutical innovation 2019" (Deloitte Center for Health Solutions, 2019), 6, *https://www2.deloitte.com/content/dam/Deloitte/uk/Documents/life-sciences-health-care/deloitte-uk-ten-years-on-measuring-return-on-pharma- innovation-report-2019.pdf.*

[122] Congressional Budget Office (CBO), "How Taxes Affect the Incentives to In- vest in New Intangible Assets" (CBO, November 2018), 22–23, *https:// www.cbo.gov/system/files?file=2018-11/54648-Intangible_Assets.pdf.*

1990 article, Grabowski and Vernon found that 70 percent of new drugs made less than their R&D costs. Entities in the third most profitable decile barely broke even; those in the second decile had discounted profits nearly twice discounted R&D costs.[123] Fifty-five percent of industry revenues came from the top 10 drugs, whose average discounted profits exceeded discounted R&D costs by a factor of five. In an updated article released in 2010, Vernon, Golec, and DiMasi found that 80 percent of new drugs made less than their capitalized R&D costs. Entities in the second most profitable decile barely broke even; those in the first decile had discounted profits more than twice their discounted R&D costs.[124] Other studies have found that of the most successful 10 percent of approved drugs, only 1 percent of those that entered clinical trials— maybe three new drugs each year—generate half of the profits of the entire drug industry.[125]

This dynamic explains why virtually all academic assessments find strong links between industry profits and R&D investments. For instance, the OECD has found that "there exists a high degree of correlation between pharmaceutical sales revenues and R&D expenditures."[126] Indeed, there exists an almost 1:1 correlation (0.97) between R&D expenditures and sales in the OECD study. (See Figure 10.) Related academic research shows a statistically significant relationship between a biopharma enterprise's profits from the previous year and its R&D expenditures in the current year.[127] Likewise, Gambardella found that sales revenue from previous periods have a significant, positive impact on current-period biopharma R&D.[128] Henderson and Cockburn find that the pharmaceutical firms with the greatest sales are also the ones with the largest R&D investments. Lastly, research by Dubois et

---

[123] Henry Grabowski and John Vernon, "A New Look at the Returns and Risks to Pharmaceutical R&D," *Management Science,* Vol. 36, No. 7. (July 1990), 804–821.

[124] John Vernon, Joseph Golec, and Joseph DiMasi, "Drug Development Costs When Financial Risk is Measured Using the Fama-French Three-Factor Model," *Health Economics* 19, (August 2010), *https://pubmed.ncbi.nlm. nih.gov/19655335/.*

[125] Jack Scannell, "Four Reasons Drugs Are Expensive, of Which Two Are False," *Forbes,* October 13, 2015, *http://www.forbes.com/sites/matthewherper/2015/ 10/13/four-reasons-drugs-are-expensive-of-which-two-are-false/#257708d948 a5.*

[126] Organisation for Economic Co-operation and Development, "Pharmaceutical Pricing Policies in a Global Market" (OECD, September 2008), 190, *http:// www.oecd. org/els/pharmaceutical-pricing-policies-in-a-global-market.htm.*

[127] Destrina Grace Simanjuntak and Raymond R. Tjandrawinata, "Impact of Profitability, R&D Intensity, and Cash Flow on R&D Expenditure in Pharma- ceutical Companies" (Social Science Research Network, April 29, 2011), *http://papers.ssrn.com/sol3/papers.cfm ?abstract_id=1824267.*

[128] Alfonso Gambardella, Science and Innovation: The US Pharmaceutical Indus- try During the 1980s (Cambridge University Press, 1995).

al. makes this dynamic crystal clear, finding that every $2.5 billion of additional bio-pharmaceutical revenue leads to one new drug approval.[129]

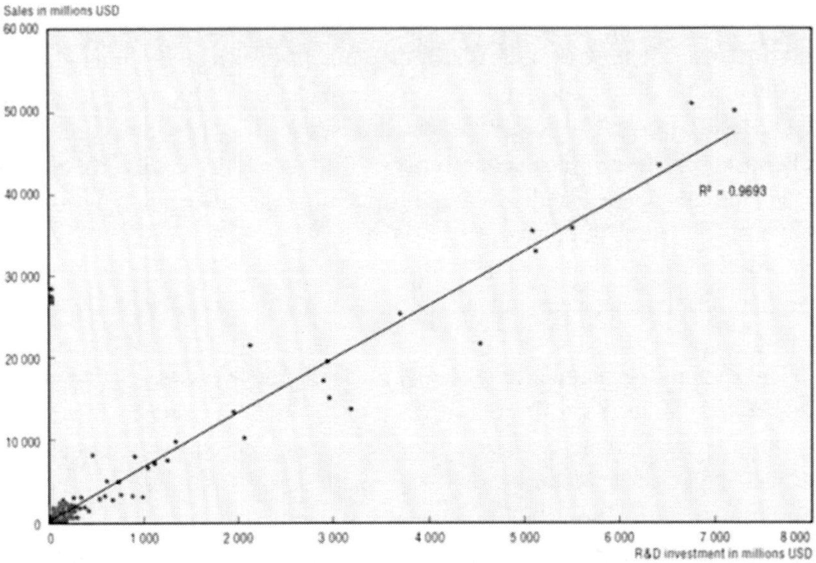

Note: The data were prepared on the basis of annual reports and consolidated accounts received up to and including 31 July 2006. Annual reports with a year-end older than 30 months from the cut-off date or a publication date older than 24 months from cut-off date are excluded.

Source: DIUS (2007).

Figure 10. R&D expenditure and sales in the pharmaceutical indistry, 2006.[130]

Drug Price Controls Inhibit R&D and Drug Discovery

This explains why academic studies consistently reveal that a reduction in current drug revenues leads to a decrease in future research and the number of new drug discoveries.[131] For instance, one study found that a real 10-percent decrease in the growth of drug prices would be associated with an approximately 6-percent decrease in pharmaceutical R&D spending as a share

---

[129] Pierre Dubois, "Market size and pharmaceutical innovation," *The Rand Jour- nal of Economics,* Vol. 46, Issue 4 (October 2015): 844–871, *https:// onlinelibrary.wiley.com/doi/full/10.1111/1756-2171.12113.*

[130] OECD, "Pharmaceutical Pricing Policies in a Global Market," 190.

[131] Joe Kennedy, "The Link Between Drug Prices and Research on the Next Gen- eration of Cures" (ITIF, September 2019), *https://itif.org/publications/2019/ 09/09/link-between-drug-prices-and-research-next-generation-cures.*

of net revenues.[132] Similarly, Lichtenberg found a 10-percent decrease in cancer drug prices would likely cause a 5- to 6-percent decline in both cancer regimens and research articles.[133] Likewise, Golec and Vernon show that if the United States had used an EU-like drug pricing system from 1986–2004, this would have resulted in a decline in firms' R&D expenditures of up to 33 percent and the development of 117 fewer new medicines.[134] Maloney and Civan found that a 50-percent drop in U.S. drug prices would result in the number of drugs in the development pipeline decreasing by up to 24 percent.[135] Similarly, Abbot and Vernon estimate that a price cut of 40 to 45 percent in real terms would reduce the number of new development projects by 50 to 60 percent.[136] Most recently, 2021 research by Tomas Philipson and Troy Durie at the University of Chicago estimates that a 1-percent reduction in pharmaceutical industry revenue leads on average to a 1.54-percent decrease in R&D investment.[137]

Applying their research to H.R. 5376 (the Build Back Better Act), Philipson and Durie find the legislation would reduce revenues by 12.0 percent through 2039, with the reduced revenues meaning R&D spending will fall by about 18.5 percent, or $663 billion. They find that this cut in R&D activity leads to 135 fewer new drugs, while this drop in new drugs is predicted to generate a loss of 331.5 million life years in the United States.[138]

Conversely, research by Schwartz et al. found that if government price controls in non-U.S. OECD countries were lifted, the number of new

---

[132] Carmelo Giaccotto, Rexford E. Santerre, and John A. Vernon, "Drug Prices and Research and Development Investment Behavior in the Pharmaceutical Industry," *The Journal of Law and Economics,* Vol. 48, Issue 1 April 2005, *https://www.jstor.org/stable/10.1086/426882?seq=1#page_scan_tab_contents.*

[133] Frank R. Lichtenberg, "Importation and Innovation," NBER Working Paper No. 12539, September 2006, *https://www.nber.org/papers/w12539.*

[134] Joseph Golec and John A. Vernon, "Financial Effects of Pharmaceutical Price Regulation on R&D Spending by EU Versus US Firms," *Pharmacoeconomics,* Vol. 28, Issue 8 (2010), 625, *https://pubmed.ncbi.nlm.nih.gov/20617857/.* All cost estimates were converted to 2019 dollars using the consumer price index.

[135] Michael T. Maloney and Abdulkadir Civan, "The Effect of Price on Pharma- ceutical R&D," *SSRN Electronic Journal,* Vol. 9, Issue 1 (2009): 1–14, *https:// ssrn.com/abstract=995175 or http://dx.doi.org/10.2139/ssrn.995175.*

[136] Thomas A. Abbott and John A. Vernon, "The Cost of U.S. Pharmaceutical Price Reductions: A Financial Simulation Model of R&D Decisions," NBER Working Paper No. 11114 (February 2005), *https://www.nber.org/papers/ w11114.*

[137] Tomas J. Philipson and Troy Durie, "Issue Brief: The Impact of HR 5376 on Biopharmaceutical Innovation and Patient Health," November 9, 2021, *https://cpb-us-w2.wpmucdn.com/voices.uchicago.edu/dist/d/3128/files/2021/08/Issue-Brief-Drug-Pricing-in-HR-5376-11.30.pdf.*

[138] *Ibid.*

treatments available would increase by 9 to 12 percent by 2030, equivalent to 8 to 13 new drugs in that year. This could potentially increase the life expectancy of someone 15 years old today by 0.6 to 1.6 years on average.[139] Instead of copying other OECD countries in a "reference-price-race-to-the-bottom," U.S. policy should instead actually be to encourage peer countries to appropriately value innovative medicines.

Analyses such as these explain why a February 2018 report by the President's Council of Economic Advisors found that while lowering reimbursement prices in the United States would reduce the prices Americans pay now for biopharmaceutical products, it would "make better health costlier in the future by curtailing innovation," thus failing to meet the goal of reducing the price of health care by reducing the incentives for innovative products in the future.[140]

Drug Price Controls Impede Access to Medicines

Stringent drug price controls don't only impede R&D and innovation, they preclude access to innovative medicines. For instance, the Department of Health and Human Services' October 2018 report, "Comparison of U.S. and International Prices for Top Medicare Part B Drugs by Total Expenditures," analyzed the price and availability of 27 drugs across 16 comparator countries.[141] It found that only 11 of the 27 drugs examined were widely available in all the comparator countries, indicating that patients in these countries were experiencing delays in access to innovative treatments. For instance, while 95 percent of new cancer drugs are available to patients in the United States, this compared to just an average of 55 percent of new drugs are available among the 16 reference countries. Further, for the cancer drugs available in the reference countries, there appears to be a 17-month average

---

[139] Taylor T. Schwartz et al., "The Impact of Lifting Government Price Controls on Global Biopharmaceutical Innovation and Population Health" (Precision Health Economics, 2018), *https://tools.ispor.org/research_pdfs/58/pdffiles/ PHP216.pdf.*

[140] Executive Office of the President, Council of Economic Advisors, "Reforming Biopharmaceutical Pricing at Home and Abroad" (Executive Office of the President, February 2018), 6, *https://www.whitehouse.gov/wp-content/ uploads/2017/11/CEA-Rx-White-Paper-Final2.pdf.*

[141] U.S. Department of Health and Human Services, "Comparison of U.S. and International Prices for Top Medicare Part B Drugs by Total Expenditures" (U.S. Department of Health and Human Services, October 2018), *https:// aspe.hhs.gov/system/files/ pdf/259996/ComparisonUSInternationalPricesTop SpendingPartBDrugs.pdf.*

lag between the time they are available in the United States and their availability elsewhere. This concords with research by Cockburn, Lanjouw, and Schankerman finding that countries that introduce drug price controls experience "significantly longer lags" in new drug introduction of 25 to 80 percent.[142]

A broad range of research suggests that Americans enjoy access to innovative medicines earlier than citizens in other nations do.[143] For instance, considering the availability of new medicines first launched globally from 2011 through year-end 2019, 87 percent were available first in the United States, a wide gap over Germany and the United Kingdom, at 63 and 59 percent respectively, with percentages declin- ing to as low as 46 percent in Canada and 39 percent in Australia. Considering the percentage of drugs available within 1 year of global first launch, again U.S. citizens enjoyed the greatest access, with 80 percent of drugs available to Americans first, followed by Germany and the United Kingdom at 47 and 41 percent, respectively, and again Canada and Australia trailing at 26 percent and 19 percent, respectively. (See Figure 11.) For these medicines, the average delay in availability in months from global first drug launch averaged 0 to 3 months in the United States, 10 in Germany, 11 in the United Kingdom, 15 in Canada, 16 in Japan, 18 in France, and 20 in Australia.

It should be noted that the earlier availability of drugs to American citizens applies to virtually every drug type. For instance, considering the availability of 356 new medicines introduced since 2011, 87 percent are now available to U.S. patients, compared to 63 percent in Germany, and that trend applies across the board, from drugs treating cancer on mental illness to those treating rare diseases.

---

[142] Iain M. Cockburn, Jean O. Lanjouw, Mark Schankerman, "Patents and the Global Diffusion of New Drugs," National Bureau of Economic Research, Working Paper 20492, *https://www.nber.org/papers/w20492.pdf.*

[143] Kevin Haninger, "New analysis shows that more medicines worldwide are available to U.S. patients," *The Catalyst,* June 5, 2018, *https://cata- lyst.phrma.org/new-analysis-shows-that-more-medicines-worldwide-are-avail- able-to-u.s.-patients;* Patricia M. Danzon and Michael F. Furukawa, "Inter- national Prices and Availability of Pharmaceuticals in 2005," *Health Affairs,* Vol. 7, No. 1 (January/February 2008), *https://www.healthaffairs.org/doi/ abs/10.1377/hlthaff.27.1.221.*

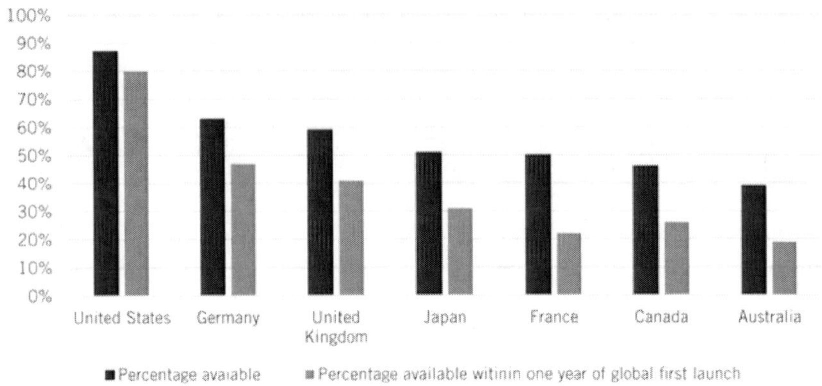

Figure 11. National availability of new medicines first launched globally from 2011 to year-end 2019.[144]

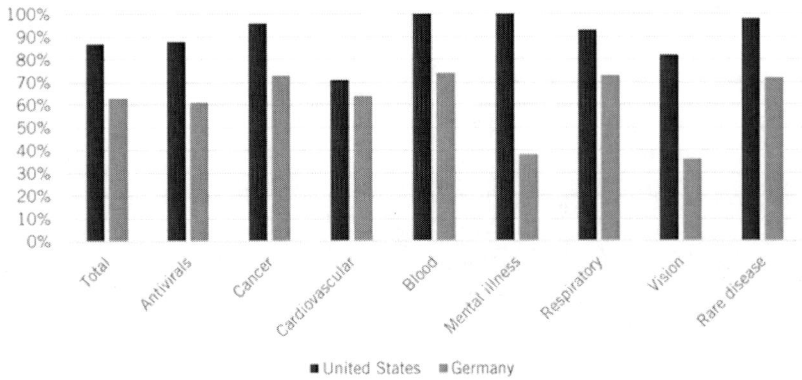

Figure 12. Compsrison of new drug availability since first launch, by thrapeutic type, Germany and the United States.[145]

Thus, the vast preponderance of evidence suggests that Americans enjoy access to innovative medicines earlier than citizens in other nations, and that produces tremendous individual and public health benefits. That's why drug price control systems that incorporate international reference pricing features

---

[144] PhRMA analysis of IQVIA Analytics Link, U.S. Food and Drug Administration (FDA), European Medicines Agency (EMA), Japan's Pharmaceuticals and Medical Devices Agency (PMDA), Health Canada and Australia's Therapeutic Goods Administration (TGA) data. June 2020. Note: New active substances approved by FDA, EMA, PMDA, Health Canada and/or TGA and first launched in any country between January 1, 2011 and December 31, 2019.

[145] *Ibid.*

would import drug availability delays every bit as much as they would import lower prices.

According to the European Union's own data from 2012, nearly 600,000 European deaths could be avoided each year if the continent's health-care systems simply offered "timely and effective medical treatments," including access to innovative drugs.[146] While that statistic certainly refers to a wide range of missing therapeutic interventions and public health gaps, it also suggests the costs of not getting innovative drugs to patients in time to make a difference. The United States shouldn't allow itself to find itself in the same position.

Drug Price Controls Undermine Nations' Biopharmaceutical Industry Competitiveness

The stringent drug price controls other regions and nations, such as the European Union and Japan, have implemented have seriously harmed the competitiveness of those nations' biopharmaceutical industries.

For instance, in the early 1990s, European and U.S. companies each held about a one-third share of the global drug market. But leadership began to shift in the 1990s. By 2004, Europe's share would fall to 18 percent, while the U.S. share jumped to 62 percent.[147] And from 1990 to 2017, pharmaceuticals R&D investment in Europe grew 4.5 times, while in the United States, it increased by more than 800 percent.[148] As Nathalie Moll of the European Federation of

---

146 Andrew Spiegel, "The tragic toll of drug price controls," *The Hill,* May 5, 2017, *https://thehill.com/blogs/pundits-blog/healthcare/332145-the-tragic-toll-of-drug-price-controls;* European Union, "Eurostats Statistics Explained: Ame- nable and preventable deaths statistics" (June 2015), *https://ec.europa.eu/ eurostat/statistics-explained/index.php?title=Archive:Amenable_and_preventable_deaths_statistics&direction =next&oldid=237655#cite_note-2;*Eurostats Statistics Explained: "Avoidable, amenable and preventable mortality in the EU28, 2012 (numbers)," *https://ec.europa.eu/ eurostat/statistics-explained/index.php?title=File:Avoidable,_amenable _and_preventable_mortality_in_the_ EU28,_2012_(numbers).png.* An updated 2021 report found "A total of 1.0 mil- lion deaths in 2016 of people aged less than 75 years could have been avoided in the EU, either through better healthcare systems and/or better public health interventions." European Union, "Eurostats Statistics Explained: Pre- ventable and treatable mortality statistics (2021)," *https://ec.europa.eu/eurostat/statistics-explained/index.php?title= Preventable_and_treatable_mor tality_statistics.*

147 Kimberly Cleaves, "Imbalanced Innovation," *Modern Drug Discovery* (July 2004): 23–24, *http://pubsapp.acs.org/subscribe/archive/mdd/v07/i07/pdf/ 704business3.pdf?*

148 Nathalie Moll, "Would the last pharmaceutical investor in Europe please turn the lights out," European Federation of Pharmaceutical Industries and Asso- ciations blog, January 3,

Pharmaceutical Industries and Associations (EFPIA) writes, "The sobering reality is that Europe has lost its place as the world's leading driver of medical innovation. Today [January 2020], 47 percent of global new treatments are of U.S. origin compared to just 25 percent emanating from Europe (2014–2018). This represents a complete reversal of the sit- uation just 25 years ago."[149] As one report explains, "the heart of pharma's problem in Europe is the market's inability to "liberate the value" from its products."[150]

European countries' extensive use of drug price controls began in earnest in the 1980s and accelerated in the 1990s. By imposing such draconian drug price controls, European regulators have severely disrupted the economics of innovation in the European life-sciences industry. As the EFPIA explained in a 2000 report, "Many European countries have driven prices so low that many new drugs can no longer recoup their development costs before patents expire."[151] As the report continues, "These policies, most of which seek only short-run gains, seriously disrupt the functioning of the market and sap the industry's ability to compete in the long run." As industry analyst Neil Turner wrote in 1999, those policies "set in motion a cycle of under- investment and loss of competitiveness that's very difficult to break out of."[152] While Europe's drug price controls certainly lead to lower drug prices and charges that Europe "free rides" off U.S. biopharmaceutical innovation, one report notes, "Europe's free ride is not free" and shows that Europe's drug price controls actually lead to considerable "social and economic costs in Europe, in the form of delayed access to drugs, poorer health outcomes, decreased investment in research capabilities, and a drain placed on high-value pharmaceutical jobs."[153]

2021 research by Schulthess and Bowen confirm that these trends continue today, finding that a 10-percent drop in the price of medicines in price-controlled European Union markets was associated with a 14-percent decrease in total venture capital funding (10 percent early stage and 7 percent late); a 7-percent decrease in biotech patents; a 9-percent decrease in biotech start-up funding relative to the United States; and an 8-percent increase in the

---

2020, *https://www.efpia.eu/news-events/the-efpia- view/blog-articles/would-the-last-pharmaceutical-investor-in-europe-please-turn-the-lights-out/.*

149 *Ibid.*

150 Neil Turner, "European Pricing Squeeze," PharmaExec.com, October 1, 2002, https:// www.pharmexec.com/view/european-pricing-squeeze.

151 EFPIA, "The Pharmaceutical Industry in Figures: 2000" (EFPIA, 2000).

152 Turner, "What's gone wrong with the European pharmaceutical industry.

153 Cleaves, "Imbalanced Innovation."

delay of access to medicines.[154] As the report observes, "the continued downward pressures on prices in Europe have led to declines in biopharmaceutical industry investments in the European Union relative to the United States."[155] For example, from 2013 to 2019, biotech investments in the United States increased sixfold even as they remained static in the European Union, while by 2020, the U.S. share of total annual biotech start-ups was roughly three times greater than the European share.[156]

Japan began introducing biennial price controls in the early 1980s, beginning with a steep, across-the-board reduction of 18.6 percent, with biennial cuts thereafter. As Cardiff University Professor Maki Umemura explains, "The biennial price reductions had a particularly severe impact on Japanese pharmaceutical firms' incentives to invest in R&D."[157] As she continues, "These reductions incentivized Japanese firms to launch a stream of new drugs with short product life and little innovative value that could recoup the costs of R&D, rather than invest in more substantial innovation. This hindered the industry's prospects of launching breakthrough drugs that would have been more competitive overseas."[158] That's because Japan's severe profit controls not only limited the potential profits from biopharmaceutical innovation (thus decreasing the incentive to invest), but they further limited drug company revenues (thus decreasing the ability to invest). Umemura's research suggests that drug prices in Japan decreased by as much as two-thirds in the decade from 1981 to 1991.[159]

Heather O'Neill and Lena Crain examined the relationship between Japan's drug prices decreases and drug innovation in their 2005 report, "The Effects of Price Regulation on Pharmaceutical R&D and Innovation," concluding:

Japan's government sets prices of new drugs based on older comparator drugs. Recently, price premiums have been permitted on truly innovative drugs, but even with the premiums in place the introductory price is not higher than that of older drugs. Following a drug launch, the government decreases

---

[154] Duane Schulthess and Harry Bowen, "The Historical Impact of Price Controls on the Biopharma Industry" (Vital Transformations, November 2021), *https://vitaltransformation.com/wp-content/uploads/2021/11/11.23-The-Im-pact-of-price-controls_Final.pdf.*

[155] *Ibid.*

[156] *Ibid.*

[157] Maki Umemura, "Unrealised Potential: Japan's Post-war Pharmaceutical In- dustry, 1945–2005," Thesis Submitted to the Department of Economic History, London School of Economics (August 2008), 89, *https://etheses.lse.ac.uk/ 2172/1/U613404.pdf.*

[158] *Ibid.,* 90–91.

[159] *Ibid.,* 89.

the price as the product matures; the highest price ever received is the first one. Prices fall by as much as two-thirds from the original price within 10 years. The low introductory prices, coupled with no inflationary price increases, discourage new product development.[160] O'Neill and Crain developed an econometric model to assess the impact of Japanese drug price regulations on pharmaceutical innovation. As the authors conclude, "the regulations in Japan create an environment that is not conducive to innovation."[161] Their econometric model found that, controlling for R&D employment and time, Japan approved 7.5 fewer new chemical entities (NCEs) than the United States on average in a given year in the years from 1980 to 2002.[162] Moreover, not surprisingly, Japan's biopharmaceutical industry has faltered significantly, with Japan's share of global value-added in the pharmaceutical industry declining by 70 percent, from 18.5 percent to just 5.5 percent, from 1995 to 2018.[163]

In summary, stringent drug price controls have wreaked considerable damage on the European and Japanese biopharmaceutical industries and would likely do the same to the United States.

Better Ways to Control Drug Prices

Instead of seeking to implement broad-based and steep drug price controls, policy- makers should focus on bolstering the R&D and innovation efficiency of America's biopharmaceutical system and lowering the costs seniors pay at the pharmacy counter.

Bolster R&D and Innovation Efficiency

Instead of trying to slash prices on the dubious theory drug companies can make do with lower profits, lawmakers should turn their attention to the other side of the industry's ledger—the costs of R&D and production, especially of

---

[160] Heather M. O'Neill and Lena Crain, "The Effects of Price Regulation on Phar- maceutical R&D and Innovation," Business and Economic Faculty Publica- tions, Ursinsus College, Vol. 5 (2005), 62, *https://digitalcommons.ursinus. edu/bus_econ_fac/5/.*

[161] *Ibid.,* 68.

[162] *Ibid.,* 67–69.

[163] OECD.Stat, "TiVA: Trade in Value Added Database 2021," accessed via *https:// stats.oecd.org/Index.aspx?DataSetCode=TIVA_2021_C1.*

large molecule biotech drugs—by spurring the kinds of innovations that can significantly improve R&D productivity and production process efficiency.[164] Indeed, capitalizing on new technologies to lower the cost of drug innovation and production is the only viable way to achieve what everyone wants—a long-term trend toward producing more cures (and more ancillary economic benefits) at less cost.

Promisingly, a new slate of technologies including artificial intelligence (AI), "big data," CRISPR gene editing, nanotechnology, and biologics manufacturing is transforming how new drugs are discovered, developed, clinically tested, and produced.[165] In particular, data-driven innovation promises to transform many aspects of medicine. In the pharmaceutical industry, better access to data can improve drug discovery, clinical review, testing, and post-market monitoring. However, these benefits require access to massive amounts of data from many people. Congress could ease drug discovery by appropriately loosening data restrictions in the health-care market, especially because current Federal policy makes the sharing of data difficult, even de-identified data individual patients are eager to share in order to help find a cure.

In order to facilitate this improved drug discovery, policymakers should enforce the publication of data from clinical trial results by directing agencies such as the FDA and NIH to be more aggressive about penalizing noncompliance. Congress should direct the Department of Health and Human Services (HHS) to create a model for data trusts that facilitates data sharing among biopharmaceutical stakeholders involved with data-driven drug development. Policymakers should also increase the availability of new kinds of data from nontraditional sources, such as biometric, lifestyle, and environmental data, while directing the FDA to develop best practices for data collection in health care to ensure equitable outcomes, such as strategies to increase coverage of underrepresented populations.[166]

Congress should also support investments that could make pharmaceutical manufacturing more efficient. One study contends that pharmaceutical manufacturing is expensive, inefficient, and non-innovative, with firms using

---

[164] Stephen Ezell, "Congress Should Double Down on Innovation to Boost Produc- tivity in Biopharmaceutical R&D," *Morning Consult,* November 22, 2021, *https://morning consult.com/opinions/congress-should-double-down-on-inno- vation-to-boost-productivity-in-biopharmaceutical-rd/.*

[165] Joshua New, "The Promise of Data Driven Drug Development" (Center for Data Innovation, September 2019), *https://datainnovation.org/2019/09/the-promise-of-data-driven-drug-development/.*

[166] Ezell, "Ensuring U.S. Biopharmaceutical Competitiveness," 48.

outdated production techniques and old plants.[167] The study attributes much of this to high regulatory barriers and inefficient intellectual-property protection of manufacturing methods. Proposed changes, such as faster regulatory approvals for manufacturing innovations that do not affect quality, and preventing other companies from immediately copying improvements discovered by others either through process patents or by administratively denying other companies from copying the innovation for a certain period of time, could result in production cost savings of $50 billion each year.

Congress could facilitate this process by expanding Federal support for joint industry-university research efforts on biopharma R&D efficiency and effectiveness, such as funding new programs through the National Science Foundation's Industry/ University Cooperative Research Centers (I/UCRC) program. American universities need more initiatives such as MIT's NEW Drug Development ParadIGmS (NEWDIGS) program, which is "a unique collaborative 'think and do' tank focused on enhancing the capacity of the global biomedical innovation system to reliably and sustainably deliver new, better, affordable therapeutics to the right patients faster."[168] Lawmakers should also expand public-private partnerships investing in biomedical R&D and technology commercialization, including by significantly expanding investments in biomedical-focused Manufacturing USA centers, such as the Na- tional Institute for Innovation in Manufacturing Biopharmaceuticals (NIIMBL).[169]

Because basic scientific research is the foundation of biomedical knowledge, Congress should make it a priority to restore funding for the National Institutes of Health to early 2000s levels as a share of GDP, which would cost about $12 billion. Lastly, the critically important Prescription Drug User Fee Act (PDUFA), which helps fund the FDA, is due for renewal in 2022. Congress should work proactively to reauthorize the legislation and ensure its innovation-supporting aspects are enhanced.[170]

---

[167] W. Nicholson Price II, "Making Do in Making Drugs: Innovation Policy and Pharmaceutical Manufacturing," *Boston College Law Review,* Vol. 55, Issue 2 (2014): 492, *https://lawdigitalcommons.bc.edu/bclr/vol55/iss2/5/.*

[168] Massachusetts Institute of Technology (MIT) Center for Biomedical Innova- tion, "Welcome to MIT NEWDIGS," *https://newdigs.mit.edu/.*

[169] The National Institute for Innovation in Manufacturing Biopharmaceuticals (NIIMBL), "About NIIMBL," *https://niimbl.force.com/s/about-niimbl.*

[170] Stephen J. Ezell, "How the Prescription Drug User Fee Act Supports Life- Sciences Innovation and Speeds Cures" (ITIF, February 2017), *http:// www2.itif.org/2017-pdufa-life-sciences-innovation.pdf.*

Medicare Part D Reforms

ITIF supports Medicare Part D reforms aimed at easing the out-of-pocket cost of medications incurred by seniors at the pharmacy counter. Part D reforms aimed at realigning plan and drugmaker incentives to constrain drug prices and limit beneficiaries' out-of-pocket costs are warranted. In particular, ITIF supports the proposal to cap at $2,000 out-of-pocket prescription drug costs on Part D beneficiaries that don't already qualify for cost-sharing protections (i.e., through low-income subsidies (LIS)). ITIF also supports the provision in the Build Back Better Act which would "smooth" beneficiaries' out-of-pocket costs over the course of a year so that a beneficiary wouldn't potentially have to pay as much as $2,000 in a single month.

Regarding a $2,000 out-of-pocket cap, a study by the Urban Institute estimates that such a cap would benefit more than 860,000 seniors while increasing Medicare drug spending by less than 1 percent.[171] The Urban Institute study found that, in 2019, 18 percent of Part D enrollees spent more than $3,500 in out-of-pocket costs, 30 percent experienced out-of-pocket costs of $2,500 to $3,000, and 40 percent had out-of-pocket costs above $2,000. The Urban Institute estimates such a spending cap would require an additional $199 million in beneficiary premium spending and $583 million in Medicare program spending in 2019.[172] ITIF further supports capping monthly patient out-of-pocket costs for drugs treating certain chronic diseases, such as a $35 monthly cap for insulin for the treatment of diabetes.

ITIF also supports the proposal to ensure that the rebates insurers and PBMs negotiate for Medicare Part D drugs are passed through to seniors at the pharmacy counter. The rebates (averaging nearly 30 percent for Medicare Part D drugs) are usually paid to PBMs in consideration of preferred placement on the insurance plan's formulary, but the PBMs tend not to share the rebates directly with beneficiaries. Changing this rule change could save older Americans as much as $83 billion at the pharmacy counter over the span of 10 years.[173]

---

[171] Robert King, "Urban Institute: Part D $2,000 out-of-pocket cost cap could ben- efit nearly 1M seniors," *Fierce Healthcare,* March 2, 2022, *https:// www.fiercehealthcare.com/ payers/urban-institute-part-d-2000-out-pocket-cost- cap-could-benefit-nearly-1m-seniors.*

[172] *Ibid.*

[173] Blake Pelzer and Paul Spitalnic, "Proposed Safe Harbor Regulation," Center for Medicare and Medicaid Services: Office of the Actuary, (August 2018), *https://aspe.hhs.gov/sites/ default/files/private/pdf/260591/OACTProposed SafeHarborRegulationImpacts.pdf.*

To be sure, implementing both the out-of-pocket cap and the rebate rule would mean some degree of insurance premium increases for seniors; however, it would rebalance the current dynamic where those who are most ill or have the most health challenges tend to be paying the most, while those who are least ill pay less. In a way, the sickest are subsidizing the healthiest, turning the principle of insurance on its head (i.e., collectively pooling risk and providing resources to those who require it in time of need). In ITIF's view, the cap, which would require some degree of sacrifice from drugmakers, insurers, taxpayers, and Part D enrollees alike, would rebalance cost structures to help seniors most in need.

Moreover, promoting affordability at the pharmacy counter for seniors will likely promote medication adherence. That matters greatly when patients' failure to adhere to their prescribed medication regimens costs our health system $289 billion annually. Moreover, non-adherence accounts for about 10 percent of hospitalizations and 125,000 annual deaths.[174] Facilitating greater adherence that could help reduce hospitalizations and other downstream costs would help circle the square with part of the increased costs that would be created by implementing the cap. In other words, considering the Urban Institute's estimate that a spending cap would require an additional $199 million in beneficiary premium spending and $583 million in Medicare program spending, if some large portion of that amount could be recaptured through reducing the $289 billion resulting from missed prescription adherence, then that dynamic produces substantial value and economic sustainability for the broader Medicate system while also improving patients' lives.

Getting these issues right is vitally important in the time and wake of the COVID–19 pandemic. For instance, according to the National Cancer Institute, missed screenings and other pandemic-related impacts on cancer care could result in about 10,000 additional deaths from breast and colon cancer (which together account for about one-sixth of all cancer deaths) alone over the next 10 years.[175] And that's just two types of cancer. COVID–19 has already put America's health-care system under tremendous strain, but the downstream effects of the pandemic: from long-COVID, from mental stress, weight gain, and lack of physical fitness opportunities for even those who

---

[174] Golin et al., "Interventions to Improve Adherence to Self-administered Medi- cations for Chronic Diseases in the United States" (*Annals of Internal Medi- cine,* December 2012), *https://www.acpjournals.org/doi/10.7326/0003-4819- 157-11-201212040-00538.*

[175] Norman E. Sharpless, "COVID–19 and Caner," *Science,* Vol. 368, Issue 6497 (June 2020): 1290, *https://science.sciencemag.org/content/368/6497/1290.*

never had the virus (one study found 42 percent of U.S. adults gained more weight than they intended during the pandemic, and of those, the amount they reported gaining averaged 29 pounds), and myriad other maladies that weren't caught earlier due to missed doctors' visits and screenings means both America's health-care and health insurance system will be placed under further strain for years to come.[176]

Conclusion

In considering drug price reform, policymakers must walk a delicate line between balancing the interests of present and future generations. We could certainly have cheaper drugs today, but the inescapable reality is that if this is done by imposing price controls (as opposed to better drug insurance coverage or other means to increase competition in PBMs), this would mean fewer new medicines and likely reduced access to them for future generations. That tradeoff is inescapable. And the reality is that the system the United States has put in place over the past 4 decades has worked more effectively than anywhere else in the world.

On September 14, 2017, the FDA approved Mvasi, the first biosimilar for Roche's Avastin, a breakthrough anti-cancer drug for lung, cervical, and colorectal cancer. In other words, a drug for forms of cancers that scarcely existed 20 years ago is now available as a generic. That's emblematic of an effective system of U.S. life-science innovation that promotes breakthrough innovation and then facilitates generic competition to help manage drug prices.

As Jack Scannell, a senior fellow at Oxford University's Center for the Advancement of Sustainable Medical Innovation (CASMI), frames it, "I would guess that one can buy today, at rock bottom generic prices, a set of small-molecule drugs that has greater medical utility than the entire set available to anyone, anywhere, at any price in 1995." He continued, "Nearly all the generic medicine chest was created by firms who invested in R&D to win future profits that they tried pretty hard to maximize; short-term financial gain building a long-term common good."[177]

---

[176] Caitlin O'Kane, "Most Americans say the pandemic has been bad for their weight," CBS News, March 23, 2021, *https://www.cbsnews.com/news/covid- weight-gain-30-pounds-pandemic/.*

[177] Scannell, "Four Reasons Drugs Are Expensive, of Which Two Are False."

It's that dynamic that explains why anti-lung cancer drugs that simply didn't exist 20 years ago are available on the market at generic prices today. And it's that dynamic that enables us to envision a future where drugs are available at generic prices in 2042 for a set of diseases that have greater medical utility than the entire set available to anyone, anywhere, at any price in 2022. But that will only be the case if policymakers preserve the conditions that have enabled the U.S. life-sciences innovation system that has become the envy of the world. In other words, Congress needs to focus on the long-term future of Americans, not simply today's outcry by some.

In conclusion, the United States enjoys a bountiful return on the roughly 14 percent of national health-care expenditures it invests in prescription drugs each year. America's market-based, private-enterprise-led, government-supported biomedical innovation system has tremendous strengths. It is both the envy of the world and the source of the majority of the world's new drugs benefiting American and global citizens alike. To be sure, some reform is needed—notably to address the pinch seniors are experiencing in out-of-pocket costs at the pharmacy counter—but radical reconstructive surgery in the form of stringent drug price controls is not.

Questions Submitted for the Record to Stephen J. Ezell Questions Submitted by Hon. Mike Crapo on Problematic Claims Regarding the House-Passed Build Back Better Act

Question. A range of claims advanced in support of the drug price controls included in the House-passed Build Back Better Act (BBBA) warrant substantial scrutiny and skepticism.

Some backers of the bill have cited a January 2022 AARP piece suggesting that gas and milk prices would be astronomical if they had grown at the rate of prescription drug prices for the past 15 years. Notably, however, the article in question relies on a June 2021 report using a dataset ending in December 2020, thus predating the recent surge in general inflation, which has coincided with far lower growth in drug prices. Moreover, the study in question focuses only on a subset of brand-name drugs, thus excluding the low-cost generics that account for 90 percent of the market, and its pricing metric fails to account for post-sale rebates and other price concessions. It also uses a 15-year window, which masks the recent slowing in even list price increases for medications.

In terms of the current wave of inflation eroding American families' finances, between February 2021 and 2022, general inflation (CPI–U) rose by 7.9 percent, while the consumer price index specific to milk increased by 11.2 percent and the gasolinespecific index surged by 38 percent. The prescription drug-specific index (CPI–Rx, which includes generics but still excludes post-sale rebates), by contrast, grew by just 2.4 percent.

What metrics and studies provide the most accurate and inclusive data on price trends for prescription drugs?

How does medication price inflation relate to general inflation and inflation specific to other goods cited by AARP, such as milk and gasoline?

Answer. The best source for data on drug prices paid by U.S. consumers is actually the U.S. Bureau of Labor Statistics (BLS) and its Consumer Price Index (CPI). And this data shows that prescription drugs have in no way been a significant contributor to the increased inflation the United States is presently experiencing. In fact, over the past 12 months, prescription drug prices increased just 2.4 percent, well below the average CPI increase of 8 percent and less than other parts of the U.S. health-care system, such as health insurance, which experienced a 4.1 percent increase. (See Figure 1.)

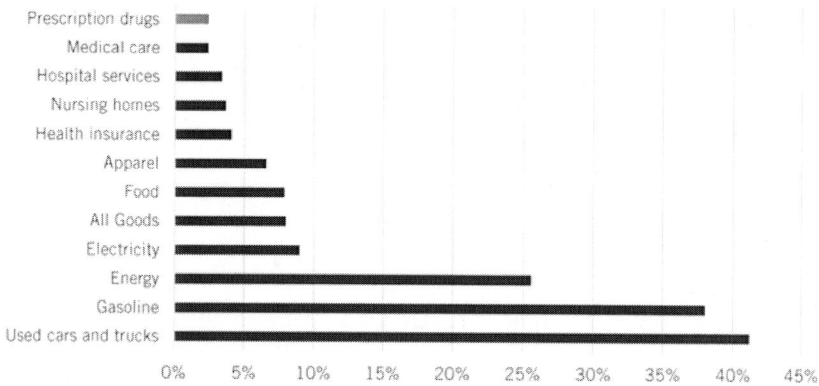

Figure 1. consumer price index by sector, 12-month change ending in February 2022.[178]

In fact, among the goods where U.S. consumers have faced dramatically increased inflation over the past year, drug prices didn't even make it within the top 100-highest price increases among the BLS itemized CPI (which tracks

[178] Bureau of Labor Statistics, Consumer Price Index (accessed March 10, 2022), *https://www.bls.gov/cpi/*.

over 300 unique consumer expenditure categories). Moreover, between 2020 and 2021, BLS recorded zero inflation on prescription drugs and only a 0.8-percent price increase on non- prescription drugs. In the 12 months ending in February 2022, the cost of gasoline in the United States increased nearly 20 times more, 38 percent, than the cost of prescription drugs, 2.4 percent. Over that period, U.S. food prices increased by 8percent, including a 6.9-increase for milk (for the 12-month period ending in January 2022).[179] Again, these price increases for food were considerably higher than the price increases for prescription drugs.

Moreover, Americans' out-of-pocket drug expenditures, as a share of their personal income, have been consistently dropping over the past 2 decades. In fact, out-of- pocket drug costs are at an all-time low relative to total U.S. health spending. In 1960, out-of-pocket drug costs made up 9.5 percent of total U.S. health expenditures; today, that number is only 1.1 percent. In fact, consumers have consistently paid a lower share of their personal incomes toward out-of-pocket drug costs every year since 1960. The share of personal incomes in the United States paid toward out- of-pocket drug costs has halved over the last 15 years, from 0.53 percent in 2005 to 0.24 percent in 2020. (See Figure 2.)

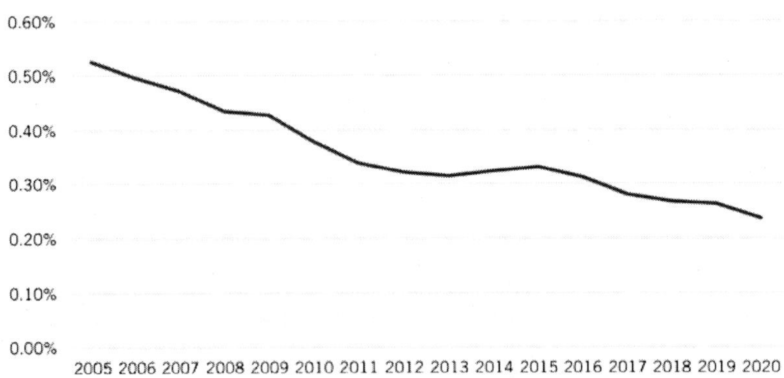

Figure 2. U.S. out- of-pocket drug expenditures, as a share of personal income, 2005-2020.[180]

[179] Scott Brown, "Dairy price inflation lags other foods," Hoard's Dairyman, February 17, 2022, https://hoards.com/article-31538-dairy-price-inflation-lags- other-foods.html.

[180] Bureau of Labor Statistics, Consumer Expenditure Survey (Healthcare ex- penditures, 2005–2020), https://www.bls.gov/cex/.

Indeed, as calculated by the U.S. Bureau of Labor Statistics, from 2005 to 2020, Americans' reported expenditures on health insurance increased by over 160 percent, and total health-care expenditures increased 94 percent, while consumer expenditures on drugs actually fell by almost 9 percent. (See Figure 3.) Of course, this does not necessarily mean overall drug expenditures fell because health insurance and hospitals also purchase drugs, but it does address consumers' out-of-pocket costs. It's reflective of a system that, broadly, both supports the creation of innovative drugs and then pathways for generic or biosimilar entrants to introduce price- decreasing competition.

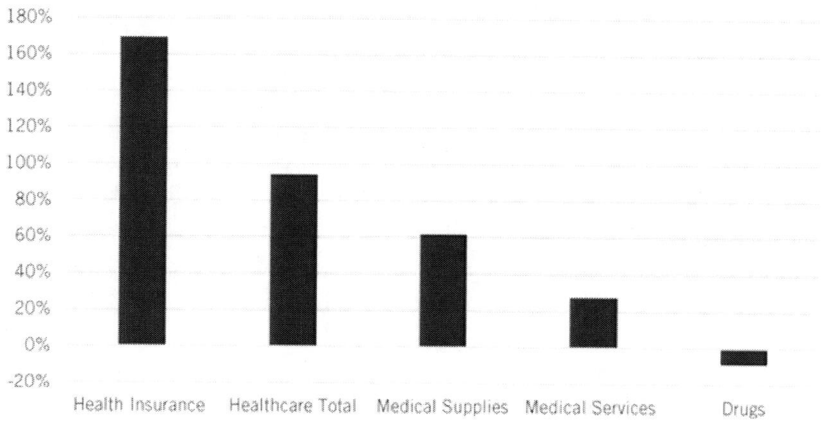

Figure 3. percent change in consumers' reported healthcare expenditures, 2005-2020.[181]

Another good source of data on U.S. health-care expenditures is the Peterson-KFF Health System Tracker.[182] Data from Peterson-KFF show that the percentage of total U.S. health-care spending going toward retail prescription drugs was consistent from 2000 to 2017, at mostly under 10 percent, and even dipped slightly to 8 percent in 2020.[183] Other good sources of data on health expenditure trends include Altarum's report "Projections of the Non-Retail Prescription Drug Share of National Health Expenditures" and

---

[181] *Ibid.*

[182] Peterson Center on Healthcare and Kaiser Family Foundation, Peterson-KFF Health System Tracker, "National Health Spending Explorer," *https:// www.healthsystemtracker.org/health-spending-explorer/.*

[183] Peterson-KFF Health Systems Tracker, (National Health Spending, accessed March 12, 2022), *https://www.healthsystemtracker.org/health-spending-ex- plorer/.*

the report by Inmaculada Hernandez et al., "Changes in List Prices, Net Prices, and Discounts for Branded Drugs in the U.S., 2007–2018."[184]

Question. In advocating for enactment of the BBBA's drug pricing provisions, some have characterized the bill's government price-setting program as market- based and fair, providing manufacturers with a say in the pricing of their products. These advocates have sought to differentiate the program from price controls and rate-setting mechanisms.

In reality, however, the legislation would allow the HHS Secretary to set any price of his or her choosing for virtually any product selected. Under the bill, non- compliance with any component of the price-setting program—including meeting bureaucratic deadlines, agreeing to participate in the program, and accepting the price that the Federal Government sets, however arbitrary or unrealistic—would trigger an unprecedented and seemingly unconstitutional noncompliance penalty of up to 95 percent of all gross sales across all markets. Manufacturers thus have no choice in the matter and no leverage in the process. The proposal would also permanently prohibit judicial and administrative review of most elements of the new program, rendering any price set by the Secretary as absolutely final and enforceable.

In short, the bill provides for negotiation in name only.

Is the government price-setting program created under the House-passed BBBA in any way negotiation? Does it, as its backers attest, rely on market forces and provide manufacturers with a meaningful say in setting prices?

To your knowledge, has Congress enacted any provision resembling the 95-percent noncompliance penalty—nondeductible and applied across gross sales for all market segments—in modern political history?

Answer. The BBBA does not establish a true "negotiation" of drug prices in Medicare; rather it's more about arbitrary price setting that would enable the HHS secretary to dictate prices to manufacturers who would have little or no power to truly negotiate. As Doug Holtz-Eakin elaborates, "The BBBA would enshrine a unique and punitive 95-percent excise tax on gross profits on a therapy if the manufacturer does not agree to the secretary's demands and set a ceiling for a drug's price. . . . Given the 95-percent excise tax the secretary would be free to wield against noncompliant innovators, 'price extortion'

---

[184] Altarum, "Projections of the Non-Retail Prescription Drug Share of National Health Expenditures," September 3, 2020, *https://altarum.org/publications/ projections-non-retail-prescription-drug-share-national-health-expenditures;* Inmaculada Hernandez et al., "Changes in List Prices, Net Prices, and Dis- counts for Branded Drugs in the US, 2007–2018," *Journal of the American Medical Association,* Vol. 323, No. 9 (2020): 856, *https://pubmed.ncbi. nlm.nih.gov/32125403/.*

would be a more honest label for the provision than 'price negotiation'."[185] Moreover, unlike past proposals, there would be no floor price below which the secretary would be unable to force further concessions. As Holtz-Eakin continues:

> While the BBBA would not apply Medicare's negotiated prices for drugs to non-Federal programs, the most significant implication of the BBBA's dollar-for-dollar penalties on price increases that exceed the rate of inflation is that, for the first time, the Federal Government would be unilaterally capping drug prices nationwide, both in Federal programs and in the private market. This shift in the Federal Government's posture toward private markets, negotiations, and competition cannot be overstated. [Thus] . . . significantly under the BBBA the Federal Government would cap the price of all drugs throughout the entire health-care system by penalizing any manufacturer who increases a drug's price faster than the rate of inflation.[186]

No, I am not aware of any instance in U.S. history where Congress has enacted any provision resembling a 95-percent non-compliance penalty. There is, however, considerable evidence of the damage that punitive excise taxes inflict on biomedical innovation. For instance, the Affordable Care Act imposed a 2.3 percent excise tax on the price of taxable medical devices sold in the United States from 2013 to 2015. A study by the Tax Foundation found that, even in the short time it was imposed, the tax resulted in higher prices as well as less research and development (R&D).[187] In fact, the Office of the Actuary for the Centers for Medicare and Medicaid Services stated that the medical device tax would ultimately increase national health-care expenditures.[188] Moreover, the Tax Foundation found that if the medical excise tax had remained imposed as originally envisioned, it would likely have

---

[185] Doug Holtz-Eakin, "Testimony on: The Build Back Better Act's Prescription Drug Policies and Their Potential Impacts" (American Action Forum, March 16, 2022), 5–6, 12, *https://www.finance.senate.gov/imo/media/doc/DHE%20SFC%20Testimony%20BBBA%20Drug%20Policies.pdf.*

[186] *Ibid.*, 6, 12.

[187] Ulrik Boesen, "Why the Medical Device Tax Should Be Repealed," Fiscal Fact No. 677 (Tax Foundation, November 2019), 1, *https://files.taxfoundation. org/20191203103452 /TaxFoundation_FF677.pdf.*

[188] Department of Health and Human Services, Centers for Medicare and Med- icaid Services, Office of the Actuary, "Estimated Financial Effects of the 'Pa- tient Protection and Affordable Care Act,' as Amended," April 22, 2010, *https://www.cms.gov/Research-Statistics-Data-and-Systems/Research/ActuarialStudies/downloads/PPACA_2010-04-22.pdf.*

resulted in a decline of 21,390 full-time equivalent jobs and a reduction in GDP of $1.7 billion.[189] But even in the mere 3 years in which the medial device tax was in place, it conflicted considerable damage on the U.S. medical device industry.[190]

The United States also has a broader history with government policies that attempt to set aggressive price controls, and their effect has generally been deleterious. For instance, in 1971, President Nixon's Cost of Living Council, led by Arnold Weber, attempted to quash inflation by temporarily blocking for 90 days increases in nearly all wages and prices. But it issued rules, such as one attempting to control prices in futures markets, that, in Weber's words, were "so contrary to established behavior that the markets simply shut down."[191] Nixon's price controls failed to stop inflation, reduced the value of the dollar by one-third, and were a significant contributor to the ensuing 1970s stagflation, as inflation persisted throughout the decade at an average annual rate of 8 percent.[192]

It's certainly true that some patients are paying more than they should for drugs at the pharmacy counter. Some reform is needed—notably to address the pinch seniors are experiencing in out-of-pocket costs at the pharmacy counter—but radical reconstructive surgery in the form of stringent drug price controls is not the solution.

Question. BBBA's defenders sometimes argue that the life sciences sector is uniquely and exceptionally profitable and could thus easily absorb the costs trig- gered by the bill's price controls. Others argue that biopharmaceutical R&D estimates overstate the sector's commitment to innovative research, pointing to studies suggesting that marketing and advertising expenses for at least some segments of the industry exceed R&D investments.

Do these arguments accurately characterize the relative profitability, R&D intensity, and marketing/advertising expenditures of the biopharmaceutical sector? Why or why not?

---

[189] Boesen, "Why the Medical Device Tax Should Be Repealed."

[190] Stephen Ezell, "Affordable Care Act Endangers Innovative U.S. Life Sciences Industries," *Innovation Files,* July 3, 2013, *https://www.innovationfiles.org/affordable-care-act-endangers-innovative-u-s-life-sciences-industries/.*

[191] James R. Hagerty, "When Nixon Froze Prices, Arnold Weber Enforced the Rules," *The Wall Street Journal,* August 27, 2020, *https://www.wsj.com/arti- cles/when-nixon-froze-prices-arnold-weber-enforced-the-rules-11598536800.*

[192] William N. Walker, "Nixon Taught Us How Not to Fight Inflation," The Wall Street Journal, August 13, 2021, https://www.wsj.com/articles/nixon-fight-in-flation-price-controls-stag flation-gas-shortages-biden-democrats-reconciliation-bill-federal-reserve-11628885071.

Answer. The U.S. biopharmaceutical industry is both America's and the world's most R&D-intensive industry—of any kind. As the U.S. Congressional Budget Office (CBO) explains, "Over the decade from 2005 to 2014, the industry's R&D intensity averaged 18 to 20 percent per year. That ratio has been trending upward since 2012, and it exceeded 25 percent in 2018 and 2019."[193] This level of R&D investment is substantially more than any other U.S. industry. As the CBO observes, "By comparison, average R&D intensity across all [U.S.] industries typically ranges between 2 and 3 percent" and even "R&D intensity in the software and semiconductor industries, which are generally comparable to the drug industry in their reliance on R&D, has remained below 18 percent."[194] (See Figure 4.) America's biopharmaceutical sector accounts for 18 percent of total U.S. business R&D investment.[195] Importantly, the CBO notes that while "Consumer spending on brand-name prescription drugs has risen, [the industry's] R&D has risen more quickly."[196]

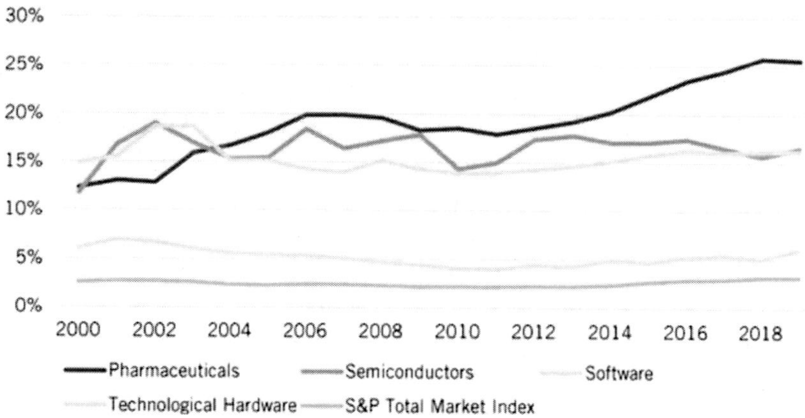

Figure 4. Average R&D intensity for publicly traded U.S. companies, by industry.[197]

[193] Congressional Budget Office (CBO), "Research and Development in the Phar- maceutical Industry" (CBO, April 2021), 4–5, *https://www.cbo.gov/publica- tion/57025.*

[194] *Ibid.*

[195] TEConomy Partners, LLC and PhRMA, "Economic Impact of the U.S. Bio-pharmaceutical Industry" (TEConomy Partners and PhRMA, December 2019), 7, *https://www.phrma.org/-/media/Project/PhRMA/PhRMA-Org/PhRMA-Org/PDF/D-F/Economic-Impact-US-Biopharmaceu* tical-Industry-December- 2019.pdf.

[196] Congressional Budget Office, "Research and Development in the Pharma- ceutical Industry."

[197] *Ibid.*, 5.

The notion that America's innovative life-science industry is spending more on advertising than R&D is fundamentally specious. For that to be the case, the industry would have to be spending more than one-quarter of its total revenues on advertising, which it is not. According to the CBO, in 2019, the pharmaceutical industry invested $83 billion dollars in R&D (which, adjusted for inflation, was an amount 10 times greater than the industry spent per year in the 1980s).[198] In contrast, totalpharmaceutical advertising spending reached $6.58 billion in 2020 (up modestly from the $4.9 billion it was in 2007).[199]

Moreover, this advertising isn't simply zero-sum, designed to gain market share over competitors. Rather, much of it is about educating consumers—and in the case of biopharma, educating health-care providers, too—about choices.[200] Moreover, the drug industry is different than say the soap or car industry where it's relatively easy for consumers to find out on their own about new products and the differences between products. Some of the marketing expenses are to educate doctors and consumers about the value and efficacy of new drugs. This is why Frosch et al. find that more than half of physicians agree that ads educate patients about health conditions and available treatments and nearly 75 percent of patient respondents agree that advertisements improve their understanding of diseases and treatments.[201]

The notion that the pharmaceutical industry is "exceptionally profitable" is also questionable. Researchers at the University of Southern California led by Professor Neeraj Sood have sought to estimate excess returns (the extent to which a firm's profits are higher than expected given the risk associated with their investments) for manufacturers and middlemen in the pharmaceutical supply chain. They found that the rate of return on investments of large firms in the pharmaceutical industry between 2013 and 2018 was just 1.7 percent once adjusted for the risk premium paid for capital and the more logical treatment of R&D expenditures as long-term investments rather than current

198 Ibid.

199 Beth Snyder Bulik, "The top 10 ad spenders in Big Pharma for 2020," FiercePharma, April 19, 2021, https://www.fiercepharma.com/special-report/ top-10-ad-spenders-big-pharma-for-2020.

200 Robert D. Atkinson, "Why Life-Sciences Innovation Is Politically 'Purple'— And How Partisans Get It Wrong" (ITIF, February 2016), 6, https://itif.org/publications/2016/02/22/why-life-sciences-innovation-politically-purple.

201 D.L. Frosch, D. Grande, D.M. Tarn., and R.L. Kravitz, "A Decade of Con- troversy: Balancing Policy with Evidence in the Regulation of Prescription Drug Advertising," American Journal of Public Health, Vol. 100, No. 1 (Janu-ary 2010): 24–32, https://www.ncbi.nlm.nih.gov/pmc/articles/PMC27912 53/.

costs.[202] For comparison, the overall S&P 500 had an excess rate of return of more than double—3.6 percent—over this period.

The authors also found that other players in the pharmaceutical supply chain re- alized higher excess returns. Specifically, for the period from 2003 to 2018, they found that wholesalers earned excess returns of 8.1 percent and that insurers, pharmacy benefit managers (PBMs), and retailers collectively earned excess returns of 5.9 percent. The authors did find that the cohort of biotechnology firms in their study realized the highest excess returns of any group, at 9.6 percent, though they note this was in part driven by several blockbuster drugs introduced from 2013 to 2015, notably new hepatitis C drugs, and that by 2018 the sector's excess rate of return had fallen to under 9 percent. More importantly, however, the authors note that, "In contrast with middlemen, monopoly power in the pharmaceutical and biotech sectors—derived through the U.S. patent system—provides [an] incentive for innovation that might not happen otherwise."[203]

But the point here should be the value these industries are delivering for society relative to their degree of profitability. America's life-sciences innovators are deliv- ering innovative drugs that have accounted for 73 percent of the increase between 2000 and 2009 in life expectancy at birth across 30 countries, including the United States (or 1.27 years of the 1.73-year increase in life expectancy).[204] Moreover, America's life-sciences companies employ approximately one-quarter of America's total R&D workforce. Meanwhile, 23 percent of the American biopharmaceutical industry's workforce can be found at the lab bench in R&D jobs seeking to create new cures, giving the industry a share of employment dedicated to R&D three times higher than the national average.[205] Those numbers represent tremendous returns and value to society, especially relative to profitability; PBMs, according to Sood's data, are more profitable than pharmaceutical firms and almost as much so as biotechnology ones, but they're not nearly employing one-quarter of America's R&D

---

[202] Neeraj Sood, et al., "Do companies in the pharmaceutical supply chain earn excess returns?", International Journal of Health Economics and Manage- ment, Vol. 21 (January 4, 2021): 99–114, https://doi.org/10.1007/s10754-020- 09291-1. (The researchers calculated the "risk adjusted rate of return" by sub- tracting capital costs, which vary with the level of risk across industries.)

[203] *Ibid.*, 110.

[204] Frank Lichtenberg, "Pharmaceutical Innovation and Longevity Growth in 30 Developing and High-income Countries, 2000–2009," *Health Policy and Tech- nology* Vol. 3, Issue 1 (March 2014): 36–58, *https://www.sciencedirect.com/science/article/abs/pii/S2211883713000646.*

[205] TEConomy Partners, LLC and PhRMA, "Economic Impact of the U.S. Bio- pharmaceutical Industry," 7.

workforce or developing products that have tremendous impacts on American and global citizens' quality and length of life.

Lastly, many BBBA proponents assert that America's life-sciences innovators aren't focused on breakthrough innovation or just focus on "me-too" drugs. But the reality is that there are currently 4,500 medicines under development in the United States, including 560 seeking to treat pediatric diseases, 537 for neurological diseases, 362 for cell and gene therapies, and hundreds more for mental illness, asthma and allergies, and other maladies.[206] Many of these are potentially "first-in-class" drugs, including 86 percent for Alzheimer's, 79 percent for various forms of cancer, 75 percent for psychiatry, 74 percent for neurology, and 73 percent for cardiovascular disease.[207] To assert that the industry, broadly, isn't working to develop breakthrough treatments is fundamentally fallacious.

And trying to make progress in many of these fields is extremely difficult. For in- stance, consider that between 1998 and 2017, there were 146 attempts to bring new Alzheimer's treatments to market, but just 4 out of those 146 were successful approvals. In other words, 97 percent proved unsuccessful.[208] (However, the value of a successful treatment would be profound: the United States could save $220 billion within the first 5 years and a projected $367 billion in the year 2050 alone if a cure or effective treatment for Alzheimer's disease could be found.)[209]

The difficulty of innovating safe and effective new drugs is further illustrated both by efforts to develop oncology drugs and to develop vaccines in response to the COVID–19 pandemic. A 2019 study by Wong, Siah, and Lo examining oncology drug development efforts from January 1, 2000 to October 31, 2015 found that oncology programs have just a 3.4 percent chance of ultimate Food and Drug Administration (FDA) approval (and yet companies continue to invest tens of billions of dollars trying to tackle

---

206 PhRMA, "Chart Pack: Biopharmaceuticals in Perspective, Fall 2020" (PhRMA, 2020), 21, *https://www.phrma.org/resource-center/Topics/Advances-in-Treat-ment/Chart-Pack-Biopharmaceuticals-in-Perspective-Fall-2020.*

207 *Ibid.*, 22.

208 PhRMA, "Why Has Research into Alzheimer's Disease Been So Hard?", *https://innovation.org/en/diseases/neurological/alzheimers/why-has-re-search-into-alzheimers-disease-been-so-hard.*

209 The Alzheimer's Association, "Changing the Trajectory of Alzheimer's Disease" (The Alzheimer's Association, 2015), *https://www.sciencedirect.com/science/article/abs/pii/S22118 83713000646.*

oncology challenges).[210] Similarly, life-sciences companies responded with great alacrity in attempting to develop COVID–19 vaccines and therapeutics. But thus far, only 2 of 58 vaccine attempts (3.4 percent) have received final approval (18 are in Phase III clinical trials). But already 26 vaccine candidates have failed, as well as 54 proposed antiviral medications and 90 different therapeutic treatments.[211]

Question. In making the case for the House-passed BBBA drug pricing policies, some have suggested that most new drugs that come to market are "me-too" products that either make modest changes to existing medications or treat conditions that already have numerous therapeutic options. These claims seem at odds with the drug development landscape, where the majority of the 50 new drugs approved last year were first-in-class treatments, and where studies regarding existing therapies can lead to new indications and uses, along with improvements that offer outsize patient benefits. One drug originally indicated to treat chronic lymphocytic leukemia, for instance, received approval as a disease-modifying therapy (DMT) for the treatment of multiple sclerosis roughly 11 years later, after a far-reaching and costly clinical development program. This type of follow-on innovation can result in major medical breakthroughs.

To what extent do we see meaningfully innovative drugs and biologics approved each year, and what potential value does follow-on innovation offer to patients?

How would the government price-setting program and other price controls included in BBBA impact incentives for follow-in innovations like new indications for existing therapies, new formulations (i.e., to mitigate or eliminate side effects, to streamline dosing regimens, etc.), and other product improvements and changes?

While the House-passed BBBA technically makes no changes to patents and exclusivities with respect to prescription drugs, the government price-setting program and multi-market price growth cap policies would affect a manufacturer's ability to derive economic value from these market

---

[210] Chi Heem Wong, Kien Wei Siah, and Andrew W. Lo, "Estimation of clinical trial success rates and related parameters," *Biostatistics,* Vol. 20, Issue 2 (April 2019): 273–286, *https://doi.org/10.1093/biostatistics/kxx069.*

[211] BIO, "COVID–19 Therapeutic Development Tracker," *https://www.bio.org/ policy/human-health/vaccines-biodefense/coronavirus/pipeline-tracker;* BIO, "Response to Federal Trade Commission: Request for Information on Merger Enforcement" (BIO, April 15, 2022), 4.

protections. How would the bill's price controls impact the incentives for innovation currently inherent in patents and exclusivities?

Answer. As just noted, contrary to critics' assertions, America's biopharmaceutical industry is an innovation-oriented one, not a me-too-oriented one.

In 2020, the FDA's Center for Drug Evaluation and Research (CDER) approved 53 novel drugs.[212] Of these novel drugs, 21 were considered first-in-class and 31 were designated orphan drug status.[213] Similarly, the FDA's Center for Biologics Evaluation and Research (CBER) approved eight biologics.[214] The year 2020 also saw the first therapeutics for COVID–19 and some forms of premature aging, such as progeria.[215]

Similarly, in 2021, CDER approved 50 novel drugs, and CBER approved 10 new biologics.[216] Despite the slight overall decrease in novel drugs, 27 were given first-in-class designation, and 26 were granted orphan drug status.[217] Although it is too early in 2022 to provide significant data, the FDA lists 10 novel drugs and 2 biologics already approved as of April 21, 2022, along with 9 new generics or biosimilars.[218]

---

[212] FDA CDER, "Novel Drug Approvals for 2020" (January 13, 2021), *https://www.fda.gov/drugs/new-drugs-fda-cders-new-molecular-entities-and-new-therapeutic-biological-products/novel-drug-approvals-2020.*

[213] Jeff Craven, "FDA approved more first-in-class drugs, gave more accelerated approvals in 2021," Regulatory Affairs Professional Society (January 27, 2022), *https://www.raps.org/news-and-articles/news-articles/2022/1/fda-ap-proved-more-first-in-class-drugs-more-with-a.*

[214] FDA CBER, "2020 Biological License Application Approvals" (August 20, 2020), *https://www.fda.gov/vaccines-blood-biologics/development-approval-process-cber/2020-biological-license-application-approvals.*

[215] Kari Oakes, "In 2020, all goal dates met for CDER's novel approvals" (January 13, 2021), *https://www.raps.org/news-and-articles/news-articles/2021/1/in-2020-all-goal-dates-met-for-cders-novel-approva.*

[216] FDA CDER, "Novel Drug Approvals for 2021" (January 6, 2022), *https://www.fda.gov/drugs/new-drugs-fda-cders-new-molecular-entities-and-new-therapeutic-biological-products/novel-drug-approvals-2021;* FDA CBER, "2021 Biological License Application Approvals" (December 20, 2021), *https://www.fda.gov/vaccines-blood-biologics/development-approval-process-cber/2021-biological-license-application-approvals.*

[217] Craven, "FDA approved more first-in-class drugs, gave more accelerated ap- provals in 2021."

[218] FDA CDER, "Novel Drug Approvals for 2021" (March 28, 2022), *https://www.fda.gov/drugs/new-drugs-fda-cders-new-molecular-entities-and-new-therapeutic-biological-products/novel-drug-approvals-2022;* FDA CBER, "2021 Biological License Application Approvals" (March 16, 2022), *https:// www.fda.gov/vaccines-blood-biologics/development-approval-process-cber/2022-biological-license-application-approvals; Drugs.com,* "New Drug Approvals" (accessed April 21, 2022), *https://www.drugs.com/newdrugs.html.*

And despite critics' assertions the reality is that new drug approvals have significantly accelerated over the past 2 decades. The FDA's Center for Drug Evaluation and Research's 5-year rolling approval average stood at 44 new drugs per year in 2019, double the lowest 5-year rolling average of 22 drugs approved, realized in 2009. (See Figure 5.) And the number of drugs in development globally increased from 5,995 in 2001 to 13,718 in 2016.[219]

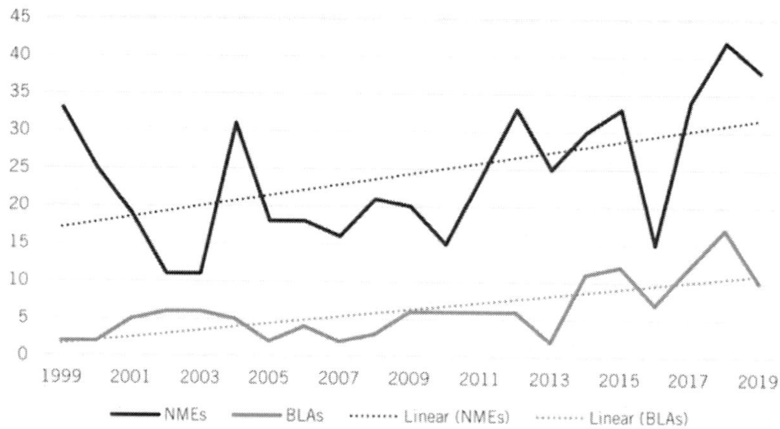

Figure 5. FDA annual approvals of new molecuar entities (NMEs) and biologic license applications (BLAs), 1999-2019.[220]

Yet, as Representative Katie Porter (D–CA) argues in her report, "Killer Profits: How Big Pharma Takeovers Destroy Innovation and Harm Patients," "Instead of taking risks to find new, critically needed drugs, large pharmaceutical companies are just repackaging the same products over and over: In 2018, only 1 in 3 new brand-name drugs that drug companies launched were 'first-in-class' drugs."[221] Similarly, Rena Conti observed in her Senate Finance Committee hearing testimony that "Sanofi testified in the

---

[219] In Vivo: The Business and Medicine Report, Vol. 34, No. 1 (January 2016), 25, https://invivo.pharmaintelligence.informa.com/outlook/industry-data/-/media/marketing/Outlook%202019/pdfs/2016.PDF.

[220] Ashley Mullard, "2019 FDA Drug Approvals," *Nature Reviews: Drug Dis- covery,* Vol. 19 (February 2020): 79, *https://www.nature.com/articles/d41573-020-00001-7.*

[221] Office of Congresswoman Katie Porter, "Killer Profits: How Big Pharma Take- overs Destroy Innovation and Harm Patients" (January 2021), 6, *https://por- ter.house.gov/uploadedfiles/final_pharma_ma_and_innovation_report_january_2021.pdf.*

Senate that only 33 of its 81 R&D projects were for new chemical entities" (again, about one-third).[222]

Is 1 in 3 low? In the 1940s and 1950s, when there were few drugs on the market and almost all were first in class, 1 in 3 would have been low. But as more drugs hit the market, the share of first-in-class drugs declined as it became harder to discover new treatments and also because of the importance of producing multiple drugs to address the same disease. Nonetheless, the share of drugs that are new has risen since the 1970s, not fallen.[223]

Moreover, criticisms of the industry for when it does invest in "me-too" drugs fails to recognize the significant clinical benefits of new drugs complementing existing drugs. Sometimes an existing drug does not perform as well as the new drug. Sometimes certain individuals have adverse reactions to an existing drug but not the new drug.[224] In addition, follow-on drugs can be better in efficacy or methodology and convenience of use and administration. DiMasi and Faden found that 32 percent of follow-on drugs have received a priority rating from the U.S. FDA, indicating that these drugs are likely to provide an important improvement over the first-to-market drug.[225] They concluded, "Overall, these results indicate that new drug development is better characterized as a race to market among drugs in a new therapeutic class, rather than a lower risk imitation of a proven breakthrough."[226] Moreover, the Government Accountability Office (GAO) found that the introduction of additional drugs lowers prices.[227]

---

222 Rena Conti, "Statement of Rena Conti: Prescription Drug Spending Reform Will Not Harm Innovation and Will Benefit the American Public at Senate Finance Committee Hearing Prescription Drug Price Inflation: An Urgent Need to Lower Drug Prices in Medicare," March 16, 2022, 6, *https://www. finance.senate.gov/imo/media/doc/Conti%20SFC%20Final%20Testimony.pdf.*

223 Mark Robberson, "An Empirical Analysis of Innovation in the Pharmaceutical Industry by Drug Class: Implications for Regulatory Policy" (Johns Hopkins Bloomberg School of Public Health, submitted for the 2019 Center of Excel- ence in Regulatory Science and Innovation and Master of Science in Regu-latory Science and Food Safety Regulation), *https://www.jhsph.edu/research/ centers-and-institutes/center-of-excellence-in-regulatory-science-and-innova-tion/Mark%20Rob berson%20CERSI%20paper%2020190505.pdf.*

224 Augustus John Rush and David J. Kupfer, "Strategies and tactics in the treat- ment of depression," in *Treatment of Psychiatric Disorders,* edited by G.O. Gabbard (Washington, DC: American Psychiatric Publishing, 2001).

225 Joseph A. DiMasi and Laura B. Faden, "Competitiveness in Follow-On Drug R&D: A Race or Imitation?", *Nature Reviews Drug Discovery,* Vol. 10, No. 1 (January 2011), *http://www.nature.com/nrd/journal/v10/n1/abs/nrd3296. html.*

226 *Ibid.*

227 United States Government Accountability Office (GAO), Drug Industry: Prof- its, Research and Development Spending, and Merger and Acquisition Deals (GAO, November 2017), *https://www.gao.gov/assets/gao-18-40.pdf.*

Indeed, follow-on innovations from original innovative drugs represent an important aspect of America's life-sciences innovation system that can bring important benefits for patients. These can include new indications (i.e., applications of an existing drug to a new disease), improvements in delivery forms (i.e., providing a medication orally as opposed to through an injection), or improvements in delivery dosages (i.e., a pill administered once a month as opposed to once daily).

For instance, in 2013, a revolutionary new treatment called Sovaldi was released that boosted hepatitis C cure rates to 90 percent. This was followed in 2014 by an improved treatment called Harvoni, which cures the hepatitis C variant left untouched by Sovaldi. By early 2020, an astonishing six new treatments for the disease had received FDA approval, opening up a wide range of treatment options that take into account patients' liver and kidney status, co-infections, potential drug interactions, previous treatment failures, and the genotype of the HCV virus.[228] Moreover, as competitors joined the market, the price of Sovaldi was cut in half.[229]

The provisions in the BBBA would likely have a deleterious impact on both follow-on and generic drug innovation. That's in no insignificant part because generic or biosimilar drugs depend, by definition, on the innovative drugs or biologics that predated them, and when drug price controls inhibit the creation of innovative medicines in the first place, they tamp down on the capacity to create the cheaper generics or biologics of tomorrow, a dynamic that would only be amplified by artificially decreasing the price of innovative drugs through price controls. As Holtz- Eakin elaborates:

> Ironically, the more successful the HHS secretary is in leveraging the BBBA's punitive excise tax to force price concessions, the fewer generic and biosimilar products are likely to come to market. Follow-on products are able to dramatically undercut name-brand drugs and biologics on price because they do not have the same R&D expenditures and because their lower prices allow them to achieve larger market shares. But if the price difference between a name-brand drug, subject to the secretary's

[228] Jocelyn Mason and Kimberly D. Boeser, "The changing HCV treatment cas- cade," *Infectious Disease News,* October 2017, *https://www.healio.com/infec- tious-disease/hepatitis-c/news/print/infectious-disease-news/{87b74536-f358-43d3-a804-f37a 98402b0b}/the-changing-hcv-treatment-cascade.*

[229] Holtz-Eakin, "Testimony on: The Build Back Better Act's Prescription Drug Policies and Their Potential Impacts," 11.

price controls, and a new generic is marginal or even non-existent, the ability of a generic to gain market share will be reduced.[230]

As to the long-term effect of the BBBA on the subsequent number of generic drugs, the University of Chicago's Tomas Philipson and Troy Durie reach a similar conclusion, writing:

> We looked at the patent life and data exclusivity of the top 20 drugs by total Medicare Part B and D spending, finding that this plan will shorten their market life by 2–4 years on average. These drugs will no longer have the advantages of exclusivity by having an artificially lower price, but cheaper generics still will not be able to be developed while they watch the government price them out of the market. This new price control scheme will lead to fewer generics and less competition which has been shown to lead to effective price reductions without undermining innovation.[231]

Question. Some have claimed that the BBBA's drug pricing provisions would exempt startups and other small biotechs from the onerous new government price-setting program included in the legislation. In reality, however, the bill includes only an extremely narrow and time-limited exemption that carves certain small biotechs out of the program for 3 years and provides them with a pricing floor for the following two, after which point the bureaucratic new system would treat these small firms like any other companies. Notably, 66 percent of biopharmaceutical companies are startups. Moreover, small businesses—many of which would not qualify for even the temporary exemption—account for 70 percent of pivotal-stage trials, and more than 90 percent of biopharmaceutical firms overall are not turning a profit.

Do the time-limited and narrow small biotech exemptions in the bill provide meaningful protection for the startups and other small businesses that comprise the majority of the life sciences sector?

If enacted, how would the government price-setting program and other price controls (such as the mandatory multi-market price growth cap) impact these small businesses and the prospects of future biopharmaceutical startups?

---

[230] *Ibid., 8.*

[231] Tomas J. Philipson and Troy Durie, "Issue Brief: The Impact of HR 5376 on Biopharmaceutical Innovation and Patient Health" (The University of Chi- cago, November 9, 2021), 20, *https://cpb-us-w2.wpmucdn.com/voices.uchicago.edu/dist/d/3128/files/2021/08/Issue-Brief-Drug-Pricing-in-HR-537 6-11.30.pdf.*

How might the imposition of the bill's price controls fuel industry consolidation, given the diversified product portfolios and compliance-related resources and staff that large multinationals often enjoy, relative to smaller businesses?

Answer. Proponents assert that life sciences could easily absorb the costs of the BBBA drug price controls. But, while that might be easier, though still deleterious, for larger firms, it forgets that start-ups account for 66 percent of U.S. biopharmaceutical enterprises.[232] Yet these startups, 90 percent of which are pre-revenue, account for 70 percent of drugs in phase III clinical trials.[233] Yet government price controls, even if there is some type of carve out for small innovators, would still sharply reduce the opportunity to earn a return. One reason is that acquisition by a larger company often represents an important, and legitimate and meritorious, exit strategy for a smaller company and to the extent the BBBA deprives larger firms of revenues, this would reverberate throughout the ecosystem. But, overall, such drug price controls would harm small and large biopharmaceutical firms alike.

Question. Therapeutic development relies heavily on high-risk investments from diverse sources. While some of the BBBA's backers anticipate that the life sciences would remain attractive to investors at every level, real-world experience tells a different story. Even under current laws and regulations, capital can—and often does—shift away from (or simply never flow into) the biopharmaceutical sector. According to one Wall Street Journal piece from last December, for instance, biotech stocks "crumbled" in 2021. Developing a new medication can take between 11.5 and 15 years, and only one in every 1,000 drug formulas ever enters preclinical trials. For the ones that do, only eight percent ever receive FDA approval. Unsurprisingly, it costs an average of $2.6 billion to develop and gain approval for a new medicine. These factors make the biopharmaceutical sector especially sensitive to the types of government price controls included in the House-passed BBBA, which University of Chicago researchers projected would lead to 135 fewer new drug approvals in the next 2 decades.

---

232 John Wu and Robert D. Atkinson, "How Technology-Based Start-Ups Promote U.S. Economic Growth" (ITIF, November 2017), 12, *https://itif.org/publications/2017/11/28/how-technology-based-start-ups-support-us-economicgrowth.*

233 Biotechnology Innovation Organization (BIO), "Research & Development: Biopharmaceutical Sector, A Driver of Innovation," *https://www.bio.org/sites/default/files/legacy/bioorg/docs/BIO_RD_one%20pager%205-9-17.pdf;* CBO, "Research and Development in the Pharmaceutical Industry," 8.

How would the price controls included in the BBBA likely impact the investment landscape with respect to biopharmaceutical innovation?

Supporters of the BBBA's government price-setting program sometimes cite the Veterans Affairs (VA) Department as a model for Part D. In practice, however, the closed formulary leveraged by the VA impairs access to many medications. Among the top 200 Part D drugs by overall spend, for instance, one study found that Part D plans covered an average of nearly three-fourths of the products, while the VA covered just over half. Among a sample of 25 first-in-class treatments, Part D plans covered more than three in every five, while the VA covered just 40 percent. The VA also integrates value assessments using quality-adjusted life years (QALYs) into its pricing practices, despite widespread criticism of these metrics by disability advocates, who argue that QALYs devalue individuals with exceptional needs, along with older individuals.

Answer. Life-sciences companies depend on profits from one generation of biomedical innovation to fund investment in the next. Research by Dubois et al. makes this dynamic crystal clear, finding that every $2.5 billion of additional biopharmaceutical revenue leads to one new drug approval.[234] Related academic research shows a statistically significant relationship between a biopharma enterprise's profits from the previous year and its R&D expenditures in the current year.[235] Likewise, Gambardella found that sales revenue from previous periods have a significant, positive impact on current-period biopharma R&D.[236] Henderson and Cockburn find that the pharmaceutical firms with the greatest sales are also the ones with the largest R&D investments.[237] Drug price controls would harm future investments in biomedical innovation.

Question. Is the VA drug pricing system an appropriate model or exemplar for Part D? Why or why not?

---

234 Pierre Dubois, "Market size and pharmaceutical innovation," *The Rand Jour- nal of Economics,* Vol. 46, Issue 4 (October 2015): 844–871, *https:// onlinelibrary.wiley.com/doi/full/10.1111/1756-2171.12113.*

235 Destrina Grace Simanjuntak and Raymond R. Tjandrawinata, "Impact of Profitability, R&D Intensity, and Cash Flow on R&D Expenditure in Pharma- ceutical Companies" (Social Science Research Network, April 29, 2011), *http://papers.ssrn.com/sol3/papers.cfm?abstract_id=1824267.*

236 Alfonso Gambardella, *Science and Innovation: The US Pharmaceutical Indus- try During the 1980s* (Cambridge University Press, 1995).

237 R. Henderson and I.M. Cockburn, "Scale, Scope, and Spillovers: The Deter- minants of Research Productivity in the Pharmaceutical Industry," *RAND Journal of Economics,* Vol. 27, No. 1 (1996): 32–59, *https://www.nber.org/pa- pers/w4466.*

Answer. The VA approach doesn't provide a satisfactory exemplar for Medicare Part D, that's especially because, unlike Medicare Part D, the VA employs a "one- size-fits all' approach that limits access to medicines. It's a closed formulary. In particular, "the VA employs a narrow, exclusionary formulary to generate savings, and comparisons of coverage between the VA and Medicare demonstrate that the VA offers fewer choices, particularly of the most cutting-edge and innovative medicines."[238] For instance, considering the top-200 Part D brand medicines, a July 2020 study found that, while 74 percent were covered by Medicare, just 52 percent were covered by the VA formulary. Likewise, the VA National Formulary covers just 40 percent of first-in-class Part D medicines, compared with more than 62 percent in Medicare Part D.[239] As the GAO explains, while "the VA can steer utilization toward a limited number of drugs within a given therapeutic class; Medicare Part D plans, on the other hand, generally have broad networks of pharmacies and as such may have broader formularies than VA's."[240] Moreover, because of limitations on the VA formulary, to acquire access to the medicines they need, more than half of all veterans supplement their VA benefits with other sources of health coverage, including Part D.[241] The VA's use of QALYs also discriminate against the disabled, seniors, the chronically ill and communities of color; for instance, a QALY for a patient with multiple sclerosis can be worth half as much as a healthy, young individual, and a person over the age of 70 is worth approximately 30 percent, simply due to their age.

Question. In defending the government price-setting program and multi-market price growth cap policies in the BBBA, some policymakers have contended that under current law, manufacturers enjoy maximal price-setting power and can charge whatever they want, while purchasers and consumers lack any leverage. In practice, however, all three of the largest pharmacy benefit managers (PBMs) exclude between 400 and 500 drugs from their standard formularies, and the number of drugs excluded by these formularies

---

[238] Nicole Longo, "Five reasons tying VA prices to Medicare Part D misses the mark," *The Catalyst,* September 22, 2021, *https://catalyst.phrma.org/five-rea- sons-tying-va-prices-to-medicare-part-d-misses-the-mark.*

[239] AmerisourceBergen, "Potential Access Implications of a National Formulary in Part D," July 16, 2020, *https://www.xcenda.com/insights/comparing-the-gen- erosity-of-drug-coverage-in-the-medicare-part-d-and-veterans-affairs-programs.*

[240] GAO, "Prescription Drugs: Department of Veterans Affairs Paid About Half as Much as Medicare Part D for Selected Drugs in 2017" (GAO, December 2020), *https://www.gao.gov/assets/gao-21-111.pdf.*

[241] Kevin Stroupe et al., "Medication acquisition across systems of care and patient-provider communication among older veterans," *Am J Health Syst Pharm,* Vol. 70, Issue 9 (May 2013): 804–13, *https://pubmed.ncbi.nlm.nih. gov/23592363/.*

increased by 676 percent from 2014 to 2020. Moreover, rebates paid by manufacturers have grown substantially in recent years, further reducing net prices and demonstrating leverage on the part of the payers extracting these price concessions.

Do drug manufacturers, as many BBBA supporters argue, enjoy absolute power to charge whatever they want?

Answer. No, drug companies do not enjoy absolute power to charge whatever they want. Drug companies face many constraints: on the innovation side they're constrained by science, which is why, on average, as many as 5,000 to 10,000 compounds may be screened to get to approximately 250 promising molecular compounds that can enter preclinical testing, with 5 entering actual clinical testing.[242] And that's just getting to the clinical trial stage, as less than 12 percent of candidate medicines that even make it into Phase I clinical trials are ultimately approved by the FDA.[243] It's why oncology drug efforts have only a 3.4 percent chance of winning FDA approval.

When drugs do make it to market, even the ones getting there first will often quickly face competition. For instance, as noted previously, as competitors joined the market, the price of Sovaldi as not just a treatment but an actual cure for hepatitis C was cut in half. Further, innovative drugs have a limited period of patent protection, and when drugs go off patent, much cheaper generic drugs often come rapidly on the scene. As noted subsequently in response to a question from Senator Sasse, for instance, once Biogen's multiple sclerosis (MS) drug Tecfidera went off-patent, generic competitors entered with drugs well over 95 percent cheaper. Lastly, of course, drug makers must negotiate with pharmacy benefit managers and other wholesalers to get their drugs listed on formularies like Medicare Part D, where the negotiations are aggressive. Some argue that there's no negotiation function for Medicare Part D, and thus the government needs to take the process over. But the issue isn't negotiation or no negotiation. There is negotiation, for instance as provided by the PBMs; policymakers should focus on helping this market-based process function better, such as through increasing scrutiny and transparency on PBMs and ensuring they meet their fiduciary obligations.

---

[242] Pacific BioLabs, "Stages of Drug Development," https://pacificbiolabs.com/ stages-of-drug-development.

[243] PhRMA, "Chart Pack: Biopharmaceuticals in Perspective, Summer 2019" (PhRMA, 2019), https://www.phrma.org/-/media/Project/PhRMA/PhRMA-Org/PhRMA-Org/PDF/P-R/PhRMA_2019_ChartPack_Final.pdf.

On List Price Growth

Question. While net prices for brand-name drugs have fallen for at least four consecutive years, according to IQVIA and others, list prices for these products have grown—albeit at a slower rate than in previous years.

What are some of the underlying factors driving list price growth for prescription drugs?

Answer. When it comes to the growing disparity between drugs' list and net prices, particular attention must be paid to the role played by rebates and discounts. Discussion of drug prices tends to focus on the annually announced increase in the list prices for prescription drugs. However, sales of prescription drugs are subject to substantial manufacturer rebates and discounts, leading to a considerable reduction in manufacturer earnings. Researchers at the University of Pittsburgh School of Pharmacy and Medicine estimate that while the average annual increase in the list price for prescription drugs between 2007 and 2018 was 9.1 percent, the net increase in drug prices after rebates was only 4.5 percent.[244]

In recent years, as list prices have been growing at a slower pace, the volume of discounts and rebates has increased. For example, in 2020, list prices grew at an average rate of 4.4 percent, but net prices decreased by 2.9 percent.[245] As The Wall Street Journal, citing data from the SSR Health Report, notes, "[A]verage U.S. list prices for prescription medicines rose in the past decade, but net prices—after rebates and discounts—rose less sharply and have recently declined."[246] (See Figure 6.)

In fact, one study found that more than one-third of drug list prices were rebated back to PBMs and other entities in the supply chain. As that report describes, "Pharmaceutical spending estimates that omit rebates and discounts do not fully reflect the underlying competitive dynamics of the pharmaceutical sector and provide a misleading impression of drug spending."[247]

---

[244] Hernandez et al., "Changes in List Prices, Net Prices, and Discounts for Branded Drugs in the US, 2007–2018."

[245] *Ibid.*, 27.

[246] Jared S. Hopkins and Peter Loftus, "Flip the Script: Drugmakers Blame Middlemen for Price Increases," *The Wall Street Journal,* February 5, 2019, *https://www.wsj.com/ articles/ flip-the-script-drugmakers-blame-middlemen-for-price-hikes-11549364401.*

[247] Aaron Vandervelde and Eleanor Blalock, "The Pharmaceutical Supply Chain: Goss Drug Expenditures Realized by Stakeholders" (Berkeley Research Group, 2017),*https://www. thinkbrg.com/media/publication/863_Vandervelde_PhRMA-January-2017_WEB-FINAL.pdf.*

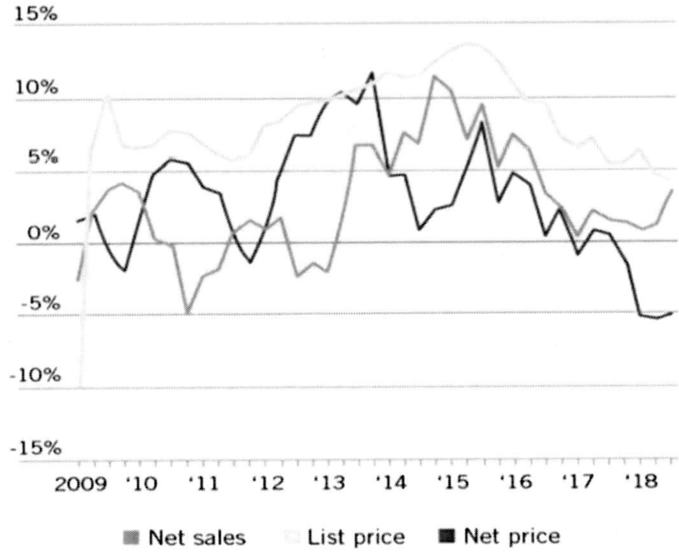

Figure 6. Change from a year earlier in U.S. prescription brand prices, 2009-2019.[248]

Fees charged by intermediaries also subtract from drug manufacturer revenues. PBMs nearly quadrupled the fees they charge biopharmaceutical companies—such as administrative and service fees—between 2014 and 2016. Total fees charged to biopharmaceutical companies by these middlemen increased from $1.5 billion in 2014 to $2.6 billion in 2015, and then doubled to nearly $5.6 billion in 2016. Along with rebates, these fees—which are typically based on the list price of a medicine— contribute to a system of misaligned incentives where middlemen make more money when the list prices of medicines increase.[249]

Despite an increase in the share of negotiated rebates shared with health plan and employer clients, total PBM revenue increased considerably between 2014 and 2016. That's in part due to the increasing administrative fees they charged biopharmaceutical companies. But PBMs aren't just charging biopharmaceutical companies more than ever before—they also brought in a record total of $22.4 billion in revenue in 2016 by charging more to others in the supply chain, such as health plans and pharmacies.[250]

---

[248] *Ibid*

[249] Robert Zirkelbach, "The PBM story you haven't heard: Hidden fees quad- rupled in two years," *The Catalyst,* March 20, 2019, *https://catalyst. phrma.org/the-pbm-story-you-havent-heard-hidden-fees-quadrupled-in-two- years.*

[250] Ibid.

For further input on the factors driving list price growth in medicines, please see the response to Senator Sasse's question on insulin pricing which follows subsequently.

On Public Funding and Innovation

Question. NIH and its grantees unquestionably conduct crucial foundational research. Through scores of strategic public-private partnerships, our current system enables research institutions and job creators of all sizes to translate and transform NIH-supported basic research into tangible biomedical breakthroughs, from diagnostic tests to treatments and cures.

That being said, proposals to replace private R&D-driven capital with taxpayer dollars raise serious concerns. Public and private research support should play complementary roles—not conflicting ones—and the Federal bureaucracy is no substitute for private-sector innovation and expertise.

According to one study, in fact, when it comes to life-sciences research resulting in a new medical innovation, the private sector invests as much as $100 in development for every $1 invested by the government. Along those lines, a survey of some of the most transformational medicines to reach the market in recent years found that whereas public funding played a critical role in achieving basic science milestones, private industry led the way for milestones related to drug discovery, production, and development, often by staggering margins.

Do you see public funding as an adequate substitute for any private-sector shortfalls that might result from government-mandated price controls?

Answer. The complementarity between the respective U.S. public and private sectors to biomedical innovation has been one of the great strengths of the U.S. approach to biomedical innovation. Public funding for basic life-sciences research, especially through the National Institutes of Health (NIH), funds basic discoveries such as into understanding the fundamental processes by which diseases develop and are transmitted or identifying novel biomarkers that signal the presence of a disease. This creates a body of knowledge which represents a platform for innovation by the private sector to try to turn novel molecules into safe drugs. Private-sector activity centers on applied R&D focused on the discovery, synthesis, testing, and manufacturing of candidate compounds intended to exploit biologic targets for the purpose of curing medical conditions. As Chakravarthy et al., note, "Without private investment in the applied sciences there would be no return on public investment in basic science."[251] Indeed, it's critical to remember that considerable investment is required to bring a drug to market even after considerable amounts of basic research have been conducted. In fact, one study by Chatterjee and Rohrbaugh found that biotechnology companies invest $100 in development for every $1 the government invests in research that leads to an innovation.[252]

Public funding would simply not be an adequate substitute for private-sector shortfalls that might result from government-mandated that price controls. That notion is as misguided as other proposals which would call for the government to take over the principal role of drug development from the private sector. Nevertheless, in their quest to shrink the for-profit drug discovery and development industry, drug populist advocates have floated a variety of such proposals, such as: having employers pay a medical research fee, which they would allocate to any research organization, including government; subjecting firms to compulsory licenses (where they must make patented discoveries available to other firms) but having the government pay patent holders directly to compensate them; having the government buy patents from firms through an auction; establishing government-funded corporations to develop and sell drugs; using prizes; and, finally, giving NIH the task.

For example, Dean Baker of the Center for Economic Policy Research writes, "We could expand the public funding going to NIH or other public institutions and extend their charge beyond basic research to include developing and testing drugs and medical equipment."[253] Knowledge Ecology International, a leading drug populist organization, has advocated eliminating drug patents and instead having the government issue prizes for drug development. It cites proposed legislation by Senator Bernie Sanders (I–VT) to create a Medical Innovation Prize Fund that would equal 0.55 percent of U.S. GDP, an amount greater than $80 billion per year, with the Federal

---

[251] Ranjana Chakravarthy et al., "Public- and Private-Sector Contributions to the Research and Development of the Most Transformational Drugs in the Past 25 Years: From Theory to Therapy," *Therapeutic Innovation and Regulatory Science,* Vol. 50, No. 6 (July 2016), *https://www.ncbi.nlm.nih.gov/pubmed/30231735.*

[252] Sabarni K. Chatterjee and Mark L. Rohrbaugh, "NIH Inventions Translate Into Drugs and Biologics With High Public Health Impact," *Nature Bio- technology* 32 (2014): 56, *https://www.nature.com/articles/nbt.2785?message- global=remove.*

[253] Dean Baker, "Malpractice" (Center for Economic Policy Research (CEPR), May/June 2009), *http://cepr.net/publications/op-eds-columns/malpractice.*

Government funding half and private health insurance companies the other half.[254]

But as the Information Technology and Innovation Foundation (ITIF) writes in "Delinkage Debunked: Why Replacing Patents With Prizes for Drug Development Won't Work," separating the cost of biopharmaceutical research and development from the final market price of medicines would misalign incentives, raise bureaucratic costs, and limit innovation.[255] Indeed, while advocates claim that "delinking" drug prices from R&D investments would make innovative medicines far cheaper, the truth is it would almost surely lead to less new drug development and slower progress in improving human health.

For instance, for prizes to work globally, governments would have to replace at least $200 billion per year in private medical R&D with taxpayer funds, which is unlikely given the budget challenges many governments face and the fact many of the benefits would flow to other countries.[256] Consider that as part of the World Health Organization's (WHO) push to increase investment in global health R&D, WHO member states in 2013 agreed to establish a Global Observatory on R&D to monitor spending and set priorities, and also to undertake a number of global health R&D demonstration projects. At the World Health Assembly in Geneva in May 2017, Marie-Paule Kieny, WHO assistant director-general for Health Systems and Innovation, remarked on the chronic underfunding of this "critically important' agenda, noting that one of the demonstration projects (on a nano-based malaria drug delivery system) is being canceled unfinished due to a lack of funding.[257]

According to the WHO, $85 million was needed between 2014 and 2017 to complete these projects, yet by the end of 2016, only $11 million had been committed by only 10 WHO member states, leaving a shortfall of $73 million.[258] WHO's website on the R&D demonstration projects has not had

---

[254] Mike Masnick, "Senator Sanders Introduces Medical Innovation Prize Bills," *TechDirt,* June 1, 2011, *https://www.techdirt.com/2011/06/01/senator-sand-ers-introduces-medical-innova tion-prize-bills/.*

[255] Philip Stevens and Stephen Ezell, "Delinkage Debunked: Why Replacing Pat- ents With Prizes for Drug Development Won't Work" (ITIF, February 2020), *https://itif.org/ publications/2020/02/03/delinkage-debunked-why-replacing-patents-prizes-drug-development-wont-work.*

[256] Matej Mikulic, "Total global spending on pharmaceutical research and devel- opment from 2010 to 2024," Statista, January 23, 2020, *https://www. statista.com/statistics/ 309466/global-r-and-d-expenditure-for-pharma- ceuticals/.*

[257] Catherine Saez, "Health R&D Still Underfunded—WHO Members Concerned, NGOs Call for More Ambition," *IP Watch,* May 29, 2017, *https://www.ip- watch.org/2017/05/2 9/health-rd-still-underfunded-members-concerned-ngos- call-ambition/.*

[258] Ibid.

any significant updates in several years.[259] A $73-million shortfall is one thing; a roughly $200-billion shortfall would be another. Put simply, if WHO members cannot agree among themselves to provide the relatively small amounts of funding for even this modest agenda, it seems highly unlikely they would stump up the hundreds of billions of dollars required to implement advocates' delinkage proposals.

Moreover, the true value of a new medicine is hard to measure before it is created, so prizes could be underfunded. That would lead to fewer companies taking the risk of investing in expensive R&D, and hence to fewer new medicines. Lastly, handing over significant control of national or global biomedical R&D flows to government bodies represent a recipe for inefficiency and for politicizing drug development. The current market-based system of drug development allows for experimentation and competition within and between therapeutic classes. Thousands of promising leads enter the drug development pathway, but only a few make it through the rigorous process of clinical trials. The cost of failures and the risks are borne almost entirely by the private sector at no cost to taxpayers. As Daniel Spulber, Professor of International Business at the Kellogg School of Management, North- western University, and an award-winning expert on innovation policy, concludes, "There is nothing wrong with awarding prizes. But replacing markets for medicines with government prizes would destroy one of the most innovative areas in the economy, and stop the endless source of life-saving medicines."[260]

On Public-Private Partnerships and Innovation

Question. You have written extensively on the importance of public-private partnerships in advancing and ensuring access to innovation, as enabled by the bipartisan Bayh-Dole Act. Some advocates and policymakers have proposed a radical re-interpretation of this framework, arguing that the Federal Government should "march in" to seize or forcibly license patents to cut costs.

---

[259] World Health Organization, "Identification of Health R&D Demonstration Projects," http://www.whogis.com/phi/implementation/phi_gtc_meeting/en/.

[260] Daniel Spulber, "Public Prizes Versus Market Prices: Should Contests Replace Patents?", Journal of the Patent and Trademark Office Society, Vol. 97, Issue 4 (2015): 690–735, https://www.scholars.northwestern.edu/en/publications/public-prizes-versus-market-prices-should-contests-replace-patent.

Both of the Bayh-Dole Act's sponsors spent decades emphatically opposing this revisionist rewriting of so-called march-in rights, which could prove particularly harmful for patients with unmet medical needs, as well as research institutions and small businesses across all of our States.

What was the original intent behind the march-in provisions in question, and how would this sweeping reinterpretation impact public-private partnerships and American innovation more broadly?

How does the current ecosystem benefit universities and nonprofit research institutions, and how might the aggressive use of march-in rights impact their financial standing, particularly with respect to royalty income?

Answer. The 1980 Bayh-Dole Act permits universities to patent their researchers' inventions, even if that research was partly funded by the Federal Government. The Act has played a pivotal role in catalyzing U.S. life-sciences innovation and creating a pathway to realize value creation from federally funded research.[261] Consider that at the end of the 1970s, the U.S. government had licensed fewer than 5 percent of its 28,000 patents, but the number of patents from government-funded research shot up over tenfold in the years since Bayh-Dole, reaching more than 40,000 in 2017.[262] And since its introduction, Bayh-Dole has enabled more than 15,000 startups launched from U.S. universities as well as 300 new medicines based on patented discoveries.[263]

The Bayh-Dole Act includes so-called "march-in rights" that permit the U.S. government, in very limited and specified circumstances, to require patent holders to grant a "nonexclusive, partially exclusive, or exclusive license" to a "responsible applicant or applicants."[264] The four circumstance in which the government is permitted to exercise march-in rights are:

1) If the contractor or assignee has not taken, or is not expected to take within a reasonable time, effective steps to achieve practical application of the subject invention;

---

[261] Stephen Ezell, "The Bayh-Dole Act's Vital Importance to the U.S. Life- Sciences Innovation System" (ITIF, March 2019), *https://itif.org/sites/de-fault/files/2019-bayh-dole-act.pdf.*

[262] Lou Berneman, "There are unintended costs of Federal efforts to control drug prices," PennLive, March 26, 2022, *https://www.pennlive.com/opinion/2022/ 03/there-are-unintended-costs-of-federal-efforts-to-control-drug-prices-opin- ion.html.*

[263] *Ibid.*; Association of University Technology Managers (AUTM), "Driving the Innovation Economy: Academic Technology Transfer in Numbers," *https:// autm.net/AUTM/media/ Surveys-Tools/Documents/FY20-Infographic.pdf.*

[264] John R. Thomas, "March-In Rights Under the Bayh-Dole Act" (Congressional Research Service, August 2016), 7, *https://fas.org/sgp/crs/misc/R44597.pdf.*

2) If action is necessary to alleviate health or safety needs not reasonably satisfied by the patent holder or its licensees;
3) If action is necessary to meet requirements for public use specified by Federal regulations and such requirements are not reasonably satisfied by the contractor, assignee, or licensees; or
4) If action is necessary, in exigent cases, because the patented product cannot be manufactured substantially in the United States.[265]

In other words, lower prices are not one of the rationales laid out in the Bayh- Dole Act as a valid justification for the use of march-in rights. In fact, as Senators Bayh and Dole have themselves noted, the Bayh-Dole Act's march-in rights were never intended to control or ensure "reasonable prices."[266] As the twain wrote in a 2002 Washington Post op-ed titled, "Our Law Helps Patients Get New Drugs Sooner," the Bayh-Dole Act:

> Did not intend that government set prices on resulting products. The law makes no reference to a reasonable price that should be dictated by the government. This omission was intentional; the primary purpose of the act was to entice the private sector to seek public-private research collaboration rather than focusing on its own proprietary research.[267]

The op-ed reiterated that the price of a product or service was not a legitimate basis for the government to use march-in rights, noting:

> The ability of the government to revoke a license granted under the act is not contingent on the pricing of a resulting product or tied to the profitability of a company that has commercialized a product that results in part from government-funded research. The law instructs the government to revoke such licenses only when the private industry collaborator has not successfully commercialized the invention as a product.[268]

---

[265] *Ibid.*, 10.

[266] Birch Bayh, "Statement of Birch Bayh to the National Institutes of Health," May 25, 2014, *http://www.essentialinventions.org/drug/nih05252004/ birchbayh.pdf.*

[267] Birch Bayh and Bob Dole, "Our Law Helps Patients Get New Drugs Sooner," *The Washington Post,* April 11, 2002, *https://www.washingtonpost.com/ar- chive/opinions/ 2002/04/11/our-law-helps-patients-get-new-drugs-sooner/d814d22a-6e63-4f06-8da3-d9698552fa24/?utm—term=.ddbf6876a380.*

[268] *Ibid.*

Rather, the Bayh-Dole Act's march-in provision was designed as a fail-safe for limited instances in which a licensee might not be making good-faith efforts to bring an invention to market, or when national emergencies require that more product is needed than a licensee is capable of producing. This is why the National Institute of Standards and Technology (NIST) report "Return on Investment Initiative: Draft Green Paper" agrees, noting, "The use of march-in is typically regarded as a last resort, and has never been exercised since the passage of the Bayh-Dole Act in 1980."[269] The report notes that, "NIH determined that that use of march-in to control drug prices was not within the scope and intent of the authority."[270] Indeed, march- in rights have never been exercised during the now-42-year history of the Bayh-Dole Act.[271]

The argument that Bayh-Dole march-in rights could be used to control drug prices was originally advanced in an article by Peter S. Arno and Michael H. Davis.[272] They contended that "[t]he requirement for 'practical application' seems clear to authorize the Federal Government to review the prices of drugs developed with public funding under Bayh-Dole terms and to mandate march-in when prices exceed a reasonable level" and suggested that under Bayh-Dole, the contractor may have the burden of showing that it charged a reasonable price.[273] While Arno and Davis admitted there was no clear legislative history on the meaning of the phrase "available to the public on reasonable terms," they still concluded that, "[t]here was never any doubt that this meant the control of profits, prices, and competitive conditions."[274]

But as John Rabitschek and Norman Latker explain, there are several problems with this analysis. First, the notion that "reasonable terms" of licensing means "reasonable prices" arose in unrelated testimony during the Bayh-Dole hearings. Most importantly, they note, "If Congress meant to add a reasonable pricing requirement, it would have explicitly set one forth in the

---

269 National Institute of Standards and Technology (NIST), "Return on Invest- ment Initiative: Draft Green Paper" (NIST, December 2018), 30, https:// nvlpubs.nist.gov/nistpubs/Special Publications/ NIST.SP.1234.pdf.

270 *Ibid, 30.*

271 Thomas, "March-In Rights Under the Bayh-Dole Act," 9.

272 Peter Arno and Michael Davis, "Why Don't We Enforce Existing Drug Price Controls? The Unrecognized and Unenforced Reasonable Pricing Require- ments Imposed upon Patents Deriving in Whole or in Part from Federally Funded Research," Tulane Law Review, Vol. 75, 631 (2001), https://engagedscholarship.csuohio.edu/cgi/ viewcontent.cgi?article =1754&context= fac_articles.

273 *Ibid.*

274 John H. Rabitschek and Norman J. Latker, "Reasonable Pricing—A New Twist for March-in Rights Under the Bayh-Dole Act," *Santa Clara High Tech- nology Law Journal,* Vol. 22, Issue 1 (2005), 162–163, *https:// digitalcommons.law.scu.edu/cgi/viewcontent. cgi?article=1399&context=chtlj.*

law, or at least described it in the accompanying reports."[275] As Rabitschek and Latker continue, "There was no discussion of the shift from the 'practical application' language in the Presidential Memoranda and benefits being reasonably available to the public, to benefits being available on reasonable terms under 35 U.S.C. § 203."[276] As they conclude, "The interpretation taken by Arno and Davis is inconsistent with the intent of Bayh-Dole, especially since the Act was intended to promote the utilization of federally funded inventions and to minimize the costs of administering the technology transfer policies. . . . [The Bayh-Dole Act] neither provides for, nor mentions, 'unreasonable prices.' "[277]

Simply put, the Bayh-Dole Act does not give the U.S. government the right to march in on the intellectual property (IP) of a company that has developed a product in whole or in part based on discoveries that may have originated in whole or in part from federally funded research simply because the government does not like the price of the resulting product. The reality is that (mis)using march-in rights or establishing new ones in order to control drug prices would result in fewer new drugs. Companies would be highly reticent to spend billions developing a drug if they knew the government could come in as long as 2 decades later and seize or compulsorily license their IP in order to control drug prices.

If the government began to use march-in rights on a regular basis to control drug prices, or the prices of other innovations, such as in the information technology (IT) or clean energy sectors, it would almost certainly have a deleterious impact on U.S. universities and their ability to earn royalties as a result of academic technology transfer activities. That matters when today many universities list technology commercialization as one of their top-five strategic priorities and university presidents often mention technology transfer as a key differentiator for their universities.[278] In 2018, U.S. universities directly generated approximately $2.94 billion in licensing revenue from the process of taking academic inventions to market. The Bayh-Dole Act has played a critical catalytic role in turning America universities into engines of innovation, a dynamic that would certainly be undermined if the government

---

[275] *Ibid,* 163.

[276] *Ibid.* Here, the Presidential Memoranda refers to memoranda produced by the Kennedy and Nixon administrations that pertained to government policy re- lated to contractor ownership of inventions.

[277] *Ibid.*

[278] Dr. Dipanjan "DJ" Nag, Antra Gupta, and Alex Turo, "The Evolution of University Technology Transfer: By the Numbers," *IPWatchdog,* April 7, 2020, *http://www .ipwatchdog.com/2020/04/07/evolution-university-technology- transfer/id=120451/.*

started to actively (mis)use Bayh-Dole march-in rights to attempt to control the prices of drugs or other products.

On Global Leadership and Competition

Question. The United States has emerged, in recent decades, as the global leader on life sciences innovation, with the world's most cutting-edge R&D, spearheaded largely by our research universities and by small businesses. Government price controls and top-down mandates, however, risk jeopardizing our position and enabling our global rivals—particularly China—to gain a competitive edge.

China, which represents the world's second-largest pharmaceutical market, has targeted its life sciences sector as a key area for strategic growth, singling the industry out in its Made in China 2025 initiative and undertaking aggressive reforms to shore up its status. With respect to active pharmaceutical ingredients, for instance, China has already established global dominance, and a range of recent reforms have substantially narrowed the country's lag-times for new drug approvals and launches.

Meanwhile, the drug price controls included in the Democrats' tax and spending package would slash domestic life sciences R&D by close to one-fifth in the years ahead, according to a University of Chicago study. In other words, as the Chinese Communist Party works to seize our global biopharmaceutical leadership, we seem poised to weaken our own sector through bureaucratic new mandates.

How do you see price controls like the ones proposed in BBBA as impacting our global life sciences leadership—particularly in relation to China—and what are some of the potential implications—both for medicine and for national security?

Answer. China rejects the foundational WTO principle of comparative advantage—that countries should specialize in production of goods and services at which they're most efficient—and instead seeks absolute advantage—dominance, or at least self-sufficiency, in virtually all advanced-technology industries, from aerospace and autos to batteries and biotechnology. That China can quickly achieve these goals is evident from looking at China's experience in rapidly coming to dominate the global market for production of solar photovoltaic cells. Indeed, China's global share of production of PV cells, the industry's core technology, surged from 14 to 60 percent between 2006 and 2013.[279] The massive industrial subsidies China's government conferred on the industry—at least $42 billion from 2010 to 2012 alone— played a key role in helping Chinese solar PV prices decrease by 85 percent from 2009 to 2017, knocking out hundreds of foreign competitors in the process. In other words, U.S. policymakers should be under no illusion that U.S. high-tech industries don't face serious threats of Chinese "innovation mercantilist" practices such as massive industrial subsidization and rampant IP theft.[280]

China certainly has ambitions to likewise become a leading, if not the leading, global player in life-sciences industries. In 2018, China's value added in the global pharmaceuticals industry was over $123 billion, 18.5 times its 1995 level and nearly equal to the contribution from the entire European Union.[281] In fact, from 2002 to 2018, China's share of the world total of global pharmaceutical industry value-added grew over four-fold, from 5.6 to 23 percent, while the United States' fell from 34 to 26 percent. (See Figure 7.) China has also become the world leader in its share of global research publications in the life-sciences, now accounting for over 70,000 annual biology and biomedicine scientific publications in 2020 and surpassing America's contribution.[282]

Meanwhile, China has become an indispensable player in the production of many active pharmaceutical ingredients (APIs). For instance, by volume, China's share of global exports of tetracycline/doxycycline reached 86 percent in 2020, and 63 percent for vitamin B1.[283] In fact, at least three WHO-identified essential medicines— capreomycin and streptomycin for treatment of Mycobacterium tuberculosis and sulfadiazine, used to treat chancroid and trachoma—rely on API manufacturers based solely in China.[284]

---

[279] David M. Hart, "The Impact of China's Production Surge on Innovation in the Global Solar Photovoltaics Industry" (ITIF, October 2020), *https://itif.org/ publications/2020/10/05/ impact-chinas-production-surge-innovation-global- solar-photovoltaics.*

[280] Sherisse Pham and Matt Rivers, "China Is Crushing the U.S. in Renewable Energy," CNN Tech, July 18, 2017, *http://money.cnn.com/2017/07/18/tech- nology/china-us-clean-energy-solar-farm/index.html;* Hart, "The Impact of China's Production Surge on Innovation in the Global Solar Photovoltaics Industry."

[281] Stephen Ezell, "Ensuring U.S. Biopharmaceutical Competitiveness" (ITIF, July 2020), https://itif.org/publications/2020/07/16/ensuring-us-biopharma-ceutical-competitiveness.

[282] National Science Foundation, "Science and Engineering Indicators: 2020," "Publications Output: U.S. Trends and International Comparisons," https://ncses.nsf.gov/pubs/ nsb20214/data.

[283] Anna Nishino, "The great medicines migration," Nikkei Asia, April 5, 2022, https://asia.nikkei.com/static/vdata/infographics/chinavaccine-3/.

[284] "Safeguarding Pharmaceutical Supply Chains in a Global Economy," before the U.S. House Committee on Energy and Commerce, Subcommittee on Health, 116th Congress

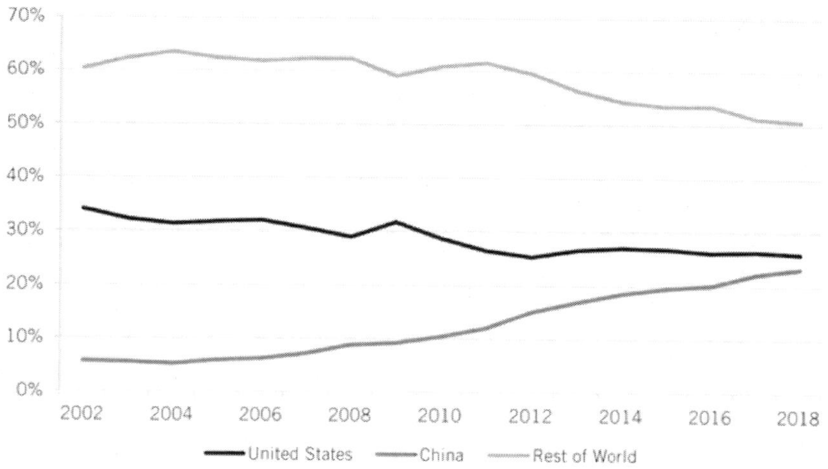

Figure 7. Country shares of value added in the global pharmaceutical industry, 2002-2018.[285]

But it's not just APIs; China is increasingly trying to compete at the frontiers of biomedical innovation. For instance, as of mid-2018, 25 Chinese companies had applied for approvals for advanced anticancer drugs based on biotechnology (PD–1/PD– L1 inhibitors).[286] Moreover, in 2017, China had 139 clinical trials with chimeric antigen receptor treatment (CAR–T) cell therapy, compared with around 118 in the United States.[287] Of just over 400 CAR–T clinical trials conducted in March of 2019, 166 were in China, and 165 in the United States.[288]

(October 30, 2019) (statement of Janet Woodcock, Director of FDA Center for Drug Evaluation and Research), https://www. fda.gov/news-events/congressional-testimony/ safeguarding-pharmaceutical- supply-chains-global-economy-10302019.

[285] National Science Foundation, "Science and Engineering Indicators: 2020," Appendix table S6–6 (accessed June 11, 2020), *https://ncses.nsf.gov/pubs/ nsb20205/data.*

[286] Jin Zhang, "The PD–1/PD–L1 Race in China," PharmExec.com, June 1, 2018, http://www. pharmexec.com/pd-1pd-l1-race-china.

[287] Fangning Zhang and Josie Zhou, "What's next for pharmainnovation in China?", McKinsey and Company Pharmaceuticals and Medical Products, September 2017, 2, *https://www.mckinsey.com/industries/pharmaceuticals-and-medical-products/our-insights/whats-next-for-pharma-innovation-in-china.* With CAR–T treatment, cell-killing T-cells are removed from the body and en- gineered to recognize the relevant cancer target. After the edited T-cells (CAR–Ts) are reintroduced to the patient, they multiply and attack the target cancer cells.

[288] Eric Ng, "Why China is going all out to invent new, stronger, cheaper drugs . . . it's not all about challenging the West," *South China Morning Post,* Octo- ber 2018, *https://www.scmp.com/news/china/society/article/2166462/why-china-going-all-out-invent-new-stronger-cheaper-drugs-its-not.*

Foreign IP theft has been a critical component of China's efforts to catch up in the global biotechnology race. Chinese actors have hacked into the IT systems of numerous U.S. biopharmaceutical companies, including Abbott Laboratories and Wyeth (now part of Pfizer).[289] Similarly, a report to the U.S. China Economic and Security Review Commission notes that Ventria Bioscience, GlaxoSmithKline, Dow AgroSciences LLC, Cargill Inc., Roche Diagnostics, and Amgen have all experienced theft of trade secrets or biological materials perpetrated by current or former employees with the intent to sell to a Chinese competitor. And in the academic sector, researchers have stolen information or samples from their employers at Cornell University, Harvard University, and University of California at Davis.[290] China has also issued compulsory licenses for the IP of particular drugs.[291]

In summary, China poses an increasingly serious threat to U.S. innovation leadership in the life sciences, both from policies that are legitimate (i.e., investing more in R&D or producing more scientific research and researchers) and those that are mercantilist (i.e., pilfering foreign IP or introducing pharmaceutical data exclusivity rules that favor companies that first launch in China).[292] To the extent price controls impede U.S. innovators' abilities to earn revenues to reinvest in future generations of biomedical innovation (as demonstrated here) then the BBBA (like other drug price control proposals) would endanger U.S. biomedical innovation leadership and open the door to foreign competitors.

---

[289] Zack Whittaker, "Justice Department Accuses Chinese Spies of Hacking into Dozens of US Tech and Industry Giants," TechCrunch, January 2019, https:// techcrunch.com/2018/12/20/us-indictment-tech-hacks-chinese/; Derek Lowe, "Chinese Pharma Espionage?", Science Translational Medicine, December 15, 2011, https://blogs.sciencemag.org/pipeline/archives/2011/12/15/Chinese_ pharma_espionage.

[290] Gryphon Scientific and Rhodium Group, "China's Biotechnology Development: The Role of US and Other Foreign Engagement" (report prepared for the U.S.- China Economic and Security Review Commission, February 2019), 104, *https://www.uscc.gov/Research/china%E2%80%99s-biotechnology-develop-ment-role-us-and-other-foreign-engagement.*

[291] Daniel C.K. Chow, "Three Major Problems Threatening Multi-National Phar- maceutical Companies Doing Business in China" (working paper, Ohio State Public Law and Legal Theory, 2017), *https://papers.ssrn.com/sol3/papers.cfm?abstract_id=3029347.*

[292] Robert D. Atkinson, "China's Biopharmaceutical Strategy: Challenge or Complement to U.S. Industry Competitiveness?" (ITIF, August 2019), *https:// itif.org/publications/2019/08/12/chinas-biopharmaceutical-strategy-challenge-or-complement-us-industry.*

Questions Submitted by Hon. Ben Sasse

Question. While we need to rein in the cost of pharmaceuticals, we also need to consider access to and creation of new therapeutics that can be potentially lifesaving. Multiple sclerosis is a good example of a disease that has benefitted from follow-on innovations. In 2020, the FDA approved Novartis' Kesimpta as a treatment for MS. This drug was originally approved 11 years earlier for the treatment of a rare form of leukemia, making this a follow-on product. It is common to find new indications for existing drugs, and we want to incentivize research and development and the multiple clinical trials that make this possible.

How would some of the lesser discussed policies in Build Back Better actually create disincentives to finding new indications for existing drugs? For example, wouldn't the bill make tax changes that disincentivize finding new indications for orphan drugs?

Can you speak to how costly the clinical trial process is, and how this might drive up prices? For example, testing a new indication for Kesimpta took 10 years and spanned 350 sites across 37 countries. This was for a drug that already existed and was approved for another use.

How might we reform this process to decrease costs?

Multiple sclerosis unfortunately lacks a cure. How would the price controls being suggested by Democrats hurt efforts to find a cure for MS?

Answer. As noted in ITIF's written testimony, a wide variety of academic studies, over time and across nations and international organizations, find that drug price controls impede biomedical innovation. Indeed, virtually all academic studies consistently reveal that a reduction in current drug revenues leads to a decrease in future research and the number of new drug discoveries.[293] The Build Back Better Act's drug price control policies would introduce the same effect.

Research in 2021 by Tomas Philipson and Troy Durie at the University of Chicago estimate that a 1-percent reduction in pharmaceutical industry revenue leads on average to a 1.54-percent decrease in R&D investment.[294] Applying their research to H.R. 5376 (the Build Back Better Act), Philipson and Durie find the legislation would reduce revenues by 12.0 percent through

---

[293] Joe Kennedy, "The Link Between Drug Prices and Research on the Next Generation of Cures" (ITIF, September 2019), *https://itif.org/publications/2019/ 09/09/link-between-drug-prices-and-research-next-generation-cures.*

[294] Philipson and Durie, "Issue Brief: The Impact of HR 5376 on Biopharmaceutical Innovation and Patient Health," 3.

2039, with the reduced revenues meaning R&D spending would fall by about 18.5 percent, or $663 billion. They find that this cut in R&D activity would lead to 135 fewer new drugs, with this drop in new drugs is predicted to generate a loss of 331.5 million life years in the United States.[295] The authors further find that therapies that treat diseases of the endocrine, cardiovascular, and respiratory systems along with treatments for cancer and neurological diseases would be most impacted by the BBBA's policies because they make up a high share of Medicare spending.[296]

Just as in other areas of life-sciences innovation, U.S. companies lead the way in innovating solutions for rare, or orphan, diseases. That's in large part because, in 1983, Congress introduced the Orphan Drug Act (ODA) and its Orphan Drug Tax Credit (ODTC), a Federal tax credit available to pharmaceutical companies working to find cures for certain rare diseases that affect patient populations of fewer than 200,000 individuals.[297] There are approximately 7,000 rare diseases, the majority of which are genetic in nature and which affect between 25 and 30 million Americans, although approximately 95 percent have no effective treatment.[298] To incent R&D of drugs for such diseases, Congress set the ODTC equal to 50 percent of qualified clinical trial costs (and also offered a seven-year period of orphan drug exclusivity). Since the law's enactment, over 500 orphan products have been approved by the U.S. FDA, whereas prior to the law's introduction fewer than 40 drugs were approved in the United States to treat rare diseases and on average only two new orphan drugs were produced each year.[299] A 2015 study by the National Organization for Rare Disorders (NORD) found that at least one-third fewer new orphan drugs would have been developed to treat rare diseases over the preceding 30 years had the act not been implemented.[300] Indeed the ODA has been widely regarded as a success, as over 600 orphan

---

295 *Ibid.*

296 Holtz-Eakin, "Testimony on: The Build Back Better Act's Prescription Drug Policies and Their Potential Impacts," 8.

297 Ray Esquivel and Rich Croghan, "How Pharmaceutical Companies Can Claim the Orphan Drug Tax Credit," Moss Adams, October 18, 2019, *https:// www.mossadams.com/ articles/2019/october/orphan-drug-pharmaceutical- credit.*

298 National Organization for Rare Disorders, "Rare Disease Day: Frequently Asked Questions," *https://rarediseases.org/wp-content/uploads/2019/01/ RDD-FAQ-2019.pdf.*

299 Jennifer Huron, "Impact of the Orphan Drug Tax Credit on Treatments for Rare Diseases" (National Organization for Rare Disorders, June 17, 2015), *https://rarediseases.org/ odtcwhitepaper/.*

300 Ibid.

drugs have been approved since the passage of the ODA, in contrast to fewer than 10 medicines for rare diseases in the decade prior to its enactment.[301]

Unfortunately, provisions in the BBBA would likely be deleterious for rare disease innovation. As Peter Saltonstall, CEO and president of The National Organization for Rare Disorders (NORD), elaborates:

> Section 138141 of the Build Back Better Act would dramatically curtail the Orphan Drug Tax Credit for qualified clinical testing expenses by removing this critical incentive for all but the first approved orphan use of a new drug. The ODTC was already diminished in 2017 in the Tax Cuts and Jobs Act when Congress reduced the total amount of the tax credit for qualifying clinical testing expenses from 50 percent to 25 percent. Given the significant time it takes to conduct clinical trials, the full impact of the changes made by the 2017 law are still unknown. To further reduce availability of the tax credit will hurt rare disease patients and hinder their ability to access treatments found to be safe and effective to treat their specific condition.[302]

The question about multiple sclerosis, and the one which follows regarding insulin prices, should focus policymakers' attention on the increasingly distortive roles that PBMs and other actors in the pharmaceutical supply chain are causing for U.S. drug prices. As ITIF noted in its written testimony, over time, drug manufacturers have lost a growing share of drug expenditures to other members of the drug supply chain, such as PBMs, health plans, hospitals, the government, and pharmacies. Since 2013, the share of drug expenditures going to manufacturers has decreased by 13 percent. Thus, while total expenditures on brand drugs grew by $268 billion between 2013 and 2020, only 31 percent of the increase accrued to manufacturers, while 69 percent accrued to other stakeholders. By 2020—for the first time ever— over half of drug expenditures accrued to non-manufacturers. (See Figure 8.)

That matters, because when patients go to the pharmacy, they're likely buying their medications from one of three pharmacy benefit managers—middlemen insurance companies that determine the final out-of-pocket cost for our medicines. In fact, just three PBMs—Caremark, Express Scripts, and

---

[301] U.S. FDA, "Developing Products for Rare Diseases & Conditions," http:// www.fda.gov/ ForIndustry/DevelopingProductsforRareDiseasesConditions/default.htm.

[302] Rohan Narayanan, "NORD Response to New Draft of the Build Back Better Act," press release, National Organization for Rare Disorders, October 29, 2021, *https://rarediseases.org/nord-response-to-new-draft-of-the-build-back- better-act/.*

OptumRx—control 76 percent of all prescription drug formularies in the United States.[303]

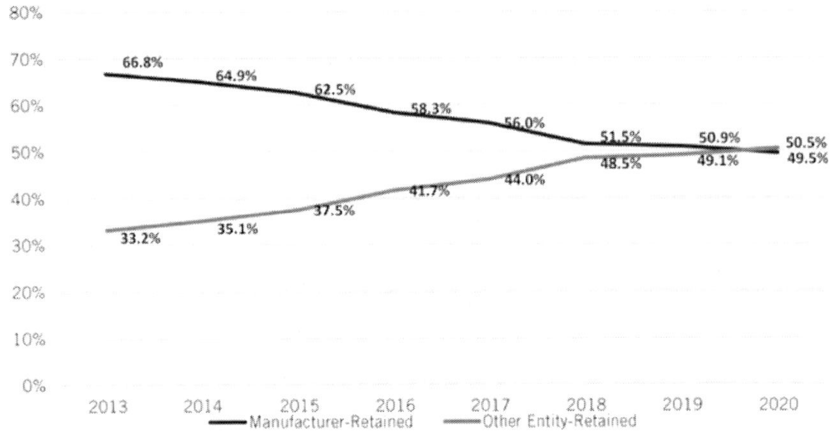

Figure 8. Total gross expenditures for brand medicines received by manufacturers and other stakeholders (2013-2020).[304]

Incidentally, this is actually a marketplace where there is significant concentration, unlike the pharmaceutical industry, as has been asserted by Congress members such as Senator Elizabeth Warren and Representative Katie Porter, the latter who cites data asserting that "between 1995 and 2015, 60 pharmaceutical companies merged into just 10."[305] But rather, the reality is that considering the combined output for firms in the United States (not imports), the sales for the top four in each industry (C4 ratio) in the Pharmaceutical Preparation Manufacturing and Biological Product Manufacturing industries (NAICS codes 325412 and 325414) increased only modestly from 2002 to 2017, from 36 percent to 43 percent, while the C8 ratio increased from 54 to 58 percent, and the C20 ratio fell slightly from 77 percent

[303] Alia Paavola, "Top PBMs by market share," *Becker Hospital Review,* May 30, 2019, *https://www.beckershospitalreview.com/pharmacy/top-pbms-by-market- share.html.*

[304] Andrew Brownlee and Joran Watson, "The Pharmaceutical Supply Chain, 2013–2020" (Berkeley Research Group, 2022), 3, *https://www.thinkbrg.com/ insights/publications/ pharmaceutical-supply-chain-2013-2020/.*

[305] Office of Congresswoman Katie Porter, "Killer Profits"; "High Drug Prices and Monopoly," *Open Markets Institute,* accessed May 10, 2021, *https://www. openmarket sinstitute.org/learn/drug-prices-monopoly.*

to 76 percent.[306] In other words, the top 20 firms in this sector have the same market share as the three leading PBMs.

Unfortunately, the PBM system has been designed in a way that is the opposite of what was originally intended: PBMs helping to lower drug costs at the pharmacy counter. Consider the case of Tecfidera (dimethyl fumarate), a blockbuster multiple sclerosis treatment manufactured by Biogen which went generic in late 2020. Within months of Tecfidera going off-patent, more than ten generic drug makers brought competing versions of dimethyl fumarate to market with "deeply discounted prices to Tecfidera."[307] Roughly one year post-generic launch, aggressive competition from generics manufacturers drove prices for a 60-count bottle of the generic equivalent today down to "a 99 percent+ discount to the brand's list price."[308] However, by Q3 2021, Medicare Part D plans covering the majority of U.S. seniors didn't even make the generic equivalent available to their members, instead only offering them brandname Tecfidera.[309] Moreover, when the generic was made available to seniors, it was largely done so at "negotiated prices" that far exceeded the lowest cost generic equivalent's.[310]

In other words, here's a case where America's life-sciences innovation system worked to support creation of an innovative drug and then a subsequent pathway for entry of much-lower-priced generic drugs, but it was the middleman system that prevented the cheaper drugs from being made available to seniors. Policymakers need to take a much closer look at the role of PBMs in America's drug payment system. That's why ITIF supports proposals calling for the imposition of greater fiduciary obligations on the activities of PBMs. ITIF also supports other proposals to increase drug price transparency, including removal of pharmacy gag clauses and requiring plan

---

306 Robert D. Atkinson and Stephen Ezell, "Five Fatal Flaws in Rep. Katie Por- ter's Indictment of the U.S. Drug Industry" (ITIF, May 20, 2021), *https:// itif.org/publications/ 2021/05/20/five-fatal-flaws-rep-katie-porters-indictment- us-drug-industry*. Source: United States Census Bureau, 2002 Economic Cen- sus Tables (accessed May 11, 2021), *https://www.census.gov/data/tables/2002/econ/census/manufacturing-reports.html;* United States Census Bureau, 2017 Economic Census Tables (accessed May 11, 2021), *https://www. census.gov/data/tables/2017/ econ/economic-census/naics-sector-31-33.html.*

307 Antonio Ciaccia, "New drug pricing report showcases highs, lows, distorted in- centives, and brokenness of Medicare Part D," 46Brooklyn, December 1, 2021, *https://www.46brooklyn.com/news/2021/12/1/wreckfidera-now-streaming.*

308 *Ibid.*

309 *Ibid.*

310 *Ibid.*

sponsors to provide patients information about drug price increases and lower-cost options.[311]

The high and increasing cost of drug R&D does affect the cost of drugs. Accordingly, one of the most important ways to better manage drug prices would be to enhance R&D efficiency in drug research, in other words, to find collaborative ways to work together to make the cost of innovating new drugs less expensive.[312] Most expensive for companies are candidate drugs that reach Phase III clinical trials and then fail; better success at weeding out those types of drugs earlier in the R&D process would make the entire drug discovery process more efficient and less expensive. One important step in this regard has actually been the PDUFA. By putting in place mechanisms that allow drug developers to have frank conversations with regulators about the technical and scientific expectations for a drug to clear certain clinical trial hurdles, it has streamlined the drug-review process to some degree and helped drug developers make better decisions about the likelihood of candidate drugs passing the clinical-trial gauntlet. Congress's 2017 reauthorization of PDUFA (PDUFA VI) also placed greater focus on supporting rare diseases and breakthrough therapies, including continued application-fee waivers and advanced reviews for medicines that can treat rare diseases, as well as prioritizing the development of breakthrough medicines for patients with life-threatening diseases. In addition, Federal support for joint industry-university research efforts on biopharma R&D efficiency and effectiveness should be expanded. For example, see MIT's NEW Drug Development ParadIGmS (NEWDIGS) program, which is "a unique collaborative 'think and do' tank focused on enhancing the capacity of the global biomedical innovation system to reliably and sustainably deliver new, better, affordable therapeutics to the right patients faster."[313]

In addition to innovative ways to enhance drug R&D efficiency, policymakers can also work to enhance drug production efficiency. For instance, One study contends that pharmaceutical manufacturing is expensive, inefficient, and non-innovative, with firms using outdated production

---

[311] Sood, et al., "Do companies in the pharmaceutical supply chain earn excess returns?", 111.

[312] Stephen Ezell, "Testimony Before the House Oversight Committee on Drug Prices, Intellectual Property, and Biomedical Innovation" (ITIF, May 2019), 14, *https://itif.org/publications/2019/05/16/testimony-house-oversight-committee-drug-prices-intellectual-property-and.*

[313] Massachusetts Institute of Technology (MIT) Center for Biomedical Innova- tion, "Welcome to MIT NEWDIGS," *https://newdigs.mit.edu/.*

techniques and old plants.[314] The study estimates modern biomanufacturing techniques could eliminate as much as $50 billion in annual production costs.

To address this, Congress should significantly expand funding for biomedical Manufacturing USA centers, including expanding funding for The National Institute for Innovation in Manufacturing Biopharmaceuticals (NIIMBL) as well as establishing other centers addressing related manufacturing technology challenges. In addition, Federal funding should be ongoing and not sunset. No other nation with similar industry-university-government precompetitive research centers sunsets funding for successful centers.

In addition, Congress should fund NSF to expand support to university-industry research centers working on biopharma production technology and potentially establish new centers. For example, the Novartis-MIT Center for Continuous Manufa turing is a partnership launched to develop continuous production technology.[315] At the same time, Congress should increase funding for NSF's Division of Engineering and target much of the increase to the Chemical Process Systems Cluster and Engineering Biology and Health Cluster.[316] Unfortunately, between 2018 and 2019, Congress increased the engineering division's budget by just 1 percent, compared with the overall NSF budget by 3 percent.

In addition, the administration should encourage the creation of the biopharma equivalent of the Semiconductor Research Corporation, a public-private consortium that, among other things, works on a long-term semiconductor technology road map. Industry should collaborate on such a production technology innovation road map, and the Federal Government should match their funding to research institutes and universities on a dollar-for-dollar basis. For example, some firms have their ownroad maps (e.g., GlaxoSmithKline's manufacturing technology road map, is focused on the use of continuous techniques).[317]

---

[314] W. Nicholson Price II, "Making Do in Making Drugs: Innovation Policy and Pharmaceutical Manufacturing," *Boston College Law Review,* Vol. 55, Issue 2 (2014): 492, *https://lawdigitalcommons.bc.edu/bclr/vol55/iss2/5/.*

[315] Rick Mullin, "Off the drawing board," Chemical and Engineering News, April 28, 2019, https://cen.acs.org/pharmaceuticals/Off-drawing-board/97/i17.

[316] National Science Foundation, "Programs: Directorate for Engineering (ENG)," https://www.nsf.gov/funding/programs.jsp?org=ENG.

[317] Mullin, "Off the drawing board."

Questions Submitted by Hon. John Barrasso

Question. As a doctor, I have seen firsthand the value innovative medicines provide to folks across Wyoming. When we make policy here in Washington, it is critical we preserve the incentives for cutting-edge therapies to come to market so folks can live longer and healthier lives.

That being said, I have concerns about the high list prices—particularly for long- established drugs. Insulin is one example. This is a life-saving drug that has been part of medical practice for decades.

Though negotiated discounts and rebates can reduce the net price for drugs like insulin, some patients' copays continue to climb as list prices tick higher.

What are the best solutions to lower the price patients pay at the pharmacy counter for insulin?

Answer. First, it's important to recognize that most Americans are able to assess their insulin at affordable prices. In fact, 76 percent of U.S. insulin prescriptions cost patients less than $35 out of pocket.[318] In fact, across all patients, the average out-of-pocket cost per month for an insulin prescription was $31 in 2019. Companies also offer affordable subscription plans for diabetic patients, such as Novo Nordisk's My$99Insulin plan, whereby eligible patients pay $99 for a monthly supply of any combination of Novo Nordisk insulin products.[319]

However, there are certainly cases where patients are paying too much for insulin. Indeed, while just 24 percent of insulin prescriptions cost patients more than $35 out of pocket, these prescriptions account for 82 percent of total patient spending on insulin.[320] For this reason, as noted in its testimony, ITIF supports capping monthly patient out-of-pocket costs for drugs treating certain chronic diseases, such as a $35 monthly cap for insulin for the treatment of diabetes.[321]

However, the more fundamental issue, for insulin or many other drugs, is that the rebates insurers and PBMs negotiate for Medicare Part D drugs need

---

[318] PhRMA, "Prescription Medicines: Insulin Costs in Context" (PhRMA, January 21, 2021), 10, *https://phrma.org/resource-center/Topics/Cost-and-Value/Prescription-Medicines-Insulin-Costs-in-Context.* Citing: IQVIA, "Medicine Spending and Affordability in the United States" (IQVIA, August 2020), *https:// www.iqvia.com/insights/the-iqvia-institute/reports/medicine-spending-and-af- fordability-in-the-us.*

[319] Novo Nordisk, "My$99Insulin," *https://www.novocare.com/insulin/my99insu lin.html.*

[320] PhRMA, "Prescription Medicines: Insulin Costs in Context," 10.

[321] Stephen Ezell, "Testimony to the Senate Finance Committee on 'Prescription Drug Price Inflation"' (ITIF, March 2022), *https://itif.org/publications/2022/ 03/16/testimony-senate-finance-committee-prescription-drug-price-inflation.*

to be passed through to seniors at the pharmacy counter. The rebates (averaging nearly 30 percent for Medicare Part D drugs) are usually paid to PBMs in consideration of preferred placement on the insurance plan's formulary, but the PBMs tend not to share the rebates directly with beneficiaries. Changing this rule change could save older Americans as much as $83 billion at the pharmacy counter over the span of 10 years.[322]

Indeed, until the rebate system is fundamentally reformed, list prices are going to continue to increase at rates well above the actual cost of drugs, with insulin a prime example. For instance, a bipartisan report by the Senate Finance Committee found that some PBMs have secured rebates on insulin as high as 70 percent in recent years.[323] In fact, in 2019, PBMs paid $52 for an insulin product that had a list price of more than $350.[324] Manufacturers often sell insulin, an essential medicine, to insurers and PBMs at deep discounts. However, many patients are forced to make out-of-pocket payments based on insulin's irrelevant list price.[325] For instance, one study found that list prices for Sanofi's insulins have grown by 140 percent over the past 8 years, while net prices have declined by 41 percent.[326] Similarly, over the past 5 years, the list price of Eli Lilly's Humalog insulin increased by 27 percent, while its net price declined by 10 percent.[327] But as Adam Fein notes, [formulary plan] "benefit designs often mask these declining net prices." As Fein notes, "Payers' drug costs and manufacturers' revenues have been dropping for the past 4 years. Despite this decline, patients' out-of-pocket costs have been rising."[328] As Fein concludes, "Third-party payers' benefit designs remain a significant barrier to addressing drug costs. Many continue to use the ever-

---

[322] Blake Pelzer and Paul Spitalnic, "Proposed Safe Harbor Regulation," Center for Medicare and Medicaid Services: Office of the Actuary (August 2018), *https://aspe.hhs.gov/sites/default/files/private/pdf/260591/OACTProposed SafeHarborRegulationImpacts.pdf.*

[323] Charles E. Grassley and Ron Wyden, "Insulin: Examining the Factors Driving the Rising Cost of a Century Old Drug" (United States Senate Finance Com- mittee, January 2021), *https://www.finance.senate.gov/imo/media/doc/Grassley-Wyden%20Insulin%20Report %20(FINAL%201).pdf.*

[324] Adam J. Fein, "Five Top Drugmakers Reveal List vs. Net Price Gaps (Plus: The Trouble With Insulin Prices)," *Drug Channels,* August 11, 2020, *https:// www.drugchannels.net/2020/08/five-top-drugmakers-reveal-list-vs-net.html.*

[325] *Ibid.*

[326] *Ibid.*

[327] *Ibid.*

[328] Adam J. Fein, "Drug Channels News Roundup, July 2020: Diabetes Costs, Regeneron's Copay Support, MA Rethinks Coupons, My Favorite Chart Updated, and ABC's Steve Collis," *Drug Channels,* July 29, 2020, *https:// www.drugchannels.net/2020/07/drug-channels-news-roundup-july-2020.html.*

growing rebate dollars of the gross-to-net bubble to offset overall plan costs rather than reducing patient's out-of-pocket spending."[329]

As the Biotechnology Innovation Organization (BIO) writes:

> The vertical consolidation of pharmacy services paired with relatively few co petitors in the space has led to some markets which exhibit monopsonist characteristics—the PBMs can represent the sole purchaser of prescription drugs for a majority of covered lives, employer plans or fully insured commercial products may have few (or no) alternatives to the dominate PBM(s) in their market if they wanted toseek out another entity to manage their pharmacy benefit, and the complexity of the pharmaceutical supply chain and scale that existing PBMs can leverage represent significant barriers for new entrants.[330]

A recent study analyzed the hypothetical distribution of $100 of spending on 32 insulin products across manufacturers, insurers, and other supply chain entities from 2014 to 2018. The authors found that while expenditures per 100 units of insulin changed little over this time, the distribution of spending changed significantly. Over this period, the share of spending retained by insulin manufacturers and health plans fell (by 33 percent and 24.7 percent, respectively), while the amounts retained by supply chain intermediaries increased substantially: wholesalers (74.7 percent), pharmacies (228.8 percent), and PBMs (154.6 percent).[331] (See Figure 9.)

Indeed, America's current drug reimbursement system can lead health plans and PBMs to favor medicines with high list prices and large rebates, making them reluctant to include lower-cost insulin and authorized generics on formularies. In fact, one study found that just one in four Medicare Part D beneficiaries, and one in five patients with commercial insurance, have access to lower-price authorized generic insulin through insurance.[332] That study finds that sharing negotiated rebates would lower Medicare Part D costs for patients, estimating that for a prototypical Medicare Part D patient with diabetes taking five medicines overall (including insulin), passing through those rebates would reduce their out-of-pocket spending by nearly $900 annually, while only increasing premiums $3 to $6 per month.[333]

---

[329] *Ibid.*

[330] BIO, "Response to Federal Trade Commission: Request for Information on Merger Enforcement," 14.

[331] *Ibid*

[332] PhRMA, "Prescription Medicines: Insulin Costs in Context," 12.

[333] *Ibid.*, 15.

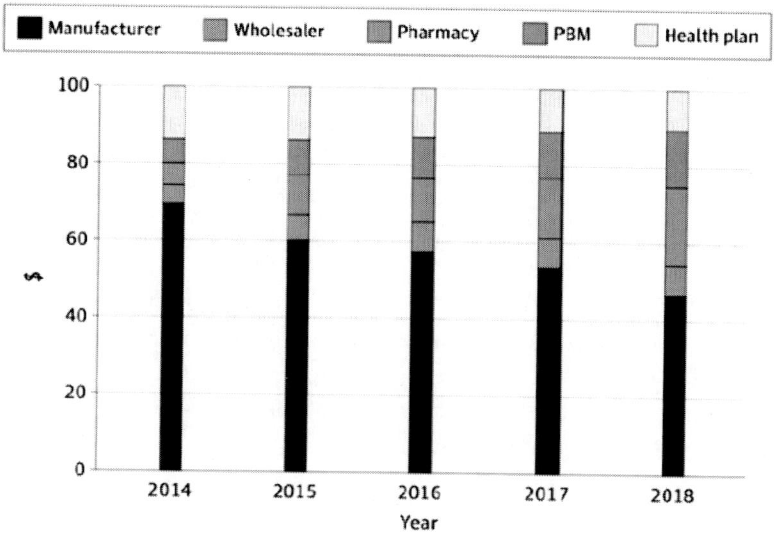

Figure 9. Average distribution of $100 in insulin expenditures for 32 insulin profucs across distrinution system participants, 2014-2018.[334]

Question. Before coming to the Senate, I practiced orthopedic surgery of over 20 years. During my surgical training, I got to know many patients with Duchenne muscular dystrophy. These young boys and their families made a lasting and personal impact on me. The sad fact was when I practiced medicine, there were no approved treatments for Duchenne's. This is why I helped host the Jerry Lewis telethon in Wyoming for many years.

In fact, the first FDA approved treatment for Duchenne's did not become available until well after I joined the Senate in 2016. For families impacted by Duchenne's, this first approval was a beacon of hope. Now, thanks to American scientific innovation, there are multiple FDA approved therapies for Duchenne's. We have not cured this disease, but we are making important progress.

As a doctor, I am passionate about ensuring the progress continues. According to the Food and Drug Administration, there are over 7,000 rare diseases that impact over 30 million Americans. While we all want to lower

[334] Karen Van Nuys et al., "Estimation of the Share of Net Expenditures on Insulin Captured by US Manufacturers, Wholesalers, Pharmacy Benefit Managers, Pharmacies, and Health Plans from 2014 to 2018," *Journal of the American Medical Association Health,* Vol. 2, Issue 11 (November 2021), *https://jamanetwork.com/journals/jama-health-forum/fullarticle/2785932.*

the price of prescription drugs, we must ensure patients can access the next generation of life-changing medications.

Can you please discuss the importance of maintaining investments in scientific research, especially with regard to supporting investments in therapies that address conditions that impact smaller patient populations?

Answer. As noted, the United States leads the world in biomedical innovation. In fact, over the past 20 years, more than 60 percent of all new drugs worldwide have been created in the United States—more than in the rest of the world combined.[335] That's in no small part because the United States has clearly been the world's largest global funder of biomedical R&D investment over the past 2 decades, a share that some analyses suggested reached as high as 70 to 80 percent over that time period.[336] Indeed, there's a direct link between the United States being the world's leading investor in biomedical R&D and the world's leading producer of innovative drugs.

And, again, it's important to remember that this wasn't always the case. Indeed, the United States once was a global "also-ran" in biomedical innovation: Europe was once the world's pharmaceuticals industry leader. Between 1960 and 1965, European-headquartered companies invented 65 percent of the world's new drugs, and in the latter half of the 1970s, European-headquartered enterprises introduced more than twice as many new drugs to the world as did U.S.-headquartered enterprises (149 to 66).[337] In fact, throughout the 1980s, fewer than 10 percent of new drugs were introduced first in the United States.[338] (See Figure 10.)

---

[335] Association of University Technology Managers (AUTM), "AUTM 2018 Licensing Survey" (AUTM, 2018), 3, *https://autm.net/AUTM/media/SurveyReports PDF/ AUTM_ FY2018_US_Licensing_Survey.pdf;* AUTM and the Biotechnology Innovation Organization: "The Economic Contribution of University/Nonprofit Inventions in the United States: 1996–2017" (AUTM and BIO, June 2019), *https://autm.net/AUTM/ media/About-Tech-Transfer/Documents/Economic_ Contribution_Report _BIO_AUTM_JUN2019_web.pdf.*

[336] Justin Chakma et al., "Asia's Ascent—Global Trends in Biomedical R&D Ex- penditures," *New England Journal of Medicine,* 370, No. 1 (January 2014); ER Dorsey et al., "Funding of US Biomedical Research, 2003–2008," *New England Journal of Medicine,* 303 (2010): 137–43, *http://www.ncbi.nlm.nih.gov/ pubmed/20068207.*

[337] Neil Turner, "What's gone wrong with the European pharmaceutical industry," *Thepharmaletter,* April 29, 1999, *https://www.thepharmaletter.com/arti- cle/what-s-gone-wrong-with-the-european-pharmaceutical-industry-by-neil-tur- ner;* David Michels and Aimison Jonnard, "Review of Global Competitiveness in the Pharmaceutical Industry" (U.S. International Trade Commission, 1999), 2–3, *https://www.usitc.gov/ publications/ 332/pub3172.pdf.*

[338] John K. Jenkins, M.D., "CDER New Drug Review: 2015 Update" (PowerPoint presentation, U.S. Food and Drug Administration/CMS Summit, Washington, DC, December 14, 2015),

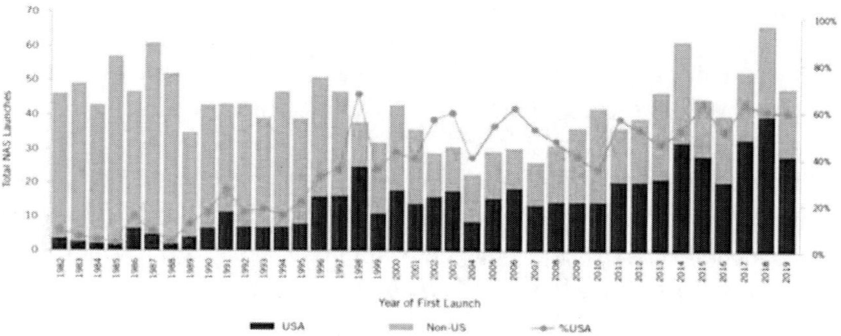

Figure 10. U.S. share of new active substances lauched on the world market, 1982-2019.[339]

And, as recently as 1990, the industry invested 50 percent more in Europe than in the United States.[340] As Shanker Singham of the Institute of Economic Affairs notes, "Europe was the unquestioned center of biopharmaceutical research and development for centuries, challenged only by Japan in the post-war period."[341] As of 1990, European and U.S. companies each held about a one-third share of the global drug market.

As Nathalie Moll of the European Federation of Pharmaceutical Industries and Associations (EFPIA) wrote in January 2020:

> The sobering reality is that Europe has lost its place as the world's leading driver of medical innovation. Today, 47 percent of global new treatments are of U.S. origin compared to just 25 percent emanating from Europe (2014–2018). It represents a complete reversal of the situation just 25 years ago.[342]

---

http://www.fda.gov/downloads/AboutFDA/CentersOffices/OfficeofMedicalProductsandTobacco/CDER/UCM477020.pdf.

339 Jenkins, "CDER New Drug Review," 23; Ian Lloyd, "Pharma R&D Annual Re- view 2020 NAS Supplement" (PharmaIntelligence, April 2020), 3. *https:// pharmaintelligence.informa.com/~/media/informa-shop-window/pharma/2020/files/whitepapers/rd-review-2020-nas-supplement-whitepaper.pdf.*

340 European Federation of Pharmaceutical Industries and Associations, "The Re- search Based Pharmaceutical Industry: A Key Actor for a Healthy Europe" (EFPIA, 2006).

341 Shanker Singham, "Improving U.S. Competitiveness—Eliminating Anti-Market Distortions" (working paper, International Roundtable on Trade and Competition Policy, 2012).

342 Nathalie Moll, "Would the last pharmaceutical investor in Europe please turn the lights out," European Federation of Pharmaceutical Industries and Asso- ciations blog, January 3, 2020, *https://www.efpia.eu/news-events/the-efpia-view/blog-articles/would-the-last-pharmaceutical-investor-in-europe-please-turn-the-lights-out/.*

By 2014, nearly 60 percent of new drugs launched in the world were first introduced in the United States, an indication both that more were being invented in the United States and that drug companies from Europe and elsewhere were introducing new drugs in America first because that's where they could recoup their investments.

This dramatic shift away from Europe serving as the "world's medicine cabinet" did not happen principally due to deficient corporate strategy or management. Instead, poor public policy in Europe and superior policy in the United States made the difference. This was particularly the case when it came to drug price controls.

As one report explained in 2002, "the heart of pharma's problem in Europe is the market's inability to 'liberate the value' from its products."[343] This was a reference to the "complex maze of government-enforced pricing and reimbursement controls" that "depressed pharma prices to the point where some companies now believe it is just not economical to launch new products in certain European countries."[344]

Europe offers a case study of the damage drug price controls inflict on the competitiveness of a nation's biopharmaceutical industry. The United States should not follow its path. Uniquely, the United States leads the world in innovating new drug and getting them to patients first while sustaining a globally competitive industry and over time making drugs broadly affordable in incentivizing competition and creating generic pathways. Policymakers should seek to improve upon this system where necessary (as ITIF noted in its testimony) but wholesale changes in the form of stringent drug policies are not needed nor warranted.

Question. The proposals put forward by congressional Democrats ignore the real challenge of ensuring that generics and biosimilars are able to launch and gain adoption quickly.

As a doctor, I strongly support both generics and biosimilars because I know they provide the same benefits as the branded products, but often at a much lower price.

What do you believe will be the impact of the policies in Build Back Better, specifically regarding the adoption and development of future generics and biosimilar medications?

---

[343] Neil Turner, "European Pricing Squeeze," *PharmaExec.com,* October 1, 2002, *https://www.pharmexec.com/view/european-pricing-squeeze.*

[344] *Ibid.*

They will be deleterious. Please see the response offered previously to Senator Crapo's question.

Prepared Statement of Douglas Holtz-Eakin, Ph.D., President, American Action Forum#

Introduction

Chairman Wyden, Ranking Member Crapo, and members of the committee, thank you for the opportunity to discuss prescription drug prices and proposals for lowering them included in the House-passed Build Back Better Act (BBBA). In this testimony, I hope to make five main points:

- The BBBA would establish an explicit government price-setting regime for pharmaceuticals, reaching into all corners of the U.S. health sector, both public and private;
- The BBBA proposals would harm consumers and negatively impact health equity through reduced innovation and higher launch prices for drugs and therapies;
- The BBBA proposals would harm and endanger the economic activity gen- erated by the biopharmaceutical industry in the United States;
- There are better ways to lower drug prices than those put forward in the BBBA; and
- Reducing drug prices should in no way be framed as addressing the consumer price inflation problem in the United States.

Let me discuss each of these in greater detail.

The views expressed here are my own and not those of the American Action Forum. I thank Christopher Holt, Tara O'Neill Hayes, and Margaret Barnhorst for their assistance.

Background

Annual health-care spending in the United States increased 9.7 percent in 2020, totaling $4.1 trillion. While the COVID–19 pandemic has played a role in recent in- creases, health-care spending and costs have both been growing rapidly for years. In 2020, 19.7 percent of the U.S. economy was devoted to health-care spending.[345] Prescription drugs, however, make up a relatively small percentage of total healthcare spending. According to the Centers for Medicare and Medicaid Services (CMS), retail prescription drug spending made up just 8.4 percent of all U.S. health-care spending in 2020.[346] While those figures do not account for therapies administered by providers in hospitals, nursing homes, or similar settings, the consulting firm Altarum estimates that non-retail prescription drug spending accounts for 4.5 percent of overall health-care expenditures annually.[347]

Though total spending on prescription therapies is not a large share of overall health spending, patients are more likely to bear the cost of medication directly due to the high coinsurance and deductibles increasingly common to drug coverage. As a result, it is widely accepted that drug prices are higher than they reasonably should be, and many argue that drugmaker profits are larger than appropriate. This thinking fails to acknowledge the high risk associated with pharmaceutical development, however. On average it takes more than a decade to bring a drug to market, and most therapies never get there. Between 2011 and 2020, only 7.9 percent of compounds that started Phase 1 clinical trials made it to market.[348] Calculating how much was spent on a particular drug's development and then calculating a "fair" percentage markup for profit fails to account for investment in unsuccessful research efforts, or the inherent risk investors take when they provide research and development (R&D) capital to innovators. A reasonable return on investment (ROI) will look different if the risk of failure is higher, and investors expect a higher ROI in exchange for the risks related to pharmaceutical development relative to other investment options. In the absence of sufficient ROI, venture capital for pharmaceutical innovation will become increasingly scarce.

---

345 https://www.healthaffairs.org/doi/10.1377/hlthaff.2021.01763.

346 https://www.cms.gov/Research-Statistics-Data-and-Systems/Statistics-Trends-and-Reports/NationalHealthExpendData/NationalHealthAccountsHistorical.

347 https://altarum.org/sites/default/files/uploaded-publication-files/Altarum%20Projections %20of%20the%20Non-Retail%20Dru.pdf.

348 https://go.bio.org/rs/490-EHZ-999/images/ClinicalDevelopmentSuccessRates2011_2020. Pdf ?ga=2.112327436.987275036.1641911607-1139759599.1641911607.

Nonetheless, there is bipartisan concern over the increasing cost of many biopharmaceutical therapies, but policymakers have differed on the best approaches to addressing prescription drug prices. While the Elijah E. Cummings Lower Drug Costs Now Act (H.R. 3) has been debated extensively,[349] far less attention has been given to the drug policies that were included in the House-passed Build Back Better Act (BBBA). The BBBA's drug price provisions are, however, no less egregious and pose no less risk to consumers and the U.S. biopharmaceutical sector than those of H.R. 3. The BBBA's drug policies would dramatically curtail future innovation and would imperil the economic benefits the United States derives from the biopharmaceutical sector.

BBBA's Overall Impact on Innovation

At the most basic level, any policies that reduce pharmaceutical industry revenue will have downward pressure on future innovation. In a recent paper from the University of Chicago, Tomas Philipson and Troy Durie estimate that a 1-percent reduction in pharmaceutical industry revenue leads on average to a 1.54-percent drop in R&D spending.[350] This does not mean that any policy that reduces industry revenue is inherently misguided, but policymakers need to be cognizant about the potential impacts of the policies they advance. Further, punitive policies aimed primarily at reducing drug company revenue—rather than those addressing specific market failures or perverse incentives enshrined in existing law—will have negative long-term impacts.

American Action Forum (AAF) researchers have documented the potential impacts on innovation of previous policies aimed at reducing pharmaceutical prices, specifically the Trump administration's International Price Index (IPI) proposal, and Speaker Pelosi's H.R. 3.[351] These proposals differ notably from the BBBA in that they tied price controls to the price of a drug in designated foreign countries. As such, these analyses cannot be directly applied to the BBBA, but they do provide some context for the potential impact of this legislation's price controls.

---

349 https://www.americanactionforum.org/testimony/testimony-on-the-lower-drug-costs-now-act- h-r-3/.

350 https://cpb-us-w2.wpmucdn.com/voices.uchicago.edu/dist/d/3128/files/2021/08/Issue-Brief-Drug-Pricing-in-HR-5376-11.30.pdf.

351 https://www.americanactionforum.org/testimony/testimony-on-the-lower-drug-costs-now-act- h-r-3/.

According to AAF analysis of the aborted IPI proposal, if that demo had been applied to all Part B drugs—expenditures for which equal roughly $30 billion—industry revenues would have been reduced approximately $9 billion per year. Considering that the cost of successfully bringing a drug to market has been estimated at approximately $2.87 billion, the $9 billion in lost revenue per year potentially attributable to the IPI proposal would be equivalent to the cost of three new medicines each year, or 30 fewer new therapies over 10 years. In the case of H.R. 3's Average International Market (AIM) price, drug prices would be capped at 120 percent of the index, rather than 126 percent in the IPI proposal, and the capped price would be applied to all U.S. payers rather than limited to Medicare Part B, which accounts for only 10 percent of all drug expenditures in the United States.[352] If the effect on drug development of the AIM price were similar to the impact of the IPI, expanding those effects to 100 percent of the U.S. market would be the equivalent of 30 fewer drugs per year or 60 percent of the total number of new drugs approved by the Food and Drug Administration (FDA) in 2021.[353] Extrapolated over 10 years, H.R. 3 would have potentially reduced industry revenue by the equivalent cost of 300 new therapies. Of course, these proposals would be unlikely to result in dollar-for-dollar reductions in R&D, so the actual number of lost therapies would be lower. These estimates are also not directly applicable to the BBBA because, whereas these past policies restrict drug prices to a limited range based on established international prices, the BBBA would implement a system of open-ended and steep price concessions based on domestic prices and enforced by a staggering 95 percent tax on gross profits of a particular therapy when a manufacturer fails to meet the Department of Health and Human Services' (HHS) price demands.

Philipson and Durie, in a robust analysis of the BBBA provisions published November 2021, estimate the legislation would reduce industry revenue by an astronomical $2.9 trillion through 2039. They attribute $1.77 trillion to the inflation rebates, $986.9 billion to government "negotiation," and $138.1 billion to the Part D reforms. Using their estimates of the impact of revenue reductions on R&D spending, the authors calculate that the BBBA would result in 135 fewer new drug approvals by 2039, and that further disincentive to researching additional indications will lead to 188 fewer new indications for existing therapies over the same period. The authors also

---

[352] https://www.americanactionforum.org/comments-for-record/comments-to-cms-on-propos ed-international-pricing-index-for-medicare-part-b-drugs/.

[353] https://www.fda.gov/drugs/new-drugs-fda-cders-new-molecular-entities-and-new-thera- peutic-biological-products/novel-drug-approvals-2021.

estimate that the policies would result in 331.5 million fewer life years through 2039. Significantly, the authors only apply the inflation limits to Medicare, but the inflation penalties will limit pricing in the private market as well, leading to even greater impacts on future innovation. They also assume that prices will be set at the absolute highest amount allowed under the BBBA, but there is no price floor, and the HHS secretary would have substantial leverage to force price concessions well below the maximum price.[354]

Rather than being more limited in its impact on innovation than previous drug pricing proposals, the BBBA's deleterious effects would be at least comparable to past proposals such as H.R. 3, and potentially even larger.

Medicare Negotiation for Drug Prices

Under the BBBA, beginning in 2025, the HHS Secretary would be authorized to "negotiate" the prices of up to 10 "negotiation-eligible drugs." In 2026 and 2027, the cap increases to 15 drugs annually, and rises to 20 drugs in 2028 and beyond. Part B drugs—those drugs administered by a medical provider in a hospital, nursing home, or similar setting—would be exempt until 2027. Additionally, all insulin products would automatically be available for negotiation beyond the yearly caps.

A negotiation-eligible drug is defined as a small-molecule or biologic (including authorized generics) treatment that has had FDA approval for at least 7 years for a small-molecule drug or 11 years for a biologic that is among the 50 single-source drugs with the highest total expenditures in Part B or Part D. Orphan drugs or "low-spend" drugs are excluded, with low-spend being defined as a drug or biologic on which Medicare spends less than $200 million annually (adjusted by the consumer price index in future years). The reduced prices would be effective after an additional 2 years, meaning small-molecule drugs would have prices reduced 9 years after approval and 13 years for biologics.

The BBBA would set a ceiling for negotiated price of between 40–75 percent of the non-Federal average manufacturer price (AMP)—the average price paid by wholesalers, net of prompt pay discounts—scaling down depending on how far the drug is past its initial exclusivity period. There would, however, be no floor below which HHS could not demand price

---

354 https://cpb-us-w2.wpmucdn.com/voices.uchicago.edu/dist/d/3128/files/2021/08/Issue- Brief -Drug-Pricing-in-HR-5376-11.30.pdf.

concessions. Unlike H.R. 3, the negotiated price would not be directly applied to the private health-care market, but the negotiated rate or "maximum fair price" would be publicized.

To provide the HHS Secretary with leverage in negotiations, the legislation would establish an excise tax specifically on sales of drugs the secretary has targeted for negotiation but for which the manufacturer has not agreed to the secretary's target price. The excise tax would be applied for any period in which the manufacturer is in "non-compliance." The tax would start out at 65 percent of sales of the therapy for the first 90 days of non-compliance, increasing at regular intervals until topping out at 95 percent for any period of non-compliance beyond 270 days.

The claim that drug prices in Medicare Part D are not negotiated misstates the reality of how Medicare pays for drugs. One might think from the rhetoric that no negotiations occur between the Medicare prescription drug program and drug manufacturers. In fact, the Medicare Part D program has robust negotiation and competition built into its very fabric.[355] Insurance companies offering drug coverage through Part D negotiate directly with manufacturers to get the best price they can for the drugs they provide. Getting a lower price benefits the prescription drug plan directly and allows it to lower premiums to attract seniors. In this way, the negotiations drive down premiums, copays, and overall drug costs. Plans are able to drive discounts by offering preferred placement on their formularies to specific therapies in exchange for lower prices. In some cases—with the exception of specific protected classes of drugs—a plan might decline to cover a particular therapy at all as part of its negotiations. This would be a problem if there were only one formulary for all beneficiaries, but beneficiaries are able to choose between a wide range of plan offerings, allowing them to select a plan that best fits their needs. In 2022, the average Medicare beneficiary has a choice of 23 stand-alone Part D plans, and 31 Medicare Advantage plans that include drug coverage.[356]

To protect this competitive environment, Federal law prohibits the HHS Secretary from interfering in the negotiations between plans and manufacturers. The Congressional Budget Office (CBO) has long held that simply removing this "noninterference" clause would not result in any savings for the program because the Secretary has no beneficiaries to negotiate on

---

355 https://www.americanactionforum.org/research/competition-and-the-medicare-part-d-program/.

356 https://www.kff.org/medicare/issue-brief/medicare-part-d-a-first-look-at-medicare-prescription-drug-plans-in-2022/.

behalf of, and no leverage for driving price concessions.[357] Giving the Secretary the legal authority to negotiate directly with manufacturers will either result in a single negotiated price for each drug— which will then have to be accepted by all insurers—thus undermining the competitive structure of Part D, or it will result in nothing.

The BBBA opts for the former, allowing the HHS Secretary to set prices that will be applied to all plans, and giving the secretary leverage to force price concessions via the draconian 95 percent excise tax on gross profits for any therapy whose manufacturer is unwilling to meet the secretary's price demands. Setting aside the negative long-term effects of the strict price controls envisioned by the BBBA, proponents should dispense with the fiction that this would resemble anything remotely like a negotiation. Given the 95-percent excise tax the Secretary would be free to wield against noncompliant innovators, "price extortion" would be a more honest label for this provision than "price negotiation."

Inflation Penalties

The BBBA would establish penalties for drugmakers if they increase the price of a particular therapy faster than the rate of inflation. For drugs covered by Part D, the AMP would be assumed as the base price of the drug for the purpose of tracking price increases. A drug's AMP would be benchmarked to October 2020, while inflation would be benchmarked to September 2021. Drugmakers could still increase their prices above inflation, but they would have to write a check for the difference. For example, if a drug's AMP was $110 per unit in October 2020, and the inflation- adjusted AMP in 2023 is $120, but the actual AMP is $130, the manufacturer would have to pay the government $10 for every unit sold in 2023. The Part D inflation cap would apply to all drugs with a price of more than $100 per patient, per year.

In Part B, the principle is largely the same with a few differences. The price of the drug to be considered would be the Average Sales Price (ASP). ASP would be benchmarked to July 2021, while inflation would be benchmarked to September 2021. While both penalties would take effect in 2023, the Part B penalty would be assessed quarterly, while the Part D penalty would be paid annually. The penalty would be applied to all single-source drugs in Part B with costs exceeding $100 per patient, per year—and biologics

---

[357] https://www.cbo.gov/sites/default/files/108th-congress-2003-2004/reports/fristletter.pdf.

would still be considered single source even if there were biosimilar competitors. Biosimilars would also be subject to penalties if their price is above that of the reference product.

While the BBBA would not apply Medicare's negotiated prices for drugs to non- Federal programs, the most significant implication of the BBBA's dollar-for-dollar penalties on price increases that exceed the rate of inflation is that, for the first time, the Federal Government would be unilaterally capping drug prices nationwide, both in Federal programs and in the private market. This shift in the Federal Government's posture toward private markets, negotiations, and competition cannot be overstated.

Additionally, the BBBA sets the inflation benchmark to a later date than the price benchmark. As a result, the legislation extracts additional revenue from drugmakers to pay for the BBBA's other provisions—reinforcing the claim that at least part of the purposes of the drug provisions is simply to generate money to pay for unrelated new spending. If the policy benchmarked both drug price and inflation to September 2021, CBO would likely have assumed that drugmakers would keep their price increases to the rate of inflation. There would be savings due to slower price growth over time, but they wouldn't be huge. By capturing the recent inflation spike and back-dating drug prices far enough to ensure that pricing decisions already made are subject to the new policy, manufacturers would have to pay for Democrats' last year of inflationary spending policies.

Faced with restrictions on future pricing flexibility, drugmakers would be incentivized to increase initial launch prices in response to inflation penalties. While these products would eventually be subject to HHS's price-setting regime, those forced price concessions would not take effect until years after the product's launch, further incentivizing manufacturers to maximize initial profits through higher launch prices.

It is worth noting that the BBBA drug provisions would be introduced in an environment of general price inflation not seen in 4 decades. The imposition of price controls on insulin and other drugs would guarantee that they will be underpriced in real terms in very short order—a recipe for further inefficiency and damage to innovation incentives. At the same time, there would be drugs that will see their prices rise at inflation—because the BBBA essentially blesses such a price rise as "legitimate"—even if no such increase is merited on the fundamentals. The result would be prices that are too high in real terms and a harm to consumers.

Insulin Price Restrictions

The House-passed BBBA specifically targets insulin prices, making all insulin products automatically subject to Medicare negotiation. The BBBA would also unilaterally limit cost sharing for insulin through Part D to $35 per month.

The BBBA would further intercede in the group and individual insurance markets to limit patient insulin costs. Starting in 2023, health insurers offering group or individual health insurance coverage would be required to provide coverage for at least one of each insulin dosage form (vial, pump, or inhaler) of each type of insulin (rapid-acting, short-acting, intermediate-acting, long-acting, and premixed). Further plans would be required to limit patient costs for insulin to no more than either $35 for a 30-day supply, or an amount equal to 25 percent of the negotiated price of the insulin product for a 30-day supply—net all price concessions—whichever is lower.

It should also be noted that the BBBA's heavy intervention in the insulin market, popular though those provisions are likely to be, will risk curtailing substantive innovation around insulin products and delivery mechanisms, as there will be little financial incentive for companies to continue to invest in their development.

Further, recent data suggests such price controls may be unnecessary. The insulin market has long suffered from the inability to sell "generic" insulins because of complicated and outdated regulatory burdens; that issue was resolved in March 2020. In anticipation, manufacturers began developing new products and accordingly, several authorized generics and a biosimilar have recently come to market and compete with some of the most popular brand-name insulin products. Following their introduction, the price per unit of insulin fell 6.8 percent from 2018 to 2020, on average, across all insulin types, except ultra-long-acting insulin.[358] This is competition at work, lowering prices. There is, however, one caveat to this point of success: Despite these new products having list prices of roughly half that of their brand-name counterparts, use among patients thus far is negligible—at least in Medicaid and Medicare Part D. It is likely that many insurers are still providing preferential treatment on the formulary to the brand-name products because such products typically come with substantial rebates—reportedly averaging between 30–50 percent.[359] This suggests rebate reform may be necessary to change this dynamic and allow the public to actually reap the benefits of these lower cost

[358] https://www.americanactionforum.org/insight/insulin-prices-an-update/.
[359] https://www.americanactionforum.org/research/insulin-cost-and-pricing-trends/.

products, as patients pay coinsurance based on list price and the use of high-priced drugs increases Federal reinsurance spending.

Health Equity and Pharmaceutical Innovation

While the costs associated with innovative therapies, particularly biologics, present access issues that can increase disparities in health equity, policies like those included in the BBBA would solve this problem, intentionally or not, by preventing new therapies from being developed in the first place. Ironically, reduced innovation could similarly impact health equity. According to Philipson and Durie, therapies that treat diseases of the endocrine, cardiovascular, and respiratory systems along with treatments for cancer and neurological diseases would be most impacted by the BBBA's policies because they make up a high share of Medicare spending. Many conditions for which treatments are lacking in these categories impact minority groups at higher rates. For example, 18.6 percent of African Americans and 14 percent of Hispanics age 65 and older suffer from Alzheimer's compared to only 10 percent of Whites.[360] African Americans are also more likely die of cancer or its complications than are Whites, 169.2 deaths per 100,000 compared to 150.3 deaths per 100,000.[361]

Given the recent focus on insulin prices, it is significant that 14.5 percent of American Indians and Alaska Natives, 12.1 percent of non-Hispanic African Americans, and 11.8 percent of Hispanics have diagnosed cases of diabetes compared to 9.5 percent of Asian Americans and 7.4 percent of non-Hispanic Whites.[362] Similar trends exist tied to educational attainment and family income. At the same time, 40.4 percent of non-Hispanic Whites with a diabetes diagnosis use insulin, compared to 33.9 percent of non-Hispanic Blacks, and 31.1 percent of Hispanics.[363] In other words, the impact of reduced innovation in insulin products will have a disproportionate impact on racial minorities, yet those same groups are more likely to struggle to access insulin therapies.

Clearly work is needed to close the pharmaceutical access gap for disadvantaged groups, however, policies that prevent new therapies from ever coming to market are a self-defeating approach.

---

[360] https://www.alz.org/media/Documents/alzheimers-facts-and-figures.pdf.

[361] https://gis.cdc.gov/Cancer/USCS/#/Demographics/.

[362] https://www.cdc.gov/diabetes/data/statistics-report/appendix.html#tabs-1-3.

[363] https://gis.cdc.gov/grasp/diabetes/DiabetesAtlas.html#.

Impact on Generic and Biosimilar Market Entry

Another under-appreciated point of concern with the BBBA is the way the legislation's provisions could disincentivize future development of generic and biosimilar therapies. Historically, flow-on products have led to significant cost savings for American patients and have been a primary driver of prescription medications' relatively small share of total health-care expenditures. Ironically, the more successful the HHS Secretary is in leveraging the BBBA's punitive excise tax to force price concessions, the fewer generic and biosimilar products are likely to come to market. Follow-on products are able to dramatically undercut name-brand drugs and biologics on price because they do not have the same R&D expenditures and because their lower prices allow them to achieve larger market shares. But if the price difference between a name-brand drug, subject to the secretary's price controls, and a new generic is marginal or even non-existent, the ability of a generic to gain market share will be reduced.

It may be that HHS is able to drive sufficient price concessions—at the cost of future innovation—to offset some of the lost savings due to a decimated generic and biosimilar pipeline, but lower prices are not the only benefit of follow-on products. Different patients respond differently to the same medication, so a robust pipeline of follow-on therapies ensures patients are more likely to have access to a therapy without unwanted side effects. Reduced market entry of generics and biosimilars could lead to fewer options for doctors to help patients avoid adverse reactions and side effects.

Economic Damage to the Biopharmaceutical Sector

The biopharmaceutical sector in the United States creates more than $1 trillion in economic activity and employs more than 800,000 workers—at an average compensation over twice the national average. More broadly, the industry supports more than 4 million jobs across the U.S. economy, and generated over $67 billion in Federal, State, and local tax revenue in 2017 alone.

The BBBA's policies aimed at reducing industry revenues put this vibrant economic engine at risk. In 1986, R&D investments by pharmaceutical firms in Europe exceeded R&D in the United States by roughly 24 percent.[364] Following the imposition of government price controls in many European

[364] https://www.nber.org/papers/w12676.

countries, and consequently the reduced return on investment, R&D spending by pharmaceutical companies grew at an annual rate of just 5.4 percent in the European Union, compared with 8.8- percent growth in the United States. As such, more than half of the world's pharmaceutical R&D investments have been made in the United States since the turn of the century, whereas less than 30 percent has been invested in Europe.[365] While shifting patterns of investment are the product of many factors, historically R&D and manufacturing investments have moved away from countries in which strict price control regimes are implemented. With countries such as India and China, among others, aggressively seeking to bolster their own biopharmaceutical industries, the BBBA would put at risk the economic benefits the United States derives from the sector and would advantage other countries in their efforts to lure away investments currently being made in this country.

Pharmaceutical Policy Options to Consider

While many—though not all—of the prescription drug pricing proposals included in the BBBA are unwise, there are worthwhile solutions for tackling drug prices in ways that promote competition and better align the incentives inherent in Federal law.

Medicare Part D Reforms

On a positive note, the House-passed BBBA does move in the right direction, undertaking a significant redesign of the Medicare Part D program, beginning in 2024, aimed at realigning plan and manufacturer incentives to constrain drug prices and to limit beneficiaries' out-of-pocket (OOP) costs. A similar proposal was included in H.R. 19 by House Republicans, and the broad framework of the proposal—originally outlined by AAF in 2018—has garnered bipartisan support, although there have been partisan differences over some of the details.[366]

---

365 https://www.abpi.org.uk/facts-and-figures/science-and-innovation/worldwide-pharma- ceutical-company-rd-expenditure-by-country/.

366 https://www.americanactionforum.org/research/redesigning-medicare-part-d-realign-incentives-1/.

Under the BBBA, brand-name and biosimilar drug manufacturers would be liable for 10 percent of costs in the initial coverage phase and 20 percent in the catastrophic phase. Government reinsurance would fall to 20 percent for brand-name drugs and biosimilars and to 40 percent for generic drugs. Insurer liability in the catastrophic phase would increase to 60 percent for all drugs. The catastrophic phase would begin at $2,000 in OOP costs, capping beneficiary costs at that point. AAF originally considered capping beneficiary OOP costs between $2,500 and $4,000 annually. The BBBA OOP cap of $2,000 is significantly below what beneficiaries are expected to pay before moving into the catastrophic phase under current law. One potential improvement, recognizing budgetary constraints and the need to balance savings for beneficiaries with costs for taxpayers, would be a slightly higher OOP cap. This could be coupled with a reduction in beneficiary coinsurance below the cap, which would benefit more enrollees—since most will never reach the OOP cap—while still providing substantial savings for taxpayers and enrollees who do reach the cap.

The BBBA would also reduce beneficiaries' coinsurance liability to 23 percent in the initial coverage phase (from 25 percent currently) and their premium liability to 23.5 percent (from 25.5 percent currently). Consequently, the Federal premium subsidy rate would rise to 76.5 percent (from 74.5 percent) and insurer liability in the initial coverage phase would be 77 percent for generic drugs and 67 percent for brand-names and biosimilars.

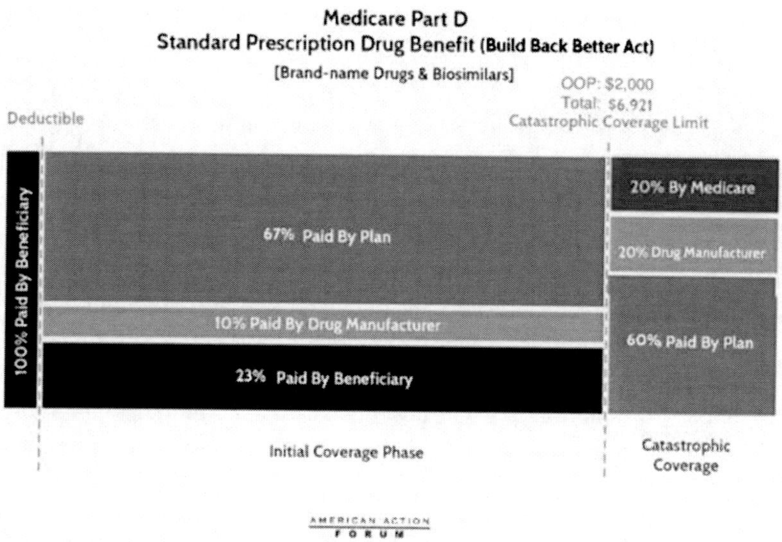

Last, the BBBA would allow for beneficiaries' OOP costs to be "smoothed" over the course of the year, rather than potentially having to pay as much as $2,000 in a single month.

While the BBBA version of the Part D redesign retains the 10-percent manufacturer share in the initial coverage phase that was added in the H.R. 3 version of the proposal, the legislation would lower the manufacturer share in the catastrophic phase from 30 percent in H.R. 3 to 20 percent, while AAF initially proposed 9 percent (note that AAF used 9 percent because that was determined to be the rate at which pharmaceutical companies would be responsible for the same level of costs at the time the original analysis was done, while AAF was neutral on whether manufacturers' share of costs should increase).

Drug Rebates

In 2019, the Trump administration proposed significant changes to the structure of drug rebates. While Congress has delayed and sought to repeal this rulemaking,[367] it would be wise to reconsider. Under current law, drug manufacturers typically provide significant rebates for drugs provided at the pharmacy counter (averaging nearly 30 percent in Medicare Part D), especially for drugs with competing alternatives. These rebates are most commonly paid to pharmacy benefit managers (PBMs) in exchange for preferred placement on the insurance plan's drug formulary. The PBMs, however, do not usually share those rebates directly with patients, instead typically using the rebates to hold down premium costs for everyone. But using rebates on high-cost drugs to broadly lower premiums instead of passing them through to beneficiaries results in the (high-cost) sick subsidizing the (low-cost) healthy, which seems counter to the intent of an insurance product.

The rebate rule, if implemented, would change that practice. Drug rebates would no longer be allowed unless they are completely passed through to the patient at the point of sale. This change would almost certainly lead to increased Part D premiums, which is why there has been opposition. Those increases are likely to be minimal, however, as the cost increase would be spread across all beneficiaries. On the other hand, the reduced cost-sharing expenses that the highest-cost beneficiaries would see should outweigh those

---

367 https://www.americanactionforum.org/weekly-checkup/a-dramatic-attempt-to-lower-drug-costs/.

premium cost increases, resulting in a net benefit to patients. Those patients with the highest costs would see the greatest benefit. The Trump administration could only propose changes to affect rebates in the Medicare program through rulemaking; if Congress were to enact a legislative version of the rebate rule, however, it could extend the policy throughout the insurance system, which is an approach worth consideration.

Competition and Increased Supply

History has proven the best way to reduce the price of a good for which there is growing demand is to increase its supply through competition. For drug pricing, that means bringing generics and biosimilars to market to compete with brand-name drugs.

A now-classic example of this phenomenon is the hepatitis C treatment, Sovaldi, which contributed over $3 billion to 2014 expenditures alone.[368] While the drug was quite expensive, it is important to note two things. First, Sovaldi—and its eventual competitors—provided a cure for what had been up until that point a costly to manage chronic disease. Second, as competitors joined the market, the price of Sovaldi was cut in half. Where there is competition, prices come down. The FDA has been doing its part by approving a record number of generic drugs and biosimilars.[369] But other barriers to unlocking robust market competition remain.

Legal Enforcement of Competition Policy

Often, once a generic drug has been on the market long enough, it acquires enough of the market share that the brand-name manufacturer stops producing its version of the drug. In many cases, the price reaches a low enough point at which other generic competitors also exit the market, leaving a sole manufacturer. In some high-profile cases we see what amounts to abuse of monopoly power—that sole manufacturer taking advantage of its position and dramatically increasing its price once there is no more competition and consumers have no choice but to purchase the now high-priced drug. In these

---

368 https://www.cms.gov/Research-Statistics-Data-and-Systems/Statistics-Trends-and-Reports/Information-on-Prescription-Drugs/index.html.

369 https://www.fda.gov/NewsEvents/Newsroom/FDAInBrief/ucm625627.htm.

cases, it should be treated as the abuse that it is and prosecuted where appropriate.

Prosecuting such monopoly abuses may require new authority for the Federal Trade Commission (FTC). The FTC's mission is "to prevent business practices that are anticompetitive or deceptive or unfair to consumers." The FTC notes that it has limited authority to take action against a company that has drastically raised the price of a drug, depending on the reason for the increase.

Drug Prices and the Challenge of Inflation

Some policymakers have touted drug pricing reforms as a way to address consumer price inflation. Inflation is a problem. As measured by the Consumer Price Index (CPI) year-over-year inflation has risen from 1.4 percent in January 2021 to 7.5 percent in January 2022. Reduced drug prices, however, has essentially nothing to do with taming the economy-wide steady rise in prices. Drug prices contribute only 1.4 percent of prices increases in the CPI, so changing drug prices will little affect the overall total. Moreover, most of the proposals in BBBA would not take full effect for years, and thus have no impact on inflation in 2022.

Conclusion

The BBBA does not establish a true "negotiation" of drug prices in Medicare; rather it would empower the HHS Secretary to dictate prices to manufacturers who would have little to no leverage. The BBBA would enshrine a unique and punitive 95-percent excise tax on gross profits of a therapy if the manufacturer does not agree to the secretary's demands and set a ceiling for a drug's price. Unlike past proposals, however, there is no floor price below which the secretary would be unable to force further concessions. Significantly, under the BBBA the Federal Government would cap the price of all drugs throughout the entire health-care system by penalizing any manufacturer who increases a drug's price faster than the rate of inflation.

The combination of price-setting by the HHS Secretary and inflation penalties would very likely reduce generic and biosimilar market entry, putting at risk potential savings and improved treatment options for millions of Americans. Price controls in the insulin market in particular will essentially eliminate future improvements in insulins and may well be unnecessary as insulin prices are beginning to drop with the emergence of greater competition. The BBBA's inflation penalties are also likely to result in higher launch prices and could drive price increases commensurate with inflation for therapies whose prices would not increase under current law.

Further, the BBBA would reduce biopharmaceutical industry revenue by $2.9 trillion through 2039 and puts at risk a U.S. biopharmaceutical sector that generates more than $1 trillion in economic activity annually, employs more than 800,000 workers, and supports more than 4 million jobs across the U.S. economy. In the mid-1980s, as European countries imposed stringent price controls, Europe saw a flight of investment in drug development and manufacturing to the United States. Under the BBBA, the United States would risk a similar loss in competitiveness to countries such as India and China that are aggressively seeking to bolster their own biopharmaceutical sectors.

The BBBA would make large-scale changes to drug policy at the Federal level and reach deep into private insurance and contracts. These policies would have widespread, negative impacts on the development of future therapies, new indications for existing therapies, and the economic benefits the United States derives from a vibrant biopharmaceutical sector. If the BBBA's policies are enacted in totality, American patients will suffer, American leadership in medical research will be diminished, and a vibrant engine of economic development for American workers and investors will be strangled. Congress should discard the majority of the BBBA's drug policies and instead focus on pursuing bipartisan reforms to Medicare Part D and enacting changes to drug rebates.

Questions Submitted for the Record to Douglas Holtz-Eakin, Ph.D. Questions Submitted by Hon. Mike Crapo

On Problematic Claims Regarding the House-Passed Build Back Better Act

Question. A range of claims advanced in support of the drug price controls included in the House-passed Build Back Better Act (BBBA) warrant substantial scrutiny and skepticism.

Some backers of the bill have cited a January 2022 AARP piece suggesting that gas and milk prices would be astronomical if they had grown at the rate of prescription drug prices for the past 15 years. Notably, however, the article in question relies on a June 2021 report using a dataset ending in December 2020, thus predating the recent surge in general inflation, which has coincided with far lower growth in drug prices. Moreover, the study in question focuses only on a subset of brand-name drugs, thus excluding the low-cost generics that account for 90 percent of the market, and its pricing metric fails to account for post-sale rebates and other price concessions. It also uses a 15-year window, which masks the recent slowing in even list price increases for medications. In terms of the current wave of inflation eroding American families' finances, between February 2021 and 2022, general inflation (CPI–U) rose by 7.9 percent, while the consumer price index specific to milk increased by 11.2 percent and the gasoline-specific index surged by 38 percent. The prescription drug-specific index (CPI–Rx, which includes generics but still excludes post-sale rebates), by contrast, grew by just 2.4 percent.

What metrics and studies provide the most accurate and inclusive data on price trends for prescription drugs?

Answer. Price trends for prescription drugs are riddled with ambiguity; list prices, net prices, out-of-pocket prices, development costs, and total spending on drugs have displayed very different patterns over time.

Concerns about increasing drug prices often refer to the narrow definition focused on sales prices (or "list price") set by drug manufacturers, though a more accurate measurement would be the net price inclusive of all discounts and manufacturer rebates. List prices for brand-name drugs, on average, increased between 5.2 and 9.3 percent between 2015 and 2019, yet the average net price of these drugs grew between 0.3 and 2.9 percent, with the trend being flat or downward sloping.[370] Additionally, while the average list price of brand name drugs rose 69 percent between 2010 and 2019, average out-of-pocket costs for those drugs declined from $27.72 in 2015 to $26.25 in 2019.[371]

Prescription drug price metrics should also consider utilization trends of certain drug types, acknowledging that the "problem" of rising prescription drug prices might not be with all drugs but driven by the high prices of select drugs. For example, the last decade has seen a significant shift toward the use

370 https://www.iqvia.com/insights/the-iqvia-institute/reports/medicine-spending-and-afford- ability-in-the-us.

371 https://www.iqvia.com/insights/the-iqvia-institute/reports/medicine-spending-and-affordability-in-the-us.

of "specialty drugs"— those that require special handling, must be administered by a doctor, require patient monitoring or follow-up care, or are used to treat complex, chronic conditions— which tend to be quite expensive.[372]

Additionally, metrics must differentiate between prescription drug spending—a function of both price and quantity—and prescription drug prices. Annual growth in pharmaceutical spending in February 2020 was 7.9 percent,[373] but annual pharmaceutical price growth was only 2.4 percent.[374] On a per capita basis, real net spending has grown by only 1 percent between 2007 and 2017 and actually declined by 2.2 percent in 2017.[375]

Ultimately, over the past 3 years, overall health-care prices have gradually increased—rising 1.3 percent between March 2018 and March 2019 and 2.5 percent from March 2020 to March 2021—though prescription drug prices have declined in two of the past 3 years: down 0.4 percent from March 2018 to 2019, rising just 1.5 percent by March 2020, and declining 2.3 percent by March 2021.

Question. How does medication price inflation relate to general inflation and inflation specific to other goods cited by AARP, such as milk and gasoline?

Answer. Inflation is a sustained rise in prices, and specific products (gasoline, drugs) or actors (oil producers, pharmaceutical manufacturers) are not responsible for economy-wide inflation. The notion that every drug price is somehow rising faster than the price of other goods is not true; as noted above, pharmaceutical price inflation in the CPI was roughly 2.5 percent over the past year, compared to 7.9 percent for the CPI as a whole. Additionally, reduced drug prices have essentially nothing to do with taming economy-wide inflation. According to the March 2022 Bureau of Labor Statistics report, pharmaceutical drug prices contributed only 1.4 percent of the price increases in the CPI, so changing drug prices will little affect the overall total.[376]

Question. In advocating for enactment of the BBBA's drug pricing provisions, some have characterized the bill's government price-setting program as market- based and fair, providing manufacturers with a say in the

[372] https://www.pcmanet.org/pcma-cardstack/what-is-a-specialty-drug/.

[373] https://altarum.org/sites/default/files/uploaded-publication-files/SHSS-Spending-Brief_ April_2021.pdf.

[374] https://altarum.org/sites/default/files/uploaded-publication-files/SHSS-Price- Brief_March_ 2021.pdf.

[375] https://www.iqvia.com/institute/reports/medicine-use-and-spending-in-the-us-review-of- 2017-outlook-to-2022.

[376] https://www.bls.gov/news.release/pdf/cpi.pdf.

pricing of their products. These advocates have sought to differentiate the program from price controls and rate-setting mechanisms.

In reality, however, the legislation would allow the HHS Secretary to set any price of his or her choosing for virtually any product selected. Under the bill, noncompliance with any component of the price-setting program—including meeting bureaucratic deadlines, agreeing to participate in the program, and accepting the price that the Federal Government sets, however arbitrary or unrealistic—would trigger an unprecedented and seemingly unconstitutional noncompliance penalty of up to 95 percent of all gross sales across all markets. Manufacturers thus have no choice in the matter and no leverage in the process. The proposal would also permanently prohibit judicial and administrative review of most elements of the new program, rendering any price set by the Secretary as absolutely final and enforceable.

In short, the bill provides for negotiation in name only.

Is the government price-setting program created under the House-passed BBBA in any way negotiation? Does it, as its backers attest, rely on market forces and provide manufacturers with a meaningful say in setting prices?

Answer. No. At a very basic level, the government would ultimately set the parameters for the negotiation. The government would determine whether a manufacturer had complied with those parameters. And the government would level substantial penalties on manufacturers who do not comply with its price concession demands. The more one drills down, the clearer it becomes that the process envisioned cannot be reasonably called a negotiation.

Question. To your knowledge, has Congress enacted any provision resembling the 95-percent noncompliance penalty—nondeductible and applied across gross sales for all market segments—in modern political history?

Answer. No.

Question. BBBA's defenders sometimes argue that the life sciences sector is uniquely and exceptionally profitable and could thus easily absorb the costs triggered by the bill's price controls. Others argue that biopharmaceutical R&D estimates overstate the sector's commitment to innovative research, pointing to studies suggesting that marketing and advertising expenses for at least some segments of the industry exceed R&D investments.

Do these arguments accurately characterize the relative profitability, R&D intensity, and marketing/advertising expenditures of the biopharmaceutical sector? Why or why not?

Answer. There are two key features to the financing of biopharmaceuticals. The first is that innovation is an inherently risky enterprise that is expensive, takes a long time, and has a very low rate of successfully bringing products to market. The second key feature is that the industry competes in capital markets with every other sector of the economy. The combination means that successful products have to be highly profitable to cover the losses from failed innovations and still provide investors with a market rate of return. In and of themselves, R&D, advertising, or other categories of expenses tell one little about the economics of the sector.

Question. In making the case for the House-passed BBBA drug-pricing policies, some have suggested that most new drugs that come to market are "me-too" products that either make modest changes to existing medications or treat conditions that already have numerous therapeutic options. These claims seem at odds with the drug development landscape, where the majority of the 50 new drugs approved last year were first-in-class treatments, and where studies regarding existing therapies can lead to new indications and uses, along with improvements that offer outsize patient benefits. One drug originally indicated to treat chronic lymphocytic leukemia, for instance, received approval as a disease-modifying therapy (DMT) for the treatment of multiple sclerosis roughly 11 years later, after a far-reaching and costly clinical development program. This type of follow-on innovation can result in major medical breakthroughs.

To what extent do we see meaningfully innovative drugs and biologics approved each year, and what potential value does follow-on innovation offer to patients?

Answer. Of the 53 new drugs approved by the FDA in 2020, 19 drugs (or roughly 36 percent) were biologics. Similarly, of the 53 drugs approved in 2019, 20 drugs (or 38 percent) were biologics. For comparison, in 1999, the FDA approved 3 biologics, making up only 8 percent of the 38 approved new drugs that year.[377]

Follow-on products are able to dramatically undercut name-brand drugs and biologics on price because they do not have the same R&D expenditures and because their lower prices allow them to achieve larger market shares. Lower prices are not the only benefit of follow-on products, however; different patients respond differently to the same medication, so a robust pipeline of follow-on therapies ensures patients are more likely to have access to a therapy without unwanted side effects.

Question. How would the government price-setting program and other price con- trols included in BBBA impact incentives for follow-in innovations

---

[377] 8 https://www.nature.com/articles/s41587-021-00814-w#Sec3.

like new indications for existing therapies, new formulations (i.e., to mitigate or eliminate side effects, to streamline dosing regimens, etc.), and other product improvements and changes?

Answer. Historically, follow-on products have led to significant cost savings for American patients and have been a primary driver of prescription medications' relatively small share of total health-care expenditures. The more successful the HHS Secretary is in leveraging the BBBA's punitive excise tax to force price concessions, the fewer generic and biosimilar products are likely to come to market. Follow-on products are able to dramatically undercut name-brand drugs and biologics on price because they do not have the same R&D expenditures and because their lower prices allow them to achieve larger market shares.

Question. While the House-passed BBBA technically makes no changes to patents and exclusivities with respect to prescription drugs, the government price-setting program and multi-market price growth cap policies would affect a manufacturer's ability to derive economic value from these market protections. How would the bill's price controls impact the incentives for innovation currently inherent in patents and exclusivities?

Answer. The BBBA would set a ceiling for negotiated price of between 40–75 percent of the non-Federal average manufacturer price (AMP)—the average price paid by wholesalers, net of prompt pay discounts—scaling down depending on how far the drug is past its initial exclusivity period. There would, however, be no floor below which HHS could not demand price concessions. Because there is a lessened ability for the manufacturer to make a profit, these price controls would have similar impacts to patent and exclusivity restrictions: a decreased profit and therefor a decreased incentive to make major investments in expensive cures.

Question. Some have claimed that the BBBA's drug-pricing provisions would exempt startups and other small biotechs from the onerous new government price-setting program included in the legislation. In reality, however, the bill includes only an extremely narrow and time-limited exemption that carves certain small biotechs out of the program for 3 years and provides them with a pricing floor for the following 2, after which point the bureaucratic new system would treat these small firms like any other companies. Notably, 66 percent of biopharmaceutical companies are startups. Moreover, small businesses—many of which would not qualify for even the temporary exemption—account for 70 percent of pivotal-stage trials, and more than 90 percent of biopharmaceutical firms overall are not turning a profit.

Do the time-limited and narrow small biotech exemptions in the bill provide meaningful protection for the startups and other small businesses that comprise the majority of the life sciences sector?

Answer. It takes an average of 15 years from the time a drug developer first begins testing a new formula until the FDA approves it.[378] Additionally, only 1 in 1,000 drug formulas will ever enter pre-clinical testing, and of those, roughly 8 percent will ultimately receive FDA approval.[379] Ultimately, it may take a long time before biotech startups develop a successful drug and offset some of their initial spending on research and development, thus, a 3-year exemption and a temporary 2-year price floor for small biotech drugs are unlikely to provide adequate protection against price controls.

Question. If enacted, how would the government price-setting program and other price controls (such as the mandatory multi-market price growth cap) impact these small businesses and the prospects of future biopharmaceutical startups?

Answer. It is clear that BBBA would be destructive to innovation in the pharmaceutical market, particularly for smaller biotech firms, as potential returns on investments diminish. Venture capital and larger pharmaceutical investors typically play a large role in supporting small biopharmaceutical startups on the leading edge of development. If the price-setting BBBA provisions are implemented, however, such investments would be less justifiable. Government price controls would erase investment incentives and upend the current market-based framework that allows investors to estimate what insurance plans might pay for a given drug, making it almost impossible for investors to secure a financial return, and thus leading investors to leave the pharmaceutical sector altogether.

Question. How might the imposition of the bill's price controls fuel industry consolidation, given the diversified product portfolios and compliance-related resources and staff that large multinationals often enjoy, relative to smaller businesses?

Answer. The less profit a business is able to make, the smaller its margin for error in choosing which products to pursue. Large multinational corporations have the margins to allow for greater experimentation in a wider range of product areas, with other profitable drugs subsidizing research and development of expensive and/ or less profitable drugs. Conversely, smaller

378 https://www.oecd-ilibrary.org/social-issues-migration-health/health-at-a-glance-2015/re- se arch-and-development-in-the-pharmaceutical-sector_health_glance-2015-70-en.

379 http://www.fdareview.org/approval_process.shtml.

drug manufacturers are already limited in the resources they can put into any given drug and have less cushion to allow for more research and development. Limiting the profits of these large multinationals will have some effect on their investments into research and innovation, but limiting the profits of smaller manufacturers will kneecap the ability of these small manufacturers to research more than just a few drugs. Industry consolidation trends have already shown a pattern in which a small company, focused on only a few products or even just one, are frequently purchased by larger corporations.

Question. Therapeutic development relies heavily on high-risk investments from diverse sources. While some of the BBBA's backers anticipate that the life sciences would remain attractive to investors at every level, real-world experience tells a different story. Even under current laws and regulations, capital can—and often does—shift away from (or simply never flow into) the biopharmaceutical sector. According to one Wall Street Journal piece from last December, for instance, biotech stocks "crumbled" in 2021. Developing a new medication can take between 11.5 and 15 years, and only one in every 1,000 drug formulas ever enters preclinical trials. For the ones that do, only 8 percent ever receive FDA approval. Unsurprisingly, it costs an average of $2.6 billion to develop and gain approval for a new medicine. These factors make the biopharmaceutical sector especially sensitive to the types of government price controls included in the House-passed BBBA, which University of Chicago researchers projected would lead to 135 fewer new drug approvals in the next 2 decades.

How would the price controls included in the BBBA likely impact the investment landscape with respect to biopharmaceutical innovation?

Answer. The United States has persisted as a global leader in biotech and biopharmaceutical development for years thanks to market-based functions of research and development, yet such a policy would effectively allow the government to dictate the price that a company may charge for a drug and immediately halt funding of drug discovery and development. Manufacturers depend on investment capital, and Federal policies that dramatically curtail return on investment will have a detrimental effect on manufacturer's ability to attract the capital necessary to continue bringing new treatments to market. Investors and venture capital firms will stop investing in new therapies and will give up on medicines that have not yet been invented. Policies in the BBBA would seek to limit drug spending through restrictive government price controls, preferencing lower spending over access to a broad range of innovative new drugs. According to Tomas Philipson and Troy Durie from the University of Chicago, BBBA provisions would reduce industry revenue by an astronomical $2.9 trillion through 2039: $1.77 trillion from inflation rebates, $986.9 billion from government inflation, and $138.1 billion from Part D reforms.[380]

Question. Supporters of the BBBA's government price-setting program sometimes cite the Veterans Affairs (VA) Department as a model for Part D. In practice, however, the closed formulary leveraged by the VA impairs access to many medications. Among the top 200 Part D drugs by overall spend, for instance, one study found that Part D plans covered an average of nearly three-fourths of the products, while the VA covered just over half. Among a sample of 25 first-in-class treatments, Part D plans covered more than three in every five, while the VA covered just 40 percent. The VA also integrates value assessments using quality-adjusted life years (QALYs) into its pricing practices, despite widespread criticism of these metrics by disability advocates, who argue that QALYs devalue individuals with exceptional needs, along with older individuals.

Is the VA drug pricing system an appropriate model or exemplar for Part D? Why or why not?

Answer. No. The decision to use government price setting based on the VA means Medicare beneficiaries will have less access to medications that will be excluded from the formulary and will either have to use less-optimal treatments or go without. Additionally, the QALY methodology for drug pricing, especially to assess the value of rare disease drugs and new therapies, is arbitrary and fails to account for societal or non-health benefits that result from improved health. Given the limitations of QALY measurements for the elderly, disabled, and terminally or chronically ill, the Affordable Care Act banned their use in Medicare formularies. QALYs make arbitrary assessments of the value of life and have the potential to further limit access to new life-saving medicines and therapies.

Question. In defending the government price-setting program and multi-market price growth cap policies in the BBBA, some policymakers have contended that under current law, manufacturers enjoy maximal price-setting power and can charge whatever they want, while purchasers and consumers lack any leverage. In practice, however, all three of the largest pharmacy benefit managers (PBMs) exclude between 400 and 500 drugs from their standard formularies, and the number of drugs excluded by these formularies increased by 676 percent from 2014 to 2020. Moreover, rebates paid by

---

[380] https://cpb-us-w2.wpmucdn.com/voices.uchicago.edu/dist/d/3128/files/2021/08/Issue-Brief-Drug-Pricing-in-HR-5376-11.30.pdf.

manufacturers have grown substantially in recent years, further reducing net prices and demonstrating leverage on the part of the payers extracting these price concessions.

Do drug manufacturers, as many BBBA supporters argue, enjoy absolute power to charge whatever they want?

Answer. No. Drug manufacturers are limited not just by what the general market is willing to pay for their products, they are also limited by negotiations with PBMs and insurers for what they can charge.

On Tying Drug Prices to Inflation

Question. Price controls reflect a tried—and failed—tool for taming inflation. They may sound appealing on paper, but in practice, they produce consistently catastrophic and counterproductive results.

Last August, William Walker, the former General Counsel and Deputy Director of the Federal Cost of Living Council under President Nixon, warned against repeating the mistakes of the past by relying on pricing mandates to reverse inflation. Writing in The Wall Street Journal, he noted that the Nixon-era price controls triggered supply shortages and economic strain, in addition to proving completely ineffective at sustainably tackling price growth, which continued to surge throughout the late 1970s.

The drug pricing provisions from the House-passed BBBA seem likely to fall into the same trap. In addition to resulting in higher launch prices for new medicines, these price controls would tie price increases to general inflation, essentially meaning that periods of high inflation would allow for the highest medicine price hikes. This approach defies basic economics, as the past year's experience has shown in stark terms.

Whereas general inflation totaled 7.9 percent from February 2021 to February 2022, the prescription drug price index grew at just 2.4 percent over the same period. This essentially means that manufacturers could have increased the scope of their average price hikes more than threefold and still fallen under the general inflation threshold. Tying drug prices to inflation, in short, would mean more volatility for working families, as well as higher prices for new products.

What factors should Congress consider as it looks at proposals like the inflation cap mandate from BBBA?

Answer. Efforts to restrict price increases to no more than the rate of inflation do not work in the long run. Instead, policies that limit the ability of a company to increase prices over time simply result in increases in the initial list price of medications when they first come to market. Such anti-market policies are punitive in nature, aimed more at punishing pharmaceutical companies for high prices than at meaningfully addressing health-care costs. The problem with seeking to punish drug companies for high prices is that in most cases the effects of these policies will simply lead to higher launch prices nationwide, passing costs on to consumers and negatively impacting patients.

It is also worth noting that the BBBA drug provisions would be introduced in an environment of general price inflation not seen in 4 decades. The imposition of price controls on insulin and other drugs would guarantee that they will be underpriced in real terms in very short order—a recipe for further inefficiency and damage to innovation incentives. At the same time, there would be drugs that will see their prices rise at inflation—because the BBBA essentially blesses such a price rise as "legitimate"—even though no such increase is merited on the fundamentals. The result would be prices that are too high in real terms and a harm to consumers.

On List Price Growth

Question. While net prices for brand-name drugs have fallen for at least four consecutive years, according to IQVIA and others, list prices for these products have grown—albeit at a slower rate than in previous years.

What are some of the underlying factors driving list price growth for prescription drugs?

Answer. List prices are in part being driven by negotiations with PBMs, who are given a certain percentage of the rebates they negotiate from manufacturers on behalf of insurance companies. The higher the list price (which now almost functions as a negotiation start point rather than being reflective of the cost of the drug), the higher the rebate, and thus the higher the cut for the PBM, incentivizing PBMs to choose drugs with higher list prices for their insurer's formulary.

On Additional Part D Plan Options

Question. While the competitive market that drives Medicare Part D has kept premiums stable and low, out-of-pocket spending has surged for some seniors in recent years, due in part to the growing inclusion of higher deductibles and coinsurance tied to the list—or sticker—price of a drug, rather than a flat copay. From 2012 to 2022, for instance, the standard Part D deductible grew by 50 percent, and the share of plans charging the maximum amount rose from 43 percent to 71 percent for 2022.

While the average senior has more than 50 different Part D plan options, tailored to a broad range of preferences and needs, plans with no or low deductible are relatively uncommon, along with options that pass drug rebates directly to patients at the pharmacy counter. Unfortunately, regulations from the Obama administration prohibit plan sponsors from offering more choices, with an arbitrary cap of three plan offerings per region.

The Lower Costs, More Cures Act would address this issue by raising that cap, as well as allowing sponsors to offer an additional two plans above the limit, so long as at least one of these new options passes a sizable share of price rebates directly to consumers at the point of sale. For some medicines, these rebates could cut costs by upward of 80 or 85 percent.

How could opening the door to additional Part D plan options allow for more innovation in benefit design, and what other incentives could we put in place to encourage choices with lower out-of-pocket spending?

Answer. Raising the cap cannot diminish innovation and options, so seniors will have a greater variety of choices among plan designs, including those with much lower out-of-pocket costs. The challenge for plan designers is to maintain these options as relatively expensive seniors migrate to plans with low out-of-pocket costs. In the absence of countervailing reforms, this will present the market with tradeoffs between the out-of-pocket costs and the level of premiums.

On Insulin Affordability

Question. Insulin affordability remains a pressing priority, particularly under Medicare, where roughly one in every three beneficiaries has diabetes, and more than 3 million use insulin. Unfortunately, even as net prices, which account for rebates negotiated by Part D plans and PBMs, have fallen for a wide range of insulin products, many seniors pay based on the list, or sticker, price, which can be as much as 86 percent higher—or even more, in some cases.

This dynamic can prove particularly problematic before reaching the deductible, as well as during the coverage gap phase, where virtually all plans charge percentage-based coinsurance.

Fortunately, thanks to a program launched by President Trump starting last year, every senior in the country now has the option of enrolling in a plan with guaranteed monthly out-of-pocket spending of no more than $35 for a wide range of insulins. More than 2,100 plans are currently participating, covering more than four in every ten Medicare beneficiaries, and plan participation grew by more than 30 percent this year.

Importantly, the program is voluntary at every level, driven by market forces and competition rather than top-down or heavy-handed government mandates.

How do you see this program—which the Lower Costs, More Cures Act would permanently extend—as impacting insulin affordability for seniors, and how does it contrast with government price controls as a cost-cutting measure?

Answer. According to CMS, seniors who enroll in a plan participating in the program will save around $446 annually, or over 66 percent, relative to their average insulin cost sharing in their current plan. Given that the program is a voluntary model, plans are allowed to join at will, relying on the power of competition, rather than government-controlled price setting, to encourage plans to join the program to attract beneficiaries. The program has grown significantly since its implementation 2 years ago, now with over 100 plan sponsors and 2,100 Part D plans participating in 2022 and is expected to continue to grow over the next couple years, further improving seniors' access to affordable insulin.

On the Value of Competition

Question. In addition to ensuring low, stable premiums and earning high satisfaction rates, Medicare Part D came in substantially under-budget, costing roughly 50 percent of what the Congressional Budget Office had initially projected. Generic drugs, which account for a staggering 90 percent of all prescriptions filled today, have played a key role in driving these resounding successes through competition. The median generic medicine has a cost roughly 60 percent below its brand-name alternative.

Biosimilars, which provide lower-cost alternatives to more complex biologic medications, have the potential to build on these achievements, as well as to inject cost-cutting competition into Medicare Part B, which covers physician-administered drugs. Between the first quarters of 2020 and 2021, average sales prices for more than half of the highest-expenditure Part B drugs declined, due in part to the ramp-up of biosimilar competition, particularly for oncology products.

Answer. What key trends have we seen in recent years with respect to the biosimilar market, and how do you see competition from these products as impacting long-run Medicare spending, under both Part D and Part B?

Answer. The number of biosimilar drugs approved per year by the FDA has steadily increased since 2017, with 31 biosimilars approved and 20 currently on the market.[381] Given that biosimilars cost, on average, 30 percent less than their reference product, biosimilar competition offers significant long-term savings for both Part D and Part B. Medicare's Oncology Care Model reported savings of between $2500-$4500 per episode in which a biosimilar was used compared to the originator product for various cancer drugs.[382]

As we've seen in the insulin market, competition will lower prices. Several authorized generic insulins and a biosimilar have come to market in recent years, leading to a 6.8-percent drop in the per-unit price of insulin on average across all but ultralong-acting insulin between 2018–2020.[383] Rebate reforms should be considered to increase uptake of these lower priced alternatives, however, and ensure long-run Medicare savings.

Question. How, in your view, would the price controls included in the House-passed drug pricing provisions impact the biosimilar market moving forward?

Answer. These price controls would likely reduce the incentive for manufactures to develop biosimilars, because their naturally lower pricing would be less attractive in the face of artificially low prices for brand name drugs. In the absence of price controls, and following some regulatory reforms in 2020, manufacturers began developing new products and accordingly, several authorized generics and a biosimilar have recently come to market and compete with some of the most popular brandname insulin products. Following their introduction, the price per unit of insulin fell 6.8 percent from 2018 to 2020, on average, across all insulin types, except ultralong-acting insulin. With price controls in effect, there is significantly less incentive for the development of biosimilar competitors to current biologics.

---

381 https://accessiblemeds.org/sites/default/files/2021-10/AAM-2021-US-Generic-Biosimilar-Medicines-Savings-Report-web.pdf.

382 https://www.ajmc.com/view/biosimilars-drive-savings-in-medicare-s-oncology-care-model.

383 https://www.americanactionforum.org/insight/insulin-prices-an-update/.

On Provider Payment Cuts

Question. The drug pricing policies included in the House-passed BBBA would impose steep Medicare cuts on physicians and hospitals through the bill's government price-setting program. A recent Avalere study found that for the providers most likely to be targeted—including oncology practices—the bill would slash Medicare addon payments by an average of 40 percent. Patients, in turn, could find their care options reduced, or erased altogether, and trends like health system consolidation could accelerate.

What would the mechanics of the BBB's drug pricing policies mean for health-care providers, and what are some preferable alternatives for containing Part B spending growth in the future?

Answer. Assuming that the BBBA's provisions work as envisioned, one would anticipate the maximum fair price would be lower than the average sales price under current law. Because both current law and the BBBA would set provider reimbursement at the cost of the drug (either the maximum fair price or the average sales price) plus 6 percent, the result would be a lower reimbursement for providers. One option for controlling Part B spending would be further movement toward bundled payments for services in lieu of fee-for-service.

On Inflation

Question. What do you see as the biggest drivers of inflation, which continues to erode Americans' financial security, and how can we reverse current trends in the prices of gas, food, cars, and a host of household needs?

Answer. The current high level of inflation is the result of both supply and demand conditions. The global impact of COVID–19 has diminished supply capacity, disrupted supply chains and raised the cost of delivering goods and services. These higher input costs have been passed along as consumer price inflation. On the demand side, the economy is suffering from sustained, loose monetary policy and excessive stimulus. The American Rescue Plan, in particular, was a major policy error, injecting \$1.9 of stimulus spending at a time when there was already stimulus in place and the economy was expanding at a rapid (6.5 percent annually) rate.

On Outcomes-Based Contracting

Question. Cutting-edge gene and cell therapies have the potential to transform the treatment landscape, personalizing care options through technologies that were— until recently—the subject of science fiction. By 2025, the FDA has projected that we could see 10 to 20 approvals of these types of innovative therapies every year. The implications for patients could be game-changing, particularly for those living with previously untreatable conditions.

As payers look to ensure access to these therapies while also managing potential cost impacts, a growing number have turned to value-based arrangements, conditioning a portion of payments on patient outcome achievements and benchmarks. A far-reaching Avalere survey of health plans and PBMs from last September found that more than half had established outcomes-based contracts of this type, and 12 percent had executed more than 10 of these arrangements.

Still, outdated statutory barriers and regulations have undermined outcomes-based contracts for public and private payers alike, particularly with respect to the Anti-Kickback Statute and Medicaid price reporting rules. While the Trump administration took a vital first step toward addressing some of these barriers, its implementation has been repeatedly delayed. Congress can advance these arrangements much further through policies like some of the provisions included in the Lower Costs, More Cures Act, which would facilitate outcomes-based contracts with greater accountability, predictability, and flexibility, better serving patients across the Nation.

What role do you see value-based arrangements playing moving forward, particularly for gene and cell therapies, and what steps could Congress take to move the needle on this front?

Answer. Paying for quality outcomes is the gold standard of program design. While at times difficult to design because of multiple co-morbidities, incomplete science, and other factors, in those situations where it is possible Congress should ensure that there is a clear safe harbor from anti-kickback and self-referral laws.

Questions Submitted by Hon. Michael F. Bennet

Return on Federal R&D Investment

Question. You have rightfully noted the important contributions made by the pharmaceutical industry in developing cutting edge drugs that have saved countless lives. But our current form of subsidizing this research and development coincides with Americans (primarily seniors and families) paying far more than their international counterparts.

Would a different form of subsidization, like advance market commitments, patent competitions, or other creative grant mechanisms, be more preferable than subsidizing pharmaceutical research and development without seniors and families reaping benefits at the pharmacy counter?

Answer. The amount of subsidies, and not the form, is the key to inducing the desired level of innovation. A logically separate issue is the degree to which those subsidies show up in retail prices; it strikes me that this has more to do with insurance design and competition than anything else.

CBO Analysis

Question. Although you are a former Congressional Budget Office (CBO) Director, a nonpartisan and data-driven agency, you are seemingly dismissive of CBO's analysis of the Build Back Better Act's drug pricing provisions' impact on innovation— which estimated one fewer drug over 10 years.

Do you believe CBO is wrong in their analysis?

If so, can you provide a description of what's wrong with CBO's estimate?

Answer. Among the key provisions of the Build Back Better Act's prescription drug reforms is an immediate imposition of the draconian "negotiation" regime on insulin products. I believe this will be sufficient to end all innovation in the insulin area. Accordingly, its strikes me that one is the lower bound of the estimate of innovative drugs foregone by BBBA.

Price Gouging and Competition

Question. During your testimony and oral response, you mentioned you are supportive of implementing legal enforcement of competition policy if a drug manufacturer takes advantage of its position and dramatically increases its price only when there is no more competition. Under this paradigm, enforcement would occur once consumers have no other choice but to purchase the now high-price drug.

Can you explain what legal enforcements of competition policy exist to compel manufacturers to lower the price of a drug that does not face market competition, but now commands high prices?

Could you explain why these enforcements would be more effective than the proposed inflation penalty combined with a limited negotiation framework?

Based on your expertise at CBO, would your alternative ultimately save taxpayers and patients money over the 10-year time horizon?

Answer. I am not a lawyer and will not move past my area of expertise. There are not now such legal powers; my answer indicated that I thought it would be desirable for Congress to develop them. Moreover, as I noted, this arises largely in the context of sole-source drugs that are off-patent. One would not expect large budget savings from this market segment.

Protecting Innovation and Access

Question. I care deeply about ensuring innovation so patients with life-threatening illnesses may one day receive the treatment they need. That's why I worked with my colleagues on the Senate HELP Committee on establishing the Breakthrough Therapies designation to provide an improved pathway to innovated treatments. I also care deeply about the roughly one-third of Americans rationing or skipping doses because of prescription drug costs. I do not believe that innovation and access to these products should exist on their own, however, today, many Americans cannot access innovative treatments because of high and rising cost.

Do you believe the current business practices by manufacturers to offer treatments at high-costs ensures access to these treatments by the one-third of Americans who cannot access medicines that these manufacturer develop?

How do we ensure these Americans rationing and skipping doses have access to innovative drugs without shifting costs to the taxpayer, through premiums or out- of-pocket costs, or the U.S. Government?

Answer. As I noted in my testimony, I believe that best first step would be for Congress to enact the Part D reforms that would cap the out-of-pocket costs for seniors, protect the taxpayer, and improve the incentives for private negotiation under the program.

Questions Submitted by Hon. Chuck Grassley

Question. According to the Department of Labor, the Consumer Price Index (CPI) rose 7.9 percent in March 2022 from the year prior. That's at a 40-year peak that hasn't been reached since 1982. Hospitals, nursing homes, and other health-care entities have raised concerns to you about low reimbursement. Additionally, healthcare providers are having difficulty finding the workforce to fill open jobs. On top of all of this, health-care providers are impacted by rising inflation to purchase goods in the workplace and at home. Rising inflation is pushing up costs including in health care. I have heard from Iowans concerned about the impact of losing health-care workers, challenges with filling open health-care jobs, and/or not having the financial resources to pay for increased competitive wages.

What impact is rising inflation having on access to health-care services?

Answer. Due to the pandemic, we have seen medical price inflation that has been somewhat, but not entirely, distinct from the general inflation the rest of the economy has been experiencing. Hospitals and health-care facilities that have been understaffed due to either workforce sickness or a rapid influx of patients have been forced to pay increasingly higher salaries to traveling nurses, which in turn affects the price of care for patients. If a hospital cannot afford to pay for the extra workforce, patients suffer through decreased access to providers and longer wait times. Similarly, as prices for basic goods and services overall have risen, health-care workers have demanded higher wages to compensate, resulting in similar effects price and access for patients.

Question. The Prescription Drug Pricing Reduction Act (PDPRA) caps out-of- pocket prescription drug costs in Part D at $3,100 for seniors. This will eliminate the donut hole. Additionally, PDPRA established a voluntary option to smooth sig- nificant up-front costs over the entire year so a beneficiary does not face a $3,100 bill in the first month of the year prior to reaching the out-of-pocket cap. This policy is called "monthly smoothing." PDPRA's monthly smoothing policy is voluntary and a beneficiary can trigger this program option if they exceed the monthly threshold divided by the remaining months in the plan year. By comparison, H.R. 3 requires a patient to accrue $2,000 in costs before they can smooth costs over month-to- month. This can hurt patient access. PDPRA allows patients to elect to smooth drug costs right away without facing a $2,000 bill first.

Should we create burdensome rules for patients to manage drug costs like in H.R. 3 or promote access by giving patients flexibility like in PDPRA?

Answer. Flexibility to allow for monthly smoothing may better enable patients to pay for their drugs by preventing the patient from being forced to spend a large amount up-front before seeing relief. However, overall higher out-of-pocket (OOP) spending present in the PDPRA may still be more of a deterrent for certain more expensive patients, given the $3,100 OOP cap would not reduce beneficiaries' OOP liability, relative to current law, until total drug spending surpassed $10,945 in total drug costs.

Question. H.R. 3 would base drug prices off an international reference pricing model that uses prices from countries with socialized medicine (i.e., Canada, France, Germany, United Kingdom). Many international reference pricing models use "quality-adjusted life year" (QALY) metrics. QALY assigns value to the patient population a drug is intended for. According to the National Council on Disability (NDC), QALY discriminates against people with disabilities and limits access to lifesaving treatment. A 2019 NCD report found "sufficient evidence of the discriminatory effects of QALYs to warrant concern and recommend its prohibition." This was based on input from bioethicists, patient rights groups, and disability rights advocates. Congress prohibited QALY use under the Affordable Care Act (ACA). H.R. 3 uses government drug price dictation based on an international reference pricing index.

Should the United States set drug prices based on models—like what H.R. 3 uses—that discriminate against people with disabilities and limits access to lifesaving treatment?

What affects will this have on patient access?

Answer. No. QALYs assign an arbitrary dollar value to a year of one's life and the QALY methodology for drug pricing, especially to assess the value of rare disease drugs and new therapies, is also arbitrary and fails to account for societal or non-health benefits that result from improved health. These valuations necessarily require judgments about the value of a year of life—or fraction thereof—or the quality of that year. Decisions about value that have traditionally been made by patients and their doctors would be turned over to bureaucrats and academics. This type of evaluation system is typical of many countries with lower drug prices, where politicians have been willing to forego access to innovative treatments for their populations in order to limit health-care costs. Given the aforementioned limitations of QALY measurements for the elderly, disabled, and terminally or chronically ill, the Affordable Care Act banned their use in Medicare formularies. QALYs attempt to standardize measurements across diverse conditions and consider the value individuals place on their health care, but the health-care system is complex and difficult to replicate in a single model. Ultimately, QALYs make arbitrary assessments of the value of life and have the potential to limit access to new life-saving medicines and therapies.

Question. In 2003, Congress passed the bipartisan Medicare Modernization Act (MMA). Twelve Democrats in the Senate voted for it, including two members currently on this Finance Committee. Medicare Part D contains the non-interference provision that expressly prohibits Medicare from: (1) negotiating drug prices, (2) setting drug prices, and (3) establishing a one-size-fits-all list of covered drugs. Getting rid of the non-interference clause would result in drug price dictation. In 2003, when Medicare Part D was created, many Democrats supported banning Medicare from negotiating drug price including: Senators Biden, Kennedy, Baucus, Reid, Schumer, Leahy, Durbin, Stabenow, and Cantwell. On the House side, this included Speaker Pelosi and Ways and Means Committee Chairman Neal. The Congressional Budget Office (CBO) has said consistently in writing that letting Medicare to negotiate drug prices does not save money unless you restrict patient access (CBO said this in 2004, 2007, again in 2007, and 2019). Additionally, an April 2021 CBO report said Speaker Pelosi's H.R. 3 would lead to 38 fewer drugs produced in the next 2 decades. A University of Chicago researcher projected H.R. 3 would lead to 342 fewer new drug approvals in the next 20 years. To put in perspective, about 30 new drugs are approved by the Food and Drug Administration (FDA) annually.

For decades, CBO, the non-partisan referee, has said government drug price dictation does not save money unless you restrict access to patients. Is that still correct?

Answer. Yes, it remains correct.

Question. Is government drug price negotiations a real negotiation or is government dictating the price?

Answer. Allowing the HHS Secretary to set prices that will be applied to all Medicare plans and giving the Secretary leverage to force such price concessions with a 95-percent excise tax on gross profits for any therapy whose manufacturer is unwilling to meet the Secretary's price demands will not resemble anything remotely like a negotiation. Through the 95-percent excise tax, the Secretary would be free to wield against noncompliant innovators, thus "price negotiation" is not an honest label for this provision.

Question. President Obama's Office of Management and Budget (OMB) Director, Peter Orszag, has said this about changes to the non-interference, "negotiating ability alone is largely feckless." Can you save money if you do not limit access like restricting the formulary or dictating prices based on a domestic or international reference index?

Answer. No. In order to save money, the HHS Secretary has to have a lever to induce concessions, whether that be a formulary or a price fixing mechanism.

Question. In a previous testimony you gave to the Finance Committee, you stated that government drug price dictation would restrict access if you want to achieve savings. Academic research has also confirmed that. Can you expand on how patients will be hurt by the proposed government drug price dictation policy?

Answer. In a recent paper from the University of Chicago, Tomas Philipson and Troy Durie estimate that, as a result of the $2.9-trillion reduction in industry revenue through 2039, the BBBA would result in 135 fewer new drug approvals by 2039, and that further disincentive to researching additional indications will lead to 188 fewer new indications for existing therapies over the same period. The authors also estimate that the policies would result in 331.5 million fewer life years through 2039. Therapies that treat diseases of the endocrine, cardiovascular, and respiratory systems along with treatments for cancer and neurological diseases would be most impacted by the BBBA's policies because they make up a high share of Medicare spending. Notably, many conditions for which treatments are lacking in these categories impact minority groups at higher rates.[384]

Question. If we disincentive the private sector to produce cures, will we give up our status as the world's leading research and development country to China?

Answer. With countries such as India and China, among others, aggressively seeking to bolster their own biopharmaceutical industries, the BBBA would put at risk the economic benefits the United States derives from the sector and would advantage other countries in their efforts to lure away investments currently being made in this country. In 1986, R&D investments by pharmaceutical firms in Europe exceeded R&D in the United States by roughly 24 percent.[385] Following the imposition of government price controls

---

[384] https://cpb-us-w2.wpmucdn.com/voices.uchicago.edu/dist/d/3128/files/2021/08/Issue-Brief-Drug-Pricing-in-HR-5376-11.30.pdf.

[385] https://www.nber.org/papers/w12676.

in many European countries, and consequently the reduced return on investment, R&D spending by pharmaceutical companies grew at an annual rate of just 5.4 percent in the European Union, compared with 8.8 percent growth in the United States. As such, more than half of the world's pharmaceutical R&D investments have been made in the United States since the turn of the century, whereas less than 30 percent has been invested in Europe.[386] While shifting patterns of investment are the product of many factors, historically R&D and manufacturing investments have moved away from countries in which strict price control regimes are implemented.

Question. Should Congress pursue policies that produce less cures?
Answer. No.

Question. It was characterized during the hearing that the bipartisan Prescription Drug Pricing Reduction Act (PDPRA) merely shifted costs. This is inaccurate. I appreciate my colleague, Senator Cassidy, correcting the record later on during the hearing, stating, "Senator Wyden has said on several occasions, with all due respect, that the Wyden-Grassley bill passed by this committee in 2019 merely shifted cost to taxpayers. That's incorrect. It saved $94 billion per the CBO. And in the Part D redesign, we shifted the cost away from the consumer, from the taxpayer to the PBM and the pharmacy. Excuse me. The pharmaceutical company. We capped out- of-pocket costs at $3,200, and we allowed an amortization of payments over 12 months." As the Congressional Budget Office (CBO) stated in a March 2020 cost estimate of PDPRA (https://www.cbo.gov/system/files/2020-03/PDPRA-SFC.pdf), taxpayers would save approximately $95 billion over 10 years with the passage of PDPRA. In addition, Medicare Part D beneficiaries would see reduced cost sharing by about $72 billion over 10 years.

Based on your experience as a former CBO director, does PDPRA merely shift costs to the taxpayer?

Answer. No, it does not. One would expect that PDPRA and the Part D redesign would have impacts on the pricing of pharmaceuticals in the commercial and individual markets as well.

Question. To date, the majority party's H.R. 3 and other partisan prescription drug pricing proposals have not advanced in the Senate. Those proposals lack robust accountability and transparency provisions to reform the prescription drug pricing industry. By contrast, the bipartisan Prescription Drug Pricing Reduction Act (PDPRA), contains several provisions to reform

---

[386] https://www.abpi.org.uk/facts-and-figures/science-and-innovation/worldwide-pharma- ceutical-company-rd-expenditure-by-country/.

the prescription drug industry, including greater accountability and transparency placed on drug manufacturers and Pharmacy Benefit Managers (PBMs). Some of the accountability and transparency provisions in PDPRA would require public disclosure of excessive of prescription drug price increases and the launch price of new high-cost drugs; public disclosure of drug discounts and PBM financial audits to account for the true net cost of a drug; public disclosure of direct and indirect remuneration (DIR) fee amounts and financial audit results; the establishment of a prescription drug pricing dashboard; improved coordination between the Food and Drug Administration (FDA) and the Centers for Medicare and Medicaid Services (CMS); and the ending of spread pricing in Medicaid managed care contracts.

Can Congress truly say it is passing prescription drug reform without the suggested accountability and transparency provisions?

Is so-called "prescription drug reform" that lacks greater/improved accountability and transparency just maintaining the existing system's shell game?

Answer. Any drug pricing reform should be evaluated by its overall impact, and not on the inclusion or exclusion of specific provisions.

Question. When Congress passed the bipartisan Medicare Modernization Act (MMA) in 2003 it was the first major improvement to the Medicare program in nearly 40 years. Today, 49 million seniors have prescription drug coverage as a result of MMA. Approximately 18 years later, we have a growing problem: prescription drug affordability. AARP says brand name drugs are going up more than twice the rate of inflation. A recent National Health Interview Survey estimates suggest 3.5 million seniors are having difficulty affording their medications. A Kaiser Family Foundation report found 50 percent of Part D drugs and 48 percent of Part B drugs had price increase greater than inflation. A recent MedPAC report indicates that 443,000 Medicare Part D enrollees in 2020, up from 33,000 in 2010 (an approximate 1,200 percent increase), filled a prescription in a single claim that met the Part D out-of-pocket threshold. The Finance Committee has made progress in the previous Congress to pass a bipartisan prescription drug pricing reform, specifically the Prescription Drug Pricing Reduction Act (PDPRA). Senator Wyden admitted such during our most recent drug pricing reform hearing, stating, "A number of these ideas were developed in this committee with bipartisan support, and that remains." Senator Wyden also said, "There is no question that the committee came together in the last Congress and came up with a number of constructive bipartisan reforms. Period. Full stop." Senator

Carper also stated during the same hearing that "Senator Grassley did, I thought, a masterful job in drafting a bill with broad bipartisan support."

If comprehensive prescription drug pricing reform, such as PDPRA, is not pursued by this Congress, I believe patients will continue to suffer due to inaction by the majority party to work in a bipartisan manner to pass prescription drug pricing reform. Do you agree?

Answer. As I noted in my testimony, I believe that that single best thing Congress can do at this juncture is the pass the Part D redesign that has bipartisan support. This would protect seniors from large out-of-pocket costs, protect the taxpayer from the cost of catastrophic drug costs, and sharpen the incentives for tough private-sector negotiations between plans and manufacturers.

Question. In 2020, the Centers for Medicare and Medicaid Services (CMS) announced a new Center for Medicare and Medicaid Innovation (CMMI) Part D model to lower out of pocket insulin expenses for beneficiaries called the Senior Savings Model. The model has enabled beneficiaries to enroll in plan options guaranteeing monthly out-of-pocket spending of no more than $35 for at least one of each dosage form and type of insulin product. I supported the model and believe it is important tool to controlling out-of-pocket insulin costs. According to Avalere, seniors may be saving 63 percent to 75 percent in out-of-pocket insulin costs per month. CMS cur- rently has 2,159 plans participating in the model in all 50 States covering 17 million Part D enrollees in Calendar year (CY) 2022). Currently, CMS is in year 2 of the 5-year model. While CMS is preparing for year 3, there is limited outcome data and analysis about the model.

As CMS and policymakers gather complete data and conduct analyses about the program, what factors, trends, conditions, and outcomes metrics should Congress consider in analyzing this model to determine successes and opportunities for improvement?

Answer. Metrics could include out-of-pocket spending by beneficiaries; Federal spending increases or decreases; and medication utilization by beneficiaries (number of seniors using insulin, frequency of skipping filling prescriptions, and frequency of insulin rationing).

Questions Submitted by Hon. John Thune

Question. You've discussed that uptake of insulin biosimilars in Medicare and Medicaid has not been as significant as one may have hoped.

How long does it normally take for the needed behavioral shift to occur for prescribers and patients to move to a non-branded alternative?

Answer. The time needed for behavioral shifts to occur in the insulin market likely varies, though based on prior AAF research, patients are typically slow or even reluctant to switch to new products. The diversity of products naturally complicates how easily new products can be substituted and new insulin products are not being widely sold at all pharmacies, further limiting the physical customer base.[387]

Question. Are there other practices in place that disincentivize this shift?

Answer. Tier placement and rebates likely discourage uptake of lower-cost options. It is likely that many insurers are still providing preferential treatment on the formulary to the brand-name products because such products typically come with substantial rebates—reportedly averaging between 30–50 percent.

Question. I've worked with multiple colleagues across the aisle on advancing the idea of value-based insurance design. This principle allows plans the opportunity to improve outcomes for patients by prioritizing high-value services for patients with specific chronic conditions.

We've had a demonstration in Medicare Advantage for several years, including for diabetes. Additionally, the Trump administration put together a program to allow for reduced cost sharing for insulin that has V–BID-like characteristics.

I think this is the kind of patient-focused approach we ought to be thinking about, rather than the heavy-handed, government-focused mandates Democrats are suggesting.

Are there other ideas policymakers should consider to reduce costs and get plans and manufacturers more invested in achieving good outcomes?

Answer. I support efforts to pay for quality outcomes and Congress should provide a clear safe harbor for such designs against the impacts of anti-kickback and self- referral laws. Also, as I noted in my testimony, I believe that that single best thing Congress can do at this juncture is the pass the Part D redesign that has bipartisan support. This would protect seniors from large out-of-pocket costs, protect the taxpayer from the cost of catastrophic drug costs, and sharpen the incentives for tough private sector negotiations between plans and manufacturers.

---

[387] https://www.americanactionforum.org/insight/insulin-prices-an-update/.

Questions Submitted by Hon. Tim Scott

Question. Thirty-seven percent of South Carolinians suffer from high cholesterol. A few years ago, manufacturers of new and innovative cholesterol lowering medicines called PCSK9s took a dramatic step to lower the list price of the medicine in an attempt to improve patient affordability; however, access challenges still exist due to high co-pays and abused utilization management tools.

Does Build Back Better do anything to address these patient access challenges in the marketplace?

Answer. No, the BBBA does not address co-pays or utilization management tools for the private market, and its price controls for Medicare Part D do not address the issue of higher list prices causing higher co-pays for Medicare beneficiaries.

Question. If the negotiation process in Build Back Better reduces the price of brand products by 35 percent to 80 percent, do you think there will still be a market for biosimilar and generic drugs?

Answer. Yes, but the decreased incentives to invest in the biosimilars market means America's slow roll-out of biosimilars, relative to the Europe's, will be even slower, and generic investment is likely to decrease as well.

Question. Are there any implications for the drug supply chain and potential shortages if the market for these products is significantly reduced?

Answer. Yes, potentially. Smaller profits for manufacturers mean less investment in their supply chain, making supply chains more vulnerable to shocks.

Question. When generics are approved, they often reach up to 90-percent savings from the list price of the brand product; however, it can sometimes take up to 3 years to add a generic drug to the CMS formulary.

How can the Part D program be modernized to ensure that patients have access to lower cost generics and biosimilars?

Answer. Instead of setting price controls that will stifle pharmaceutical innovation and further limit the creation of biosimilars, Congress should seek to increase utilization of biosimilars over higher-cost alternatives, by increasing patient and provider awareness of biosimilars and their associated benefits, as well as incentivizing providers to prescribe biosimilars through temporary reimbursement increases, both of which have historically garnered bipartisan support. Reforms to drug rebates, such as the rebate rule, could also be considered to pass costs to patients at the point of sale and reduce cost-sharing expenses for the highest-cost beneficiaries.

Questions Submitted by Hon. Ben Sasse

Question. While we need to rein in the cost of pharmaceuticals, we also need to consider access to and creation of new therapeutics that can be potentially lifesaving. Multiple sclerosis is a good example of a disease that has benefitted from follow-on innovations. In 2020, the FDA approved Novartis' Kesimpta as a treatment for MS. This drug was originally approved 11 years earlier for the treatment of a rare form of leukemia, making this a follow-on product. It is common to find new indications for existing drugs, and we want to incentivize research and development and the multiple clinical trials that make this possible.

How would some of the lesser-discussed policies in Build Back Better actually create disincentives to finding new indications for existing drugs? For example, wouldn't the bill make tax changes that disincentivize finding new indications for orphan drugs?

Answer. Yes, one study[388] found that disincentives in the BBBA to research additional indications will lead to 188 fewer new indications for existing therapies over the same period.

Question. Can you speak to how costly the clinical trial process is, and how this might drive up prices? For example, testing a new indication for Kesimpta took 10 years and spanned 350 sites across 37 countries. This was for a drug that already existed and was approved for another use.

How might we reform this process to decrease costs?

Answer. According to a report submitted to HHS by the Eastern Research Group, the average cost of Phase 1, Phase 2, and Phase 3 clinical trials is $4 million, $13 million, and $20 million, respectively, though there are significant variations in trial costs between medical specialties and therapeutic areas.[389] Other studies have esti- mated the total cost of bringing a new therapy to market at approximately $2.87 billion.[390]

Inherently, clinical trials for expensive, innovative drugs will be more costly. It will be difficult to pursue reforms that decrease costs without also decreasing the value of the drug or forgoing necessary studies on drug efficacy and safety.

---

388 https://cpb-us-w2.wpmucdn.com/voices.uchicago.edu/dist/d/3128/files/2021/08/Issue-Brief-Drug-Pricing-in-HR-5376-11.30.pdf.

389 https://aspe.hhs.gov/sites/default/files/private/pdf/77166/rpt_erg.pdf.

390 https://www.centerwatch.com/articles/15357?v=preview.

Question. Multiple sclerosis unfortunately lacks a cure. How would the price controls being suggested by Democrats hurt efforts to find a cure for MS?

Answer. The price controls in the BBBA would lead to reduced profits and therefor reduced ability to research complex and difficult diseases and reduced incentive to develop expensive cures that are targeted at a relatively small population. Rare disease populations in particular would lose out.

Question. We have seen the U.S. lose its competitive advantage in places where we were once the global leader as a result of policies that harm innovation and competitiveness. One such example is the semiconductor industry, where we have ceded leadership to China despite being the creator of the industry. I worry that we are now in a similar moment with the pharmaceutical industry. While prices are too high and we need to address that problem, we lead the world in biopharmaceutical innovation thanks to R&D investments, strong IP protections, and a market-driven pricing system. I worry that the price controls being suggested will erode our competitive advantage, leading to fewer cures.

What have studies found about the corresponding cuts to research and development that happen as a result of price controls?

Answer. In a recent paper from the University of Chicago, Tomas Philipson and Troy Durie estimate the BBBA legislation would reduce industry revenue by an astronomical $2.9 trillion through 2039. They attribute $1.77 trillion to the inflation rebates, $986.9 billion to government "negotiation," and $138.1 billion to the Part D reforms. These cuts to research and development would result in 135 fewer new drug approvals by 2039, and that further disincentive to researching additional indications will lead to 188 fewer new indications for existing therapies over the same period. The authors only apply the inflation limits to Medicare, but the inflation penalties will limit pricing in the private market as well, leading to even greater impacts on future innovation. They also assume that prices will be set at the absolute highest amount allowed under the BBBA, but there is no price floor, and the HHS secretary would have substantial leverage to force price concessions well below the maximum price.[391]

Question. Why is there such a disparity between what outside economists have predicted about the number of drugs that will never come to market as a

[391] https://cpb-us-w2.wpmucdn.com/voices.uchicago.edu/dist/d/3128/files/2021/08/Issue-Brief-Drug-Pricing-in-HR-5376-11.30.pdf.

result of these price controls and what the Congressional Budget Office has predicted?

Answer. I have not done a detailed comparison of the alternative estimates and their underpinnings. CBO might be better-positioned to answer this question.

Question. Hasn't China also recognized this problem and actually moved to lift price controls on pharmaceuticals in recent years?

Answer. I am unfamiliar with these domestic China issues.

Question. Why does so much of our active pharmaceutical ingredient come from China and India and should this concern us?

Answer. In reality, U.S. supply chains are well-diversified, with China supplying only 18 percent of total active pharmaceutical ingredient imports, 9 percent of total antibiotic imports, and less than 1 percent of total vaccine imports. Moreover, U.S. production of pharmaceutical goods is often understated: 70 percent of essential medical equipment is manufactured in the United States, and 70 percent of total antibiotic spending and 50 percent of total vaccine spending is on U.S.-made product.

Question. A large pillar of the Democrats' drug pricing plan includes punishing companies for drug prices that rise faster than the rate of inflation.

With current inflation at 7.9 percent over the last 12 months, how many drugs have net prices rising faster than that?

Answer. CMS has not yet released its comprehensive datasets with 2021 or 2022 prices for Medicare covered drugs, though from 2019 to 2020, before the recent surge in inflation, 17 percent of all Medicare covered drugs had price increases of 7.5 percent or higher, though this was based on the average spending per dose, and for Part D drugs, did not account for discounts or rebates.

Given that the BBBA drug provisions would be introduced in an environment of general price inflation not seen in 4 decades, there would be drugs that will see their prices rise at inflation—because the BBBA essentially blesses such a price rise as "legitimate"—even though no such increase is merited on the fundamentals.

Question. Haven't net prices on a whole declined over the last several years? I believe even list prices have increased only marginally (1.3 percent in 2020 according to BLS data), and this doesn't take into account rebates or discounts, isn't that correct?

Answer. Based on data from SSR Health, Drug Channels Institute found con- sistent declines in the net prices of brand-name drugs from 2018 to 2020: In 2020, brand-name list prices grew by 4.2 percent, while brand-name net prices declined by 2.2 percent. Similarly, in 2019, brand-name list prices grew by 4.6 percent, while brand-name net prices declined by 2.3 percent.[392]

According to BLS data, overall prescription drug prices fell 2.4 percent from December 2019 to December 2020, remained unchanged from December 2020 to December 2021, and increased 2.4 percent from February 2021 to February 2022.

It is correct that the list price, or the wholesale acquisition cost, does not account for rebates or discounts. In contrast, a drug's net price equals the manufacturer's revenues after accounting for all rebates and discounts.

Question. What is causing the disparity between list price and net price, and how might we address this problem?

Answer. The increasing difference between list and net price points to the growing use of discounts and rebates. To address this problem, discounts and rebates should be passed on to the consumer by calculating co-pays and coinsurance based on the net price, rather than the list price as it is now. While this change would almost certainly lead to increased premiums Part D premiums, those increases are likely to be minimal as the cost increase would be spread across all beneficiaries. On the other hand, the reduced cost-sharing expenses that the highest-cost beneficiaries would see should outweigh those premium cost increases, resulting in a net benefit to patients. Those patients with the highest costs would see the greatest benefit.

Question. Does capping the annual rise in the price of a drug despite market fluctuations create a perverse incentive for companies to introduce new products at a higher list price?

Answer. Yes. Faced with restrictions on future pricing flexibility, drug makers would be incentivized to increase initial launch prices in response to inflation penalties. While these products would eventually be subject to HHS's price-setting regime, those forced price concessions would not take effect until years after the product's launch, further incentivizing manufacturers to maximize initial profits through higher launch prices.

Questions Submitted by Hon. John Barrasso

Question. As a doctor, I have seen firsthand the value innovative medicines provide to folks across Wyoming. When we make policy here in Washington,

---

392 https://www.drugchannels.net/2021/01/surprise-brand-name-drug-prices-fell.html?msclkid=a3589045b9c411ec98796a22a1fffbde.

it is critical we preserve the incentives for cutting-edge therapies to come to market so folks can live longer and healthier lives.

That being said, I have concerns about the high list prices—particularly for long- established drugs. Insulin is one example. This is a life-saving drug that has been part of medical practice for decades.

Though negotiated discounts and rebates can reduce the net price for drugs like insulin, some patients' copays continue to climb as list prices tick higher.

What are the best solutions to lower the price patients pay at the pharmacy counter for insulin?

Answer. Copays should be decoupled from the list price and rebate reforms should be considered to pass savings to patients at the point of sale. The reduced cost-sharing expenses that the highest-cost beneficiaries would see should outweigh premium cost increases, resulting in a net benefit to patients.

Question. We have heard some discussion about the impact of inflation today. Inflation is at a 40-year high, and there is no question it is hurting families in Wyoming and across our country. The cost of everything people buy from the food at the grocery store to the gasoline in their cars has gone through the roof.

At the beginning of this week, a gallon of gas sold for the highest price ever.

I'm a doctor, and I want patients paying less for their prescription drugs and all their medical care.

But right now the biggest worry for families in Wyoming is how will they buy food and fill up their tank.

Can you discuss the impact of rising energy prices on inflation?

Answer. Rising energy prices (currently 32 percent year-over-year) are a direct component of increases in the Consumer Price Index (CPI) and show up in inflation. However, rising energy costs are an important supply shock that makes the provision of goods and services more costly in general. These additional costs are passed along to consumers as well, leading to broad-based inflationary pressures.

Question. Before coming to the Senate I practiced orthopedic surgery for over 20 years. During my surgical training, I got to know many patients with Duchenne muscular dystrophy.

These young boys and their families made a lasting and personal impact on me. The sad fact was when I practiced medicine, there were no approved treatments for Duchenne's. This is why I helped host the Jerry Lewis telethon in Wyoming for many years.

In fact, the first FDA approved treatment for Duchenne's did not become available until well after I joined the Senate in 2016. For families impacted by Duchenne's, this first approval was a beacon of hope.

Now, thanks to American scientific innovation, there are multiple FDA approved therapies for Duchenne's. We have not cured this disease, but we are making important progress.

As a doctor, I am passionate about ensuring the progress continues. According to the Food and Drug Administration, there are over 7,000 rare diseases that impact over 30 million Americans. While we all want to lower the price of prescription drugs, we must ensure patients can access the next generation of life-changing medications.

Can you please discuss the importance of maintaining investments in scientific research, especially with regard to supporting investments in therapies that address conditions that impact smaller patient populations?

Answer. A historic example that demonstrates this is the hepatitis C treatment, Sovaldi. While the drug was quite expensive—it contributed over $3 billion to 2014 expenditures alone—Sovaldi (and its eventual competitors) provided a cure for what had been up until that point a costly to manage chronic disease. Second, as competitors joined the market, the price of Sovaldi was cut in half. Policies in the BBBA aimed specifically at drugs with particularly high prices threaten to upend incentives for the most innovative new medical treatments, which often by their very nature are more expensive to develop and produce, and increasingly serve smaller patient populations. According to Philipson and Durie, therapies that treat diseases of the endocrine, cardiovascular, and respiratory systems along with treatments for cancer and neurological diseases would be most impacted by the BBBA's policies because they make up a high share of Medicare spending.[393]

Question. We have heard a lot of discussion about the government negotiating prices for prescription medications. Many Democrats on this committee seem to believe they can lower prescription drug cost by giving more control over prescription drugs to the Department of Health and Human Services.

As a former Director of the Congressional Budget Office (CBO), could you please help us move past the rhetoric and understand how the Medicare Part D program actually works.

---

[393] https://cpb-us-w2.wpmucdn.com/voices.uchicago.edu/dist/d/3128/files/2021/08/Issue-Brief-Drug-Pricing-in-HR-5376-11.30.pdf.

Specifically, can you discuss what kinds of negotiations currently take place between prescription drug plans and pharmaceutical companies right now?

Answer. In Part D, direct negotiation by the HHS Secretary has been expressly forbidden, yet the program nevertheless sees aggressive negotiation over the prices of medications between Part D plan sponsors and drug manufacturers. This competitive process is the key factor in the program's success to date. Today, Part D beneficiaries have access to 54 plans, on average, enabling individuals to choose a plan that is tailored to their needs.[394] Because there are a number of plan options for beneficiaries, individual plans have the ability to use preferential tiering strategies to negotiate discounts for specific drugs. If a beneficiary requires or desires a specific medication that is not on the preferred formulary (or covered at all) for one plan, they can choose to sign up for a different plan that provides the medication at a more desirable price.

Question. Historically, can you review the impact these negotiations have had on the overall cost of Medicare Part D, especially compared to the original cost estimates of the program?

Answer. Total program expenditures for Part D came in far lower than initial CBO projections by about 48 percent. That being said, Medicare Part D is still in need of reform to realign incentives by placing greater financial risk on insurers and drug manufacturers and protecting beneficiaries from catastrophic financial risk.

Question. Finally, can you discuss how the Congressional Budget Office has viewed the removal of the so-called "noninterference" clause in terms of its overall budgetary impact?

Answer. The CBO has long held that simply removing this "noninterference" clause would not result in any savings for the program because the secretary has no beneficiaries to negotiate on behalf of, and no leverage for driving price concessions. Giving the HHS Secretary the legal authority to negotiate directly with manufacturers will either result in a single negotiated price for each drug—which will then have to be accepted by all insurers—thus undermining the competitive structure of Part D, or it will result in nothing.

---

[394] https://www.kff.org/medicare/issue-brief/medicare-part-d-a-first-look-at-medicare-prescription-drug-plans-in-2022/.

Question. The proposals put forward by congressional Democrats ignore the real challenge of ensuring that generics and biosimilars are able to launch and gain adoption quickly.

As a doctor, I strongly support both generics and biosimilars because I know they provide the same benefits as the branded products, but often at a much lower price.

What do you believe will be the impact of the policies in Build Back Better, specifically regarding the adoption and development of future generics and biosimilar medications?

Answer. The policies do not incentivize the adoption of generics and biosimilars; in fact, they reduce the incentive for these drugs to even be developed because the artificially lowered price of brand-name drugs would make naturally low-cost generics less competitive.

Prepared Statement of Steffany Stern, MPP, Vice President of Advocacy, National Multiple Sclerosis Society

Chairman Wyden, Ranking Member Crapo, and members of the committee, thank you for the opportunity to testify at this important hearing. My name is Steffany Stern, and I am the vice president of advocacy for the National Multiple Sclerosis Society. I joined the Society as a staff member 7 years ago, but have been part of the MS community since I was a year old, in 1981, when my mom, Joan, was diagnosed with MS.

My mom's diagnosis has shaped nearly all aspects of my life. I watched as she dealt with the physical challenges of this devastating disease, the emotional ramifications of living with constant uncertainty about her future, and decades of financial burden. MS, like so many other chronic health conditions, is a family disease, and it hasn't been easy for any of us.

We have come a long way since my mom was diagnosed, on her 24th birthday. My family is incredibly grateful for research innovation and the collaboration of research that has been funded by the public, the Society, and industry that led to it. In the 1980s and half of the 90s, all my mom could do to treat her MS was take vitamins, try to take care of herself, and hope that her relapses didn't take too much away from her life, in the short term or the long term. But once the MS disease-modifying therapies (which we refer to as DMTs) came to market, she's been able to take four of them, all of which have helped her manage the course of her disease.

Today, evidence shows that early and ongoing treatment with a DMT is the best way to manage the MS disease course, prevent accumulation of disability, and protect the brain from damage due to MS. There are now more than twenty DMTs on the market, including generic options, and these medications have transformed the treatment of MS over the last 29 years. When a person is diagnosed with relapsing forms of MS, they can choose between several effective medications to manage the course of their disease. Or, more accurately—they can make that choice if they can afford it. It is unconscionable that in 2022, people with MS and other health conditions who cannot pay for their medications would be in the same position my mom was in during the 1980s: left with no treatment option. For those who cannot afford their medications, all this innovation is simply meaningless.

The Society's vision is a world free of MS and our mission is that we will cure MS while empowering people affected by MS to live their best lives. To achieve this mission, we work with all companies, organizations and individuals that share our goal. On average, financial support from pharmaceutical companies over the last 5 years has accounted for less than 5 percent of Society income. The Society independently develops public policy positions on issues that are important to people affected by MS, and we do not accept pharmaceutical support for our advocacy work. Additional detailed information on our financial relationships with the pharmaceutical sector can be found on the Society's website (https://www.nationalmssociety.org/About-the-Society/Financials/Sources-of-Support/Pharmaceutical-Support).

Every day the Society hears from people struggling to afford their medication, making hard choices as families and too often going without medication for days, or months, or even stopping their treatment all together. I am grateful for the chance to share some of their experiences with you today.

What Is Multiple Sclerosis (MS)?

MS is an unpredictable, often disabling disease of the central nervous system that disrupts the flow of information within the brain, and between the brain and body. Symptoms vary from person to person and range from numbness and tingling, to walking difficulties, fatigue, dizziness, pain, depression, blindness, and paralysis. Nearly 1 million Americans live with this disease, and most people are diagnosed between the ages of 20 and 50, when they are in their prime working years. The progress, severity and specific symptoms of MS in any one person cannot yet be predicted but advances in research and treatment are leading to better understanding and moving us closer to a world free of MS.

MS is a highly expensive disease. The average total cost of living with multiple sclerosis is $88,487 per year.[395] The total estimated cost to the U.S. economy is $85.4 billion per year.[396] Disease-modifying therapies are the biggest cost of living with the disease, with individuals with MS spending an average of $65,612 more on medical costs than individuals who don't have MS.

Prices are too high and still rising—even for drugs that have been on the market for decades.

The full range of MS DMTs represent various mechanisms of action and routes of administration with varying efficacy, side effects and safety profiles. No single agent is "best" for all people living with MS[397] and, as MS presents differently in each person, every person's response to a DMT will vary. It is common for people with MS to move through several different DMTs throughout their life with MS, as they may "break-through" on a medication, or have disease activity, and need to try a different DMT.

With all this progress, people diagnosed today have the potential of a better course of MS than my mom. Yet, the price of these medications makes them out- of-reach for a growing number of people in the MS community.

While not identical, most brand MS DMTs have seen similar pricing trajectories. The price of MS therapies has dramatically risen since the first MS disease-modifying therapy was approved in 1993. When the first MS DMT came to market, the price range was $8,000 to $11,000 for one year of treatment. The annual median price for MS DMTs has increased nearly $34,000 in less than 10 years. As of February 2022 (see appendix), the median annual price of the brand MS DMTs is close to $94,000. Six of the MS DMTs have increased in price more than 200 percent since they came on market, with nine now priced at over $100,000. This trajectory is not sustainable for people with MS or the U.S. health-care system as a whole. Recent analysis of the MS

---

[395] B. Bebo et al. "A Comprehensive Assessment of the total economic burden of multiple sclerosis in the United States." ECTRIMS 2021. 15, October, 2021. *https://ectrims2021.abstract server.com/program/#/details/presentations/557.*

[396] B. Bebo et al. "A Comprehensive Assessment of the total economic burden of multiple sclerosis in the United States." ECTRIMS 2021. 15, October, 2021. *https://ectrims2021 .abstract server.com/program/#/details/presentations/557.*

[397] MS Coalition. "The Use of Disease Modifying Therapies in Multiple Sclerosis: Principles and Current Evidence." *http://www.nationalmssociety.org/getmedia/5ca284d3-fc7c-4ba5-b005-ab 537d495c3c/DMT_Consensus_MS_Coalition_color.* Accessed December 26, 2018.

DMTs shows that price increases of brand name drugs are largely driven by year-over-year price increases of drugs that are already in the market versus new products.[398]

My mom's first medication, Betaseron, came on the market in 1993 priced at $11,532. That same medication is now priced at $111,721. It has increased in price by $100,000 since it came to market. And this medication is nearly 30 years old and has not been improved, and is the same medication it was back then.

Generics alone will not improve the affordability of or access to MS medications.

Generic medications play a critical role in prescription drug affordability, yet generics for specialty drugs, like MS DMTs, are still unaffordable for many patients. These generics are often covered by health plans, including Medicare plans, more like specialty medications rather than other generics, still resulting in high cost sharing for people with MS. The brand product, despite its higher price, can receive favorable or equal treatment in specialty tiers, which disincentives the use of the lower-cost generic alternatives.

Generics are relatively new to the MS market, but the addition of generics to the MS class has not driven down the cost of DMTs substantially, as would be expected in a normal competitive market. When including generics, the median price of MS DMTs only falls to $80,412 a year and our experience with MS generics has demonstrated that they present their own unique set of access issues. Our experience has solidified our belief that we cannot rely on generics alone to improve affordability for people with MS. Congress must play a role in ensuring access to these lower-cost medications.

As detailed in the 46brookyn report "Wreck-fidera: How Medicare Part D has hidden the benefits of generic competition for a blockbuster Multiple Sclerosis treatment," in the third quarter of 2021, Medicare Part D plans covering most U.S. seniors didn't even make the generic equivalent to Tecfidera available, and only offered them the brand-name Tecfidera.[399] The generic system worked as it should have, and within a few months of Tecfidera going generic, more than 10 generic drug manufacturers were able to bring

---

[398] Hernandez, Inmaculada et al. "The Contribution of New Product Entry Versus Existing Product Inflation in the Rising Cost of Drugs." *Health Affairs.* Vol. 38, No. 1. *https://doi.org/ 10.1377/hlthaff.2018.05147.*

[399] 46brooklyn. "Wreck-fidera: How Medicare Part D has hidden the benefits of generic competition for a blockbuster Multiple Sclerosis treatment." December 1, 2021. *https://www.46brooklyn.com/research/2021/12/1/tecfidera.* Accessed March 10, 2022.

generic equivalents to the market; however, incentives within Part D made access to these lower-cost alternatives challenging at best.

The Society has seen this same dynamic play out in private plans as well. We have heard directly from people with MS and MS health-care providers that some people do not have access to MS generics or are unable to afford the cost-share of their generic MS DMT—which may still be several hundred dollars each month. It can also be more difficult to obtain patient assistance funds for generic medications, which leaves people with MS and health-care providers few choices. When generics are unaffordable, people with MS may switch to a different DMT, one that is higher cost to the system but may have a lower out-of-pocket cost for the person with MS due to insurance design or available patient assistance supports. *The Part D redesign proposed by Congress is the right first step in addressing the distorted incentives for prescription drug plans that leads to lower generic uptake.* Additionally, as there is still limited evidence around real-world utilization of specialty generics, we urge Congress to ensure access to lower cost generics and biosimilars by creating a specific generic and biosimilar formulary tier in Medicare Part D and prescription drug plans.

MS DMT prices are staggering, and are directly linked to unaffordable out-of-pocket costs for people living with MS.

As the prices of MS DMTs increase, health plans and pharmacy benefit managers (PBMs) with little ability to negotiate better prices employ increasingly strict utilization management practices (prior authorization, step therapy and formulary restrictions) to minimize their use and cost liability for these therapies instead. These practices present significant hurdles for prescribers and real barriers for people with MS. Utilization management tools can result in delays or disruptions in treatment as patients wait for their health plan to determine whether they will cover care as prescribed. Any delay or disruption in treatment is particularly problematic for people with MS as delays may result in worse health outcomes, increased health-care costs over time and disease progression that cannot be reversed.

Every day, people with MS and other chronic conditions must make impossible decisions when their doctor prescribes them a medication that is high-priced.

Since I joined the Society 7 years ago, I have heard too many stories about the hardships associated with drug costs to possibly be able to count. I have heard of people making excruciating choices that affect not only their lives, but the lives of everyone they care about—just to be able to pay what they owe to take their medications. I'm not exaggerating when I say that for many people with MS, the thought

of being without their medication is terrifying. Any time that lapses because a person is not taking their medication could mean disease progression, and that could mean a loss of mobility that becomes permanent. It could mean losing the ability to walk, to run, to live independently, to remember the moments you want to re- member, to live your life the way you want to live it.

People with MS take numerous medications, in addition to their DMTs, to manage their MS symptoms. The increasing costs of prescription drugs create numerous access challenges for people with MS, which can be financially devastating, and creates constant stress for people who already live with the uncertainty and challenges of a chronic health condition.

Like Laurie from Oregon, who had to change her MS medication twice after joining Medicare because the out-of-pocket cost of her original DMT would have bankrupted her and her husband. During these changes, Laurie's MS symptoms increased substantially, and she transitioned from the relapsing form of MS to a progressive form of the disease. In Laurie's words, "I'm furious about this. I've been living in fear about access to my DMTs in the future, at a time I am losing ground with my disease."

Therese in Indiana was forced to change DMTs after the costs for hers soared to $6,000 a month. But the next DMT didn't work for Therese; her MS progressed, bringing lingering cognitive issues, some dizziness and tingling in her hands and feet. By the time Therese had to switch to a different DMT, she had already burned through her savings.

Or Kenya in Louisiana, who occasionally rations medicine or skips it all together if she can't cover her Medicare out-of-pocket cost.

Every day, Bob in Minnesota and Diane in Wisconsin roll the dice. They each made the difficult decision to completely stop taking their MS DMT once they went on Medicare because they didn't want to financially devastate their fami- lies. For several years now, each has been without a DMT.

Sadly, these stories are not unique. In a 2019 survey of people with MS about their experience with their DMTs, more than half of those surveyed said they were concerned about being able to afford their DMT over the next few years and 40 percent had altered the use of their DMTs due to cost, with some skipping or delaying treatment.[400]

---

[400] National Multiple Sclerosis Society. "Quantifying the Effect of the High Cost of DMTs." Mar- ket Research Report. August 2019. *https://www.nationalmssociety.org/National*

Additionally, 40 percent stated that they experience stress or other emotional impact due to high out-of-pocket costs and are making lifestyle sacrifices to be able to pay for their DMT. This snapshot of real-world experiences shows why 85 percent of those surveyed said that the Federal Government should do more to control the high costs of MS DMTs.[401]

What does it really mean when we say people are making lifestyle sacrifices? It can range quite a bit, but in our survey[402] people reported:

- Spending less on entertainment and dining out,
- Saving less for future (college or retirement),
- Using a credit card more often,
- Spending less on their family,
- Spending less on groceries,
- Postponing paying other bills,
- Postponing retirement, and
- Working a second job.

A couple of real-life examples of these sacrifices include:

Lisa in Michigan told us her out-of-pocket medication expenses average approximately $9,000/year, and on a fixed income, these expenses are quite debilitating. She often uses her charge cards to cover the costs and relies on her family to pay for her food as well as other living expenses. She could not get coverage for the new, efficacious DMT she was prescribed and had to switch to a more financially accessible medication because she could not afford her copay.

And Wayne, a senior in South Carolina, who still owns and operates a small business, now takes around $13,000 out of his 401(k) account every year to pay his Medicare out-of-pocket costs.

Holly in New Mexico, who doesn't want to have to choose whether her family eats or she gets her medication.

MSSociety/media/MSNationalFiles/Advocacy/NMSS-Research-Report-Full-Access-to-MS-Medications.pdf. (Accessed April 27, 2021).

401 National Multiple Sclerosis Society. "Quantifying the Effect of the High Cost of DMTs." Market Research Report. August 2019. *https://www.nationalmssociety.org/ National MSSociety/media/MSNationalFiles/Advocacy/NMSS-Research-Report-Full-Access-to-MS-Medications.pdf.* (Accessed April 27, 2021).

402 National Multiple Sclerosis Society. "Quantifying the Effect of the High Cost of DMTs." Mar- ket Research Report. *https://www.nationalmssociety.org/NationalMSSociety/media/MSNationalFiles/Advocacy/NMSS-Research-Report-Full-Access-to-MS-Medications.pdf.* August 2019. (Accessed March 10, 2022.)

Many people with MS must rely on financial assistance from drug manufacturers to pay their out-of-pocket costs so they can afford to get their medication.

A key piece of the prescription drug access puzzle for many people with MS comes in the form of patient assistance funding. Seventy percent of people with MS have relied on patient assistance programs to be able to afford and stay on their disease-modifying treatment. The Society believes that the current status quo which makes medications largely unaffordable without patient assistance programs is unsustainable and in many ways, harmful to people with MS.

Reliance on patient assistance programs places undue stress and burden on people who rely on life-changing medications. Individuals are particularly challenged when they transition to Medicare, where patient assistance programs from manufacturers are not allowed. Charitable foundations exist for Medicare beneficiaries to apply to for some assistance affording their medication, but the need is far greater than supply. From 2018 to 2020, the various nonprofit programs serving Medicare beneficiaries with MS opened only 16 to 20 times for just a total of 87 to 98 days out of the entire year—approximately 25 to 30 percent of the year. In 2021, these funds opened only four times, for just 25 days out of the year. And to date in 2022, the funds opened only once in January, for just 3 days.

This is a nerve-wracking process for Medicare beneficiaries with MS, as an individual has to apply every year for the assistance, and it is never guaranteed even if life circumstances remain constant. People with MS often experience debilitating fatigue and cognitive challenges as common symptoms, setting them up to fail in a system that requires them to repeatedly call different assistance programs and hope to get through on a day where funds are available. This process compounds the stress and anxiety people with MS face on top of already managing a lifelong chronic condition.

Ms. Dixon from Ohio relies on these nonprofit foundations to help cover her Medicare out-of-pocket expenses—about $2,000 for a monthly supply of her DMT. She describes having to call the various 1–800 numbers each year and ask if they are helping people. In 2019, she didn't get there in time, and went several months without her DMT until she was finally able to find assistance. She is frustrated by the system, saying "I didn't ask for this disease. Why should we, as people who worked all our lives, pay so much for medicine, when we're on a fixed income and you know that we can't pay for it?"

Kenya from Louisiana calls out the need to reapply each year, and since it can take several months for approval, she has to remember to apply early or risk a disruption in her treatment. Kenya says it is challenging because she has to have the energy and mental clarity to navigate and track the complex approval process.

My mom is among the group of people living with MS who could not access her medication without charitable assistance. Her current medication has a list price of nearly $104,000. I talked to my parents, and they said that right away in January, they face a bill of $5,000 a month for my mom's medication. Her Medicare Advan- tage Part D plan pays $2,600 of that and charitable assistance pays $2,400, and the charitable assistance continues covering her out-of-pocket throughout the year. My parents painstakingly select their plans every year to find one with the best cov- erage for their medications and health-care providers and yet somehow, this is their best option. They cannot pay thousands of dollars a month, for months on end, between my mom's Social Security Disability Insurance, my dad's Social Security check, and the hourly wage he makes driving a city bus to make ends meet. When my mom went onto this medication she now takes, my parents called and called through a list of charitable funds I got from the National MS Society, finding them all to be closed and not accepting new patients; my dad remained persistent and with some good timing, he finally got the assistance they needed. The process of seeking and finding assistance is immensely stressful and uncertain, requiring time and diligence. Luckily, my dad got through and got what they needed to access my mom's drugs. People like my parents should not have to face this process just to fill her most-necessary prescription. The patient assistance should not be necessary in the first place. If my parents cannot secure that assistance, my mom is unable to continue to take her drug. They also struggle to afford the medications my dad— a 40+ year care partner and now senior with chronic health conditions—takes each month; he anticipates having to pay around $4,000 out of pocket for his medications this year.

Health-care costs have been a cause of stress and a burden for my parents since my mom was diagnosed. They were small-business owners for decades and my mom's care has always been a major line-item in their budget. I'll never forget the day he started looking at the costs he would have to pay out-of-pocket as he was transitioning to Medicare; he told me over the phone, "Steffany, I can't afford Medicare." My parents are on a fixed income and live in a very small town, but even in a low cost-of-living area, their health-care costs are unsustainable for them on Social Security. My dad is 69 years old with his own health challenges and had to get a job driving a city bus in their town, to pay their bills, and they have had to cut every possible corner—even moving to a smaller home and getting less- expensive cars. I try to help out however I can, but this is a situation no one should have to be in—health care and drug costs making retirement security out of reach.

It is not enough to only address out-of-pocket costs. People with MS need drug pricing reform.

Congressional action to address drug pricing would have the real-life impact of reducing what people with MS pay for medicines. An out-of-pocket cap and smoothing mechanism would be transformative for people who rely on Medicare to get their medications. Right now, too many people with MS and other health conditions pay much more than they can afford, and some even make the decision to go off their life-changing medications. Recent analysis confirms their experience. Cumulative annual out-of-pocket spending for Medicare beneficiaries with MS just for their MS DMT was $6,894 in 2019, including an average of $352 in out-of-pocket cost per month for those already in the catastrophic coverage phase.[403] We strongly support the concept of capping out-of-pocket costs and restructuring the Medicare Part D program to reduce beneficiaries' out-of-pocket costs. As noted above, Medicare beneficiaries living with MS have high out-of-pocket costs and typically reach the catastrophic phase early in the year. Under current law, once they reach the catastrophic phase in Part D, they are still responsible for 5 percent of the costs of their medications. These reforms would have an immediate impact on improving affordability of medications, upon implementation.

But to truly improve affordability and access to MS medications, we believe that the price of the medications must be addressed. Given the escalating prices of the MS DMTs, we support provisions that would limit how much pharmaceutical companies can increase drug prices each year. Last year, when the Society was analyzing drug prices of MS therapies, we found that five MS DMTs had increased in price by more than 30 percent. MS therapies are also incredibly expensive, so even smaller increases of 3 or 4 percent have a noticeable impact. With co-insurance very common for specialty medications like the MS DMTs, the list prices are directly linked to increased out-of-pocket costs for people with MS. Medicare is the single

---

403 Daniel M. Hartung, Kirbee A. Johnson, Adriane Irwin, Sheila Markwardt, and Dennis N. Bourdette, "Trends in Coverage for Disease-Modifying Therapies for Multiple Sclerosis in Medi- care Part D." *Health Affairs*. February 2019, Vol. 38, No.2.

largest payer of MS-related costs in the United States, and as such the high prices for the DMTs mean higher costs across the entire system.[404]

The Society has had a comprehensive set of recommendations on actions to address the high cost of MS DMTs since 2016, and one of those recommendations is to allow Medicare to negotiate the prices of prescription drugs. The Medicare program consistently spends around $5 billion on MS DMTs.[405] Allowing Medicare to potentially negotiate for lower DMT prices could result in significant cost savings for both the program and people affected by MS, who would pay lower out of pocket costs and less for their premiums.

The Society supports—and people with MS need—meaningful innovation.

There is a narrative that drug prices reflect innovation and allowing Medicare to negotiate drug prices will result in fewer new products on market. This narrative is flawed. We believe that people with MS should not have to face a choice between unaffordable medications and supporting innovation.

The innovation argument cannot explain why six MS DMTs have increased in price more than 200 percent since coming to market, nor can it justify medications still increasing in price more than 20 years after entering the market. Rather, these experiences directly point to the need for inflationary rebates. Further, the innovation narrative does not align with direct statements from biotech leaders who were involved in MS DMT pricing or marketing in an article published in 2019.[406]12 This Society-funded study suggested that the price ecosystem, overall corporate growth, international pricing disparities and supply chain-related distortions may play a more central role in drug pricing decisions than innovation. Those interviewed indicated that strategy related to initial list pricing focused on the prices of competitors in the therapeutic area. While one participant described the need to recoup development costs and incentive investments as reasons for price increases, more common responses cited corporate growth as more of a driver for price increases.

Follow-on products that simply build on previous products should not be priced as first-in-class therapies. We have seen this first-hand in MS where there are multiple treatment options, many of which have little or no

---

[404] Hartung D.M. "Economics and Cost-Effectiveness of Multiple Sclerosis Therapies in the USA." *Neurotherapeutics*. 2017;14(4):1018–1026. doi:10.1007/s13311–017–0566–3.

[405] 2019 Data from Medicare Part D and Part B Spending Dashboard. (Accessed May 7, 2021.

[406] Daniel Hartung, Lindsey Alley, Kirbee Johnston, and Dennis Bourdette. "Qualitative study on the price of drugs for multiple sclerosis." *Neurology*. 2019; 00:1–8. Doi: 10.1212/WNL.0000 000000008653.

innovation associated with the agent, but are all priced similarly. We believe there is a place for improved products to provide additional options for patients, but they must be priced appropriately and not as "first-in-class" innovation.

Despite the influx of successful DMTs in the MS space in the past 29 years, more is needed because we still don't have a cure for this disease. While we have more than 20 DMTs to treat relapsing forms of MS, we have limited options for treating progressive MS. The Society is leading collaboration in this space. In 2014, we partnered with five other MS organizations to establish what is known today as the International Progressive MS Alliance, which has advanced the development of treatment for progressive MS by removing scientific and technological barriers. Currently, this Alliance includes members of MS organizations from Australia, Belgium, Canada, Denmark, Germany, Italy, the Netherlands, Spain and the United Kingdom, as well as the MS International Federation.

It will take continued partnership from all stakeholders to move us to "best-in- class" products for both relapsing forms of MS and progressive MS. This type of innovation is happening every day and people with MS need true innovation to develop a cure. Innovation will allow for more treatments with different mechanisms, will provide novel solutions and drive better outcomes for people with MS. These are the incentives that must drive the development of novel solutions for people with MS—not supply-chain distortions or international pricing disparities. It is vital that we maintain an environment that creates opportunities to take the scientific and financial risks needed to drive development of treatments that can have life- changing benefits.

We believe Medicare negotiation will not limit innovation but has the potential to drive innovation and make space for the next wave of innovative treatments. For example, an exciting development in the MS therapy pipeline is a group of treatments known as Bruton's tyrosine kinase inhibitors, or BTKi. BTKi is important for the activity and survival of antibody-producing B-cells. These immune cells are thought to be one of the key drivers of brain and spinal cord inflammation in people living with MS. This is a brand-new line of treatment, and this class of inhibitors can act on immune cells in peripheral circulation, but also directly on cells within the brain and the spinal cord to reduce inflammation. The treatments have shown great promise in Phase 2 clinical trials and now there are multiple Phase 3 clinical trials for various BTKi molecules in both relapsing and progressive forms of MS. There's optimism that this approach may stop MS progression, but we won't know until the trials are completed. This is the kind of innovative therapies we need in the MS space and this type of innovation should be rewarded in the market. As stated previously, people must be able to afford and access innovation for it to have impact. In our health-care system, as products reach the end or pass their life cycle, prices should stagnate and decrease to free health-care dollars for the next wave of innovation. We believe that Medicare negotiation has a role in this cycle and the potential to promote uptake of truly innovative products.

My mom is one of the 85 percent of people with MS across the United States who want the Federal Government to do more to control the high cost of MS medications.

The Society urges the members of this committee to work together in a bipartisan fashion and pass meaningful reform that will lower the price of medications and out-of-pocket costs for people with MS. We appreciate that there are fundamental differences of opinion in the role of government to help facilitate lower drug prices, as well as the impact of those policies on innovation and the U.S. health-care system—but we believe that now is the time for Congress to act to make meaningful change for people with MS and millions of others who struggle to afford the medications they need to live their lives.

Medications must be affordable, and the process for getting them simple and transparent. We urge Congress to act now and allow Medicare to negotiate for prescription drugs, redesign Medicare Part D to better work for Medicare beneficiaries by capping out of pocket costs and allowing beneficiaries to smooth costs within the plan year and enact an inflationary rebate that would prevent the cost of medications from rising over the cost of inflation.

No single solution will fully address the multiple factors that work together to contribute to the high prices of medications in the U.S. We believe these policies are a good first step and will make an immediate impact on people with MS and others. *The current system does not work in the best interest for people with MS and other chronic health conditions and the status quo is not sustainable.* Medications cannot change the lives of people who need them if they cannot access them.

Patients have waited long enough. We look forward to working with Congress as it works towards enacting meaningful change for people affected by MS.

Appendix

Trends in annual price for disease-modifying therapies for multiple sclerosis; 2017 to 2022

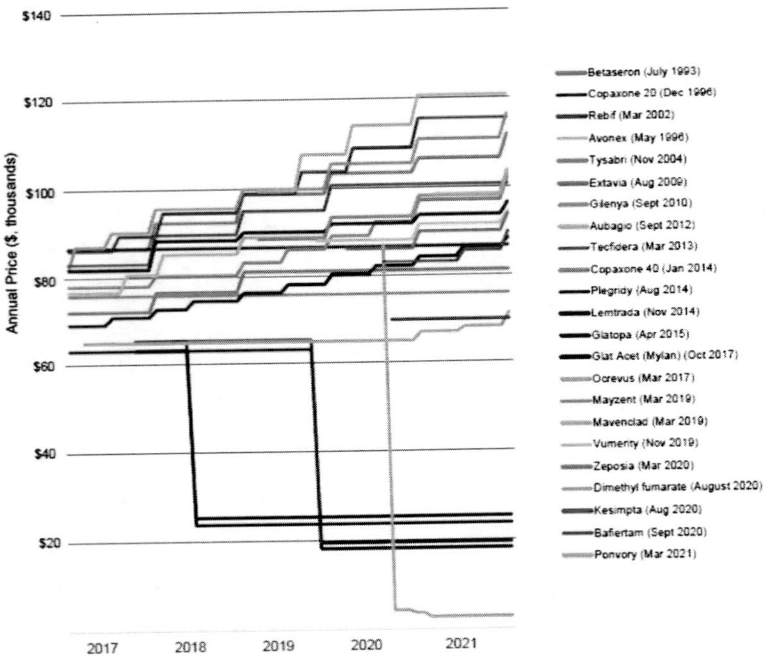

Drug (manufacturer)	5 Year Change*	5 Year CAGR**	Annual Price 2022
Self-administered Injections			
Betaseron (Bayer)	29.3%	5.2%	$111,721
Avonex (Biogen)	18.0%	3.3%	$96,482
Rebif (EMD Serono)	33.9%	5.9%	$115,359
Extavia (Novartis)	12.4%	2.3%	$81,079
Plegridy (Biogen)	18.0%	3.3%	$96,482
Kesimpta (Novartis)		5.4%	$89,765
Glatiramer Acetate			
Copaxone 20 (Teva)	0.0%	0.0%	$86,554
Copaxone 40 (Teva)	0.0%	0.0%	$75,816
Glatopa (Sandoz)	-71.1%	-21.7%	$18,250
Glatopa 40 (Sandoz)		-26.7%	$19,500
Glat Acet (Mylan)		-20.4%	$23,725
Glat Acet 40 (Mylan)		-19.8%	$25,350
S1P Receptor Modulators			
Gilenya (Novartis)	41.6%	7.1%	$116,193
Mayzent (Novartis)		5.3%	$102,938
Zeposia (Celgene)		4.7%	$93,914
Ponvory (Janssen)		5.9%	$103,660
Fumarates			
Tecfidera (Biogen)	21.3%	3.9%	$100,690
Vumerity (Biogen)		3.1%	$94,265
Bafiertam (Banner)		0.0%	$69,770
Dimethyl fumarate***		-90.0%	$2,738
Other Oral DMT			
Aubagio (Genzyme)	35.3%	6.1%	$103,643
Mavenclad (EMD Serono)		6.9%	$120,742
Infusions			
Tysabri (Biogen)	30.9%	5.4%	$102,126
Lemtrada (Genzyme)	27.7%	4.9%	$88,343
Ocrevus (Genentech)		1.9%	$71,187

Notes: Annual price estimated from wholesale acquisition costs (First Databank)
Market entrance date in parenthesis
Lemtrada is based on four 12 mg vials (Package insert dosing: 12 mg/day (5 vials) for five consecutive days in first year; 12 mg/day (3 vials) for three days in year 2)
*January 2017 to January 2022; **Compound annual growth rate (January 2017 to January 2022); ***lowest price dimethyl fumarate reported
Updated 2.15.2022 (Data through January 2022)

Questions Submitted for the Record to Steffany Stern, MPP
Question Submitted by Hon. Thomas R. Carper

Question. One population I am extremely concerned about is Medicare-only beneficiaries—especially those who are middle income and want to age in place rather than a nursing home. Programs of All-Inclusive Care or PACE should be good options for that population enabling these older adults to remain safely at home. However, the price for the PACE Part D premium is unaffordable except for the most affluent at $1,015 per month on average. I am working on a bill to reduce that cost on which I hope to work with you, Mr. Chairman.

Wouldn't this change go a long way in enabling those living with MS that are only eligible for Medicare to stay at home?

Answer. We share your concern and support Medicare beneficiaries who want to stay in their homes. Many people with MS experience a progression of symptoms throughout their disease course that results in loss of function and increasing disability over a time span of many years. We believe that the best health outcomes are achieved when people are at the center of their health care decision-making and have access to a comprehensive network of providers and health-care services that are focused on producing the best health outcomes at an affordable cost. It's essential that any care programs are able to meet all three of those elements to truly be patient-centric, and we hope your bill will address all these elements.

Question Submitted by Hon. Robert P. Casey, Jr.

Question. What alternative methodologies can lawmakers and the Secretary of HHS use, instead of QALYs, to determine drug cost and coverage?

Answer. We believe that cost-effectiveness methodologies cannot accurately measure value if they do not include patient experiences, preferences and outcomes, and QALYs are not designed to take these vital elements into account.

We would urge HHS to work with all stakeholders to develop alternative value assessment methodologies that ensure the vital elements of patient experiences, preferences and outcomes are considered.

Questions Submitted by Hon. Ben Sasse

Question. Patients are understandably more concerned with high copays for their medicines than with high list prices, which often don't reflect their actual costs.

How do you see MS patients using copay accumulator and maximizer programs?

Answer. In the Society's experience, copay accumulator and maximizer programs shift costs to people living with MS, and jeopardize their access to care. We support policies that allow copay assistance to count towards a person's deductible. Because patients are responsible for all of their health costs until their annual deductible is met, prolonging the deductible period by not counting copay assistance funds can put other medical needs financially out of reach.

Question. What impact would losing these programs have on patients' out-of- pocket costs?

Answer. As mentioned in my written testimony, many people with MS have come to rely on patient assistance funding to gain access to their medications. Seventy percent of people with MS have relied on patient assistance programs to be able to afford and stay on their disease-modifying treatment (DMTs). The out-of-pocket costs people with pay for their DMTs are simply prohibitive for many people in the MS community. If nothing is done to address the high prices of medications, out-of-pocket costs will continue to be a barrier to care for people with chronic conditions like MS. Without assistance to cover out-of-pocket costs, people with MS can struggle to adhere to their treatment plan—which can lead to worse health outcomes for them, and higher health-care costs for the system. However, assistance funding is far from a perfect solution to the problem, given how challenging it is to get into and retain access to these programs, year to year.

Question. How are you considering these patient assistance programs in the framework of broader reforms to insurance benefit design?

Answer. We believe that the system should be reformed so people with MS and other chronic health conditions do not have to rely on financial assistance to afford access their medications. However, we believe that reforms to the prescription drug and health-care system must come first, before making any changes that affect financial assistance. Jeopardizing patient access to financial assistance would mean more people are unable to access their medications. Until real solutions are put into place, this assistance must remain available.

Prepared Statement of Hon. Ron Wyden, U.S. Senator from Oregon

The Finance Committee meets this morning because there is nothing in our health-care system as broken as the way America pays for lifesaving medications like insulin. That failed system has forced millions of Americans to make daily gut-wrenching decisions between medicines or other necessities of life.

Drug companies have got Americans over a barrel. With Medicare barred from ne- gotiating better prices, this program that represents tens of millions of seniors and even more taxpayers has to take on big pharma with both hands tied behind its back. The consequences become clear when you contrast the prices Americans pay with the prices in other countries.

In preparation for this hearing, the Finance Committee investigated pricing data for several of the most commonly prescribed brand-name drugs in Medicare. We looked at list prices of top-selling drugs in the U.S. and in comparable Western countries, and we compared the figures from 2015 and 2020. The list includes medi- cations for conditions such as arthritis, diabetes, and cancer. In every case, the U.S. price in 2015 started higher than the international price. In every case, from 2015 to 2020, the U.S. price went up while the international price remained flat.

In 2015 Americans had been paying 2, 3, or 4 times as much as international pa- tients paid for these same medications. By 2020 that gap had roughly doubled for many of the most expensive drugs.

Here's a specific example. I'm holding a Humira pen that contains one dose. Humira is primarily a treatment for rheumatoid arthritis, Crohn's disease, and other autoimmune conditions—painful diseases that afflict millions of Americans. Patients typically inject one of these pens every 2 weeks. As of 2020, the price per pen in Quebec, Canada was $563. List price in the U.S. was $2,778.

Americans see this infuriating price gouging, and it's clear that big pharma is treating Medicare like they've cracked an ATM. Prescription drugs in Medicare may be the only case across the entire government where negotiating a better price is legally prohibited. It is long past time for that to change.

Democrats have a plan that would finally allow Medicare to negotiate for lower prices for brand-name drugs, focusing on the costliest products that monopolize the market. In addition, our plan would cap co-pays for insulin at

$35 a prescription. It would set a $2,000 out-of-pocket cap for seniors' medications in Medicare Part D and spread those costs over the year instead of front-loading them in January. It would also create a tough new price-gouging penalty for drug companies that raise prices faster than inflation.

A number of these ideas were developed in this committee with bipartisan support, and that remains. There's no substitute for the number one reform, allowing Medicare to negotiate like any other payer. Without negotiation, the job's not done.

For example, setting out-of-pocket caps without negotiation just passes the high prices on to somebody else, usually taxpayers. That's not sustainable, and it just puts more pressure on Medicare's finances in the long run. Unfortunately for American patients, Mitch McConnell has blocked any changes, even the proposals with bipartisan support, and repeated big pharma's talking points against them.

The drug companies say that allowing negotiation is bad for the market and will spell the end of pharmaceutical innovation, but that claim doesn't hold up to scrutiny.

First of all, it's true that pharmaceutical companies do develop breakthrough treatments. It's also true that most of the so-called "new" drugs released at higher and higher prices are actually old drugs repackaged in new ways. A relatively minor tweak to an old drug—a different syringe or a change in dosage—keeps the profits rolling in.

And second, a large and growing percentage of American seniors either ration their medications or skip them entirely because they're too expensive. Almost half of cancer patients, many of them Medicare enrollees, burn through all their savings within 2 years. If the prescription drug market prices out millions of patients and bankrupts many others, how can anybody consider it to be healthy or functional?

The scandal is what's legal. Today, big pharma has a legal right to set whatever prices they wish and expect Medicare to pay them. Drug companies can game the system to maintain monopolies and protect their cash cows. And without fail, the Republican leadership controlling the agenda for their party in Congress protects the status quo. That is a recipe to stifle innovation, not promote it.

As we meet today, there are people all over the country who know they're going to get mugged every time they go to the pharmacy counter. Higher drug prices force people to have to make terrible choices. Far too often, choosing your health also means choosing hunger.

The American people have waited long enough for Congress to act. Democrats have a plan, and we need to act quickly.

Communications

AARP

601 E Street, NW Washington, DC 20049 https://www.aarp.org/.

AARP, on behalf of our 38 million members and all older Americans nationwide, appreciates the opportunity to submit testimony on this important hearing of the Senate Finance Committee, "Prescription Drug Price Inflation: An Urgent Need to Lower Drug Prices in Medicare."

High prescription drug prices hit older Americans particularly hard. On average, Medicare Part D enrollees take between four and five prescriptions per month, often for chronic conditions that will require treatment for the rest of their lives. At the same time, Medicare beneficiaries have a median annual income of just under $30,000. One-quarter have less than $8,500 in savings. This population simply does not have the resources to absorb rapidly escalating prescription drug prices and many are facing the very real possibility of having to choose between their medication and other basic needs such as food or housing.

In the case of one of our members—Larry Zarzecki from Maryland—high prescription drug prices have forced him to use his retirement savings and sell his home to afford his medications. Larry suffers from Parkinson's disease and had to retire from law enforcement 10 years ago. He first shared his story in an AARP ad three years ago. In the absence of meaningful Congressional action, his situation has only deteriorated since that time without any relief from the high cost of his treatments. Larry states, "I shouldn't have to decide between my home or my medicine because Congress refuses to act. I'm tired of waiting for Congress."

Unfortunately, Larry isn't alone. Every day we hear from older Americans who are forced to choose between paying for the medicines they need and paying for other essentials like food and heat. We know the number one reason someone does not fill a prescription is because of the cost.

For years, prescription drug price increases have dwarfed even the highest rates of general inflation. If consumer prices had risen as fast as drug prices over the last 15 years, gas would now cost $12.20 a gallon, and milk would be $13 a gallon. Just in January, the drug industry raised prices on over 800 prescription medications— just as they have increased prices for decades— including three-quarters of the top 100 spend drugs in Medicare Part D. It is wrong, particularly in the midst of a pandemic and financial crisis, that drug companies remain free to raise the prices of their products unhindered, including those for chronic conditions that people over age 50 depend on. Moreover, it is not fair or right to ask patients and taxpayers to continue spending billions of dollars on exorbitantly priced prescription drugs in a broken U.S. market.

As we look at prescription drug prices, it is important to keep in mind that high launch prices are just the beginning; drug prices typically continue to grow even after the drugs enter the market. AARP Public Policy Institute's latest Rx Price Watch report found that the retail prices for 180 widely used specialty prescription drugs increased at more than three-and-a-half times the rate of inflation in 2020.[1] And to be clear—this isn't a one-time problem. The average annual increase in retail prices for the products that we study has exceeded the corresponding rate of inflation every year since at least 2006.

Our report also found the average annual cost of therapy for a single specialty prescription drug is now over $84,000 per year. This average annual cost was almost $20,000 higher than the median US household income ($65,712); nearly three times the median income for Medicare beneficiaries ($29,650); and more than four-and-a- half times higher than the average Social Security retirement benefit ($18,530). In other words, we are now facing prescription drug prices that exceed what most people make in a year. Notably, our analysis also found that the average annual cost for a single specialty prescription drug would have been just under $40,000, or more than $45,000 lower, if retail price changes had been limited to the general inflation rate between 2006 and 2020.

AARP is also mindful that high and growing prescription drug prices are affecting all Americans in some way. Their cost is passed along to everyone with health coverage through increased health care premiums, deductibles, and other forms of cost sharing. We have also seen massive increases in prescription drug spending under public programs like Medicare and Medicaid. These escalating costs will eventually affect all of us in the form of higher health care costs, higher taxes, cuts to Medicare or Medicaid, or all of the above.

---

[1] http://www.aarp.org/rxpricewatch.

In other words: every single American taxpayer is paying for high prescription drug prices, regardless of whether you are taking medicine yourself.

Fortunately, there is action the Senate can take right now. There is long-standing and overwhelming bipartisan support among voters for allowing Medicare to negotiate with drug companies for lower prices.[2] The policies before the Senate—including Medicare negotiation, capping out of pocket costs under Medicare Part D, and penalizing drug companies that increase their prices faster than inflation—will provide long-overdue relief to older Americans across the country. These policies, taken together, will help reduce drug prices and out-of-pocket costs. This is important because real relief for seniors and all Americans must include policies that get to the root of the problem: the high prices set by drug companies.

America's seniors aren't the only ones who stand to benefit. Lowering prescription drug prices will also save the Medicare program and taxpayers hundreds of billions of dollars. Every year, Medicare spends more than $135 billion on prescription drugs. Yet it is prohibited by law from using its buying power to negotiate with drug companies to get lower prices.

Congress must not fail to achieve this historic opportunity to finally lower prescription drug prices and bring much-needed relief to seniors across the country. The nonpartisan Congressional Budget Office (CBO) estimates that the latest drug pricing provisions passed by the House would save nearly $300 billion over 10 years— this includes provisions to penalize excessive price hikes and to allow Medicare to negotiate lower drug prices.[3] The high cost of American drugs is not only unfair to seniors and families across the country, it is flagrantly fiscally irresponsible for Congress to allow the status quo to continue.

Industry lobbyists allege that lower drug prices will come at the cost of innovation. Let us be clear—AARP has no interest in solutions that will hamper true innovation. However, research has consistently demonstrated that there is no correlation between drug prices and innovation[4] and that many new drugs could be described as innovation in name only.[5] In addition, taxpayers fund much of the initial research that can lead to new drugs, and they should

---

[2] https://www.aarp.org/research/topics/health/info-2021/drug-prices-older-americans-concerns.html.

[3] https://www.cbo.gov/publication/57626.

[4] https://www.healthaffairs.org/do/10.1377/hblog20190228.636555/full/.

[5] https://www.ncbi.nlm.nih.gov/pmc/articles/PMC6534750/;https://www.gao.gov/assets/gao-18-40.pdf; and https://www.healthaffairs.org/doi/pdf/10.1377/hlthaff.2020.00328.

not be priced out of the benefits of those drugs when they come to market. Most of the important new drugs from the past 60 years were developed with the aid of public sector research.[6] For example, NIH-funded research played a role in all 210 new drugs approved between 2010 and 2016.[7] More recently, public funding helped in the development of vaccines for COVID–19, which the government was able to purchase and make affordable to the public. Finally, it is also notable that the public does not accept the drug industry's long-standing threat of reduced innovation.[8] An AARP survey found that 83 percent of Democrats, 78 percent of Republicans and 81 percent of independents said that drug prices could be lowered without harming innovation.

Current prescription drug price trends are not sustainable and action is needed now. It is unfair that Americans continue to pay the highest drug prices in the world—three times what other nations pay for the same prescription drugs. The drug industry has been price gouging seniors for too long. Enacting the policies before this committee, including allowing Medicare to negotiate, will finally deliver on the promise of lower drug prices that will help ensure that all patients have affordable access to the drugs that they need to get and stay healthy.

Alliance for Retired Americans

815 16th Street, NW, 4th Floor Washington, DC 20006
(202) 637–5399
www.retiredamericans.org

The Alliance for Retired Americans appreciates the opportunity to submit comments to the Senate Committee on Finance regarding the committee hearing entitled "Prescription Drug Price Inflation: An Urgent Need to Lower Drug Prices in Medicare." We thank Chairman Wyden and Ranking Member Crapo for holding this hearing, and are most appreciative of the witnesses for providing insightful testimony.

---

[6] https://www.cbo.gov/publication/57126 which cites to https://aspe.hhs.gov/system/files/aspe-files/263451/2020-drug-pricing-report-congress-final.pdf.

[7] https://www.pnas.org/content/115/10/2329.

[8] https://www.aarp.org/politics-society/advocacy/info-2021/survey-voters-lower-drug- prices.html.

Founded in 2001, the Alliance is a grassroots organization representing more than 4.3 million retirees and seniors nationwide. Headquartered in Washington, DC, the Alliance and its 39 state chapters work to advance public policy that strengthens the health and retirement security of older Americans.

The Alliance strongly supports efforts to eliminate waste and reduce drug costs in Medicare's prescription drug benefits plans and the system's finances overall, and opposes proposals that shift any additional costs to beneficiaries. We categorically support the fundamental goals of this hearing, namely, to demonstrate the harm that exorbitantly high prescription drug prices have on senior citizens and the American economy, and to underline the urgency of passing legislation that would permit Medicare to negotiate drug prices.

Prescription Drug Prices

Americans pay the highest prices in the world for prescription drugs, and prices on hundreds of drugs have already increased by 5% in 2022, far outpacing inflation. According to a March 29, 2021 report by the Government Accountability Office (GAO), in 2020 Americans paid two to four times more for 20 brand-named drugs than people in Canada, France and Australia. Seniors, who take the most prescription drugs to stay healthy, bear the brunt of these high prices. The Alliance disagrees with comments made by a number of Republican committee members and witness Dr. Holtz-Eakin, who stated that when compared to recent price increases on goods and services, they do not perceive prescription drug prices to be unnecessarily high.

The Alliance believes that unacceptably high prescription drug prices are unrelated to recent inflationary price spikes caused by supply chain disruptions or the war in Ukraine. Rather, excessively high drug pricing is an ongoing problem that has existed for far too long, and is exemplified by the recent Aduhelm debacle, which shows that there is no justification for such high prices. After initially launching its Alzheimer's drug, Adulhelm, at $96,000 per year, Biogen cut the price in half after controversy over the drug approval process and concerns over the safety of the drug resulted in low sales. The drug's exorbitant cost was the chief factor contributing to the highest increase in Medicare Part B premiums in recent history. The basic monthly Medicare Part B premiums jumped from $148.50 to $170.10 thus far in 2022, an unprecedented increase of 14.5%. This is obviously a most terrible burden for Medicare beneficiaries. The Alliance has called on CMS to reduce the 2022 premium rates. The Abuhelm example is a case study on how unchecked prescription drug prices affect the entire health care system, especially for older Americans who rely on Medicare.

While drug companies have defended their high launch prices and yearly price increases as needed to fund research and development, the House Oversight and Reform Committee found in a July 2021 Staff Report that the world's leading drug companies actually spent more on payouts to investors than in research and development.

Because of the terribly high cost of prescription drugs, nearly a quarter of Americans and 20% of seniors report not being able to afford their prescriptions. As a result, millions of Americans do not take their prescriptions as prescribed by their doctor and are instead not filling them, skipping doses, or taking fewer doses than directed. One poignant example was provided to the committee by Ms. Steffany Stern, who testified that her mother faced prescription drug costs of over $5,000 per month for multiple sclerosis medicine, and highlighted in her testimony that her mother is only able to afford medicine because of assistance from charities. Clearly, her mother's situation and that of the numerous Americans who find themselves in similar circumstances should not be not tolerated in a nation as wealthy and resourceful as the United States.

Allowing Medicare to Negotiate Prescription Drug Prices

In accordance with the opening statement given by Finance Committee Chairman Wyden and brilliantly laid out by Dr. Rena Conti in her testimony, the Alliance strongly believes that it is of utmost importance that the Secretary of Health and Human Services is allowed to negotiate lower drug prices under Medicare. Without prescription drug price negotiation, the status quo, where far too many senior citizens are unable to afford their prescription drugs will continue.

As Senator Wyden pointed out, "with Medicare barred from negotiating better prices, this program that represents tens of millions of seniors and even more taxpayers has to take on Big Pharma with both hands tied behind its back." Indeed, unlike the VA and Medicaid, "prescription drugs in Medicare may be the only case across the entire government where negotiating a better price is legally prohibited, and it is long past time for that to change," the Chairman continued.

According to the Congressional Budget Office and Joint Committee on Taxation's 2019 analysis,[9] Medicare price negotiation would not only assist seniors to afford their medicine, it would also save the U.S. government billions of dollars. In fact, it would lower spending by $456 billion, which would be enough to allow Medicare to cover critical needs such as dental, vision and hearing coverage.

Counter arguments frequently offered by Republicans and Pharma, which claim that allowing for price negotiations would lead to dramatic decreases in innovation, as well as government drug price controls, are terribly misguided. In reality, as Dr. Conti demonstrated in her testimony, allowing for Medicare negotiation "would not result in material reductions in innovation in the next decade and would have small effects over 30 years—one less drug the next decade and four less drugs over the subsequent decade," she points out. Moreover, there is no indication that any of the "forgone" drugs would have become innovative cures, given that only one in eight drugs generates a new therapeutic benefit. Additionally, Dr. Conti added that "most of the new pharmaceutical products (excluding generics) provided by the U.S. FDA are not new drugs at all (but rather) only 32% were new molecular entities, while the rest represent new versions of old drugs."

Patent Abuses

Another contributing factor to the causal effect of high drug prices is the abusive practice of drug companies that take advantage of the U.S. patent system. The Alliance strongly agrees with Chairman Wyden and Finance Committee Democrats, as well as Republican members who mentioned the issue of patent abuse during the hearing, and believe that legislation needs to be enacted urgently to curb these often-egregious abuses. Pharmaceutical companies use numerous tactics to extend patent terms, including the use of patent thicket, pay-for-delay agreements, parking exclusivity, evergreening and other measures that reduce competition and keep prices inflated.

Indisputably, patent extensions cost the Medicare program billions of dollars. For example, AbbVie Pharmaceutical filed over 250 patents on Humira and used patent thicket—a group of overlapping patents—to extend its patent on the drug. The extension of Abbie's patent from 2016–2019 cost the Medicare program over $2 billion. In addition, since AbbVie's patents on

[9] https://www.cbo.gov/publication/55936.

Humira were set to expire in 2017, the company reached an agreement through a pay-for-delay deal with its competitors, Novartis and Amgen, to delay the entry of those companies' biosimilars in the United States until 2023, a delay agreement that is costing American taxpayers $19 billion.

Additional Items

Lastly, the Alliance for Retired Americans strongly supports meaningful reform items in the House passed Build Back Better Act, all of which have been mentioned during this hearing and supported by Finance Committee Democrats. The most salient of these include:

- Capping co-pays for insulin at $35.
- Setting a $2,000 out of pocket cap for seniors' medications in Medicare Part D.
- Creating a new price gouging penalty for drug companies that raise prices faster than inflation.

On behalf of our more than 4.3 million members, the Alliance for Retired Americans appreciates the opportunity to submit testimony on this vitally important issue.

American College of Clinical Pharmacy

Office of Government and Professional Affairs
1455 Pennsylvania Ave., NW, Suite 400
Washington, DC 20004
(202) 621–1820
www.accp.com

The American College of Clinical Pharmacy (ACCP) appreciates the opportunity to provide the following statement to the Senate Finance Committee related to the March 16, 2022 hearing on "Prescription Drug Price Inflation: An Urgent Need to Lower Drug Prices in Medicare."

ACCP is a professional and scientific society that provides leadership, education, advocacy, and resources enabling clinical pharmacists to achieve excellence in patient care practice and research. ACCP's membership is composed of more than 17,000 clinical pharmacists, residents, fellows, students, scientists, educators and others who are committed to excellence in clinical pharmacy practice and evidence-based pharmacotherapy.

ACCP's members practice in a variety of team-based settings, including ambulatory care environments, hospitals, colleges of pharmacy and medicine, the pharmaceutical industry, government and long-term care facilities, and managed care organizations. Our focus is the optimization of medication regimens to achieve patient-centered therapeutic goals,

ACCP welcomes the growing recognition in Congress of the unique opportunity that prescription drugs offer to improve health and enhance the quality of life for millions of American patients, and the unique challenges we face in ensuring affordable access to these vital therapies.

We look forward to working with you to incentivize integration of qualified clinical pharmacists into value-based patient-care teams in order to achieve better outcomes from the medication therapies our entire health delivery system is so heavily invested in.

Achieving Medication Optimization

ACCP believes that in order to achieve a health care system that delivers better care, smarter spending, and healthier people and communities, it is vital to establish a truly team-based, patient-centered approach to health care consistent with evolving delivery and payment models currently available under private and commercial health plans.

It is estimated that $528 billion a year,[10] equivalent to 16 percent of total health care spending, is consumed due to inappropriate or otherwise ineffective medication use. Given the central role that medications play in care and treatment of chronic conditions, combined with the continuing growth in the range, complexity and cost of medications—and greater understanding of the genetic and physiologic differences in how people respond to their medications—the nation's health care system consistently fails to deliver on the full promise medications can offer.

---

[10] Watanabe, J., McInnis, T., and Hirsch, J. (2018). Cost of Prescription Drug-Related Mor- bidity and Mortality. The Annals of Pharmacotherapy, 52(9), 829–837. http://dx.doi.org/10.1177/1060028018765159 Retrieved from https://escholarship.org/uc/item/3n76n4z6.

Comprehensive medication management (CMM) is a direct patient care service, provided by clinical pharmacists working as formal members of the patient's health care team that has been demonstrated to significantly improve clinical outcomes and enhance the safety of medication use by patients.

Optimizing Specialty Drug Use

The rapidly increasing cost of many existing and newly approved specialty drugs is a major and growing concern to patients, the American public, commercial and federal payers, and health policy economists and regulators.

Specialty prescription drugs can be defined as a prescription drug that "has a total average prescription cost greater than $1,000 per prescription; or has a total average cost per day of therapy greater than $33 per day."[11] The Centers for Medicare and Medicaid Services definition of specialty drugs is also based on price—pharmaceuticals costing $600 or more per month are considered specialty drugs.[12]

ACCP believes that a patient-centered, team-based, and evidence-driven approach to CMM must be paired with emerging value-based pricing approaches to better ensure that the rational and economical use of specialty drugs is optimized both for patients and for the health care system. CMM, applied through standardized clinical practice processes is a cornerstone of interprofessional, patient-centered care that can better ensure optimized, economical specialty drug use.

ACCP urges the Committee to pursue specialty drug pricing models that ensure patients and health systems receive commensurate value from the appropriate use of specialty drugs, employ rational and transparent pricing practices, and enable pharmaceutical manufacturers to sufficiently recoup research and development (R&D) investments.[13]

---

[11] Schondelmeyer S.W., Purvis L. Rx price watch report. Trends in retail prices of specialty prescription drugs widely used by older Americans, 2006 to 2013 [research report], 2015. Available from *www.aarp.org/content/dam/aarp/ppi/2015/rx-price-watch-specialty-prescription-drug- prices-continue-to-climb-final.pdf.*

[12] Centers for Medicare and Medicaid Services (CMS). Medicare Part D specialty tier [guidance document], 2014. Available from *www.cms.gov/Medicare/Prescription-Drug-Coverage/PrescriptionDrugCovGenIn/Downloads/SpecialtyTierMethodology.pdf.*

[13] ACCP Position Statement, 2017. Optimizing Specialty Drug Use, Pharmacotherapy, 37: 973–975. *https://doi.org/10.1002/phar.1945.*

Value-based pricing models might include indication-specific pricing, bundled payments, and explicit investigations of cost, value, comparative effectiveness and safety of specialty drugs.

Implementation of Pharmacogenomics (PGx) to Achieve Medication Optimization

Pharmacogenomics (PGx) allows clinicians to assess how a patient's genetic profile determines their responses to specific medications. Appropriate diagnosis and access to advanced diagnostics like PGx testing is essential to ensure safe and effective therapy for each patient. When applied as a component of CMM, PGx ensures that a patient's medications are individually assessed to determine that each is indicated, effective, consistent with patient expectations, and safe, in view of the comorbidities present, other concurrent medications, and the patient's ability to adhere to the prescribed regimen.

When integrated into CMM, PGx testing allows for targeted treatment decisions based on the unique characteristics of the patient's unique genetic profile. The integration of PGx within CMM reduces costs, improves outcomes and access to care, and enhances patient and provider quality of life and satisfaction. To ensure medication optimization, pharmacogenomics (PGx) should be integrated into CMM.

"Cures 2.0" legislation (H.R. 6000) currently being considered by the House Committee on Energy and Commerce includes Section 408: Medicare Coverage for Precision Medicine Consultations. Section 408 would require the Secretary of Health and Human Services to create a pilot grant program within the Center for Medicaid and Medicare Innovation (CMMI) to test approaches to delivering personalized-medicine PGx consultations by qualified clinical pharmacists.

We thank the Finance Committee for tackling these serious issues related to the increasing cost of prescription medications, Medicare coverage and payment for digital health and personalized medicine infrastructure. We urge you to advance payment policy to support the integration of evolving team-based, quality-focused payment and care delivery models that shift Medicare payment policy for providers toward value of care and away from volume of services.

About "Qualified Clinical Pharmacists"

Clinical pharmacists are practitioners who provide CMM and related care for patients in all health care settings. They are licensed pharmacists with specialized, advanced education and training who possess the clinical competencies necessary to practice in team-based, direct patient care environments. Accredited residency training or equivalent post-licensure experience is necessary for entry into direct patient care practice. Board certification is also expected once the clinical pharmacist meets the eligibility criteria specified by the Board of Pharmacy Specialties (BPS). In providing CMM, they establish a valid collaborative drug therapy management (CDTM) agreement with the patient's provider or are formally granted clinical privileges within a health care practice/institution.

We would welcome the opportunity to provide additional information, data, and connections to successful practices that provide CMM/PGx services as part of this effort to optimize the use of medications in the U.S.

Summary

We thank you for the opportunity to provide input on the Finance Committee's efforts to address prescription drug price inflation and its impact on the long-term sustainability of the Medicare program.

As part of this effort, we urge you to consider efforts to modernize access to and coverage of innovative therapies and we encourage you to utilize the unique contributions of clinical pharmacists in the area of medication optimization. We welcome the growing understanding in Congress of the unique value that qualified clinical pharmacists provide in the therapeutic management of complex conditions.

ACCP is dedicated to advancing a quality-focused, patient-centered, team-based improvement in health care delivery that (1) helps assure medication optimization, (2) enhances patient safety, (3) promotes value-based rather than volume-based care, and (4) contributes to greater affordability and sustainability for the Medicare program. We look forward to working with you to help achieve these goals.

American College of Physicians

25 Massachusetts Avenue, NW, Suite 700
Washington, DC 20001–7401
202–261–4500
800–338–2746
www.acponline.org

On behalf of the American College of Physicians (ACP), we are grateful for this opportunity to share our views with the Senate Finance Committee regarding its recent hearing on the rising cost of prescription drugs and the need to lower drug prices in Medicare. We appreciate that over the past several years the Finance Committee has conducted multiple hearings and developed polices on prescription drug reforms, but we urge the Congress to act now to approve legislation to lower drug costs that may be signed into law. Our nation and patients can no longer afford to wait for Congress to act as the high cost of prescription drugs continues to strain the budget of federal and state governments and compels our patients to resort to cutting back or skipping doses of their medicines to save money, which can lead to more serious health complications. Our statement will provide this Committee with ACP's recommendations to increase access to prescription drugs in Medicare through policies that would: allow Medicare to negotiate drug prices; impose caps on out-of-pocket spending in Medicare Part D; increase competition in the prescription drug marketplace; eliminate tax deductions for direct-to-consumer drug advertising; and improve transparency regarding drug costs.

ACP is the largest medical specialty organization and the second largest physician membership society in the United States. ACP members include 161,000 internal medicine physicians (internists), related subspecialists, and medical students. Internal medicine physicians are specialists who apply scientific knowledge, clinical expertise, and compassion to the preventive, diagnostic, and therapeutic care of adults across the spectrum from health to complex illness. Internal medicine specialists treat many of the patients at greatest risk from COVID–19, including the elderly and patients with pre-existing conditions like diabetes, heart disease and asthma.

ACP remains committed to developing polices to lower the cost of prescription drugs and has published a series of papers that provide Congress with multiple options to address this issue. These papers include policy recommendations on the following topics:

- Stemming the Cost of Prescription Drugs through policies to Improve Transparency, Value, and Competition in the Marketplace[14]
- Reducing the Cost of Prescription Drugs in Public Health Plans[15]
- Recommendations for Pharmacy Benefit Managers to Stem the Escalating Cost of Prescription Drugs[16]
- Improving Competition in the Prescription Drug Marketplace.[17]

Because the topic of prescription drug pricing continues to be of interest to patients, physicians, and government officials, ACP believes policymakers should act immediately to address current issues in the Medicare and Medicaid programs that add costs to the health care system, may inadvertently incentivize higher prices for prescription drugs, and increase out-of-pocket costs for consumers.

Prescription Drug Costs Continue to Rise

The cost of prescription drugs continues to rise, which greatly affects access to life-saving treatments for patients who are unable to afford high out-of-pocket costs. Patients increasingly face higher co-pays, more drug tiers and prescription drug deductibles, adding to the burden they face in affording high-cost medications. Many Americans face the difficult choice of filling their prescriptions or paying for necessities such as food or housing.

According to a report[18] published by the Congressional Budget Office (CBO) "nationwide spending on prescription drugs increased from $30 billion in 1980 to $335 billion in 2018. (All estimates of drug spending and prices in this report are expressed in 2018 dollars.") As outlined in ACP's 2019 position paper,[19] Policy Recommendations for Public Health Plans to Stem the Escalating Costs of Prescription Drugs, the United States spends more on prescription drugs than other high-income countries, with average annual spending of $1,443 per capita on pharmaceutical drugs and $1,026 per capita

---

14 https://www.acponline.org/acp_policy/policies/stemming_rising_cost_prescription_drugs_2016.pdf.

15 https://www.acpjournals.org/doi/pdf/10.7326/M19-0013.

16 https://www.acpjournals.org/doi/10.7326/M19-0035.

17 https://www.acpjournals.org/doi/pdf/10.7326/M19-3773.

18 https://www.cbo.gov/publication/57050.

19 https://www.acpjournals.org/doi/pdf/10.7326/M19-0013.

on retail prescription drugs. In a 2021 study[20] by the RAND Corporation, it was further affirmed that prices in the United States were 256 percent higher, on average, than in 32 other countries with comparable economies and when only comparing brand-name drugs, prices in the United States were 344 percent higher.

Reports show that although use of prescription drugs in the United States is high, it is not an outlier[21] compared with nine other high-income nations. The primary differences between health care expenditures in the United States versus other high-income nations are pricing of medical goods and services and the lack of direct price controls or negotiating power by centralized government health care systems.

Allow Medicare to Negotiate Drug Prices

We appreciate that during this hearing a significant portion of the debate was devoted to examining the impact of allowing Medicare to directly negotiate the price it pays for drugs in the Medicare Part D program. According to a Kaiser Family Foundation tracking poll,[22] granting Medicare Part D the authority to negotiate drug prices is favored by a bipartisan majority of the public, with more than 90 percent of Democrats, Republicans, and Independents agreeing with this approach. Negotiating authority was also endorsed in a report[23] by the National Academies of Sciences, Engineering, and Medicine on improving the affordability of prescription drugs as part of a package of broader reforms for consolidating and leveraging pur- chasing power and strengthening formulary design.

ACP has longstanding policy supporting the ability of Medicare to leverage its purchasing power and directly negotiate with manufacturers for drug prices. We supported a provision in H.R. 3, the Elijah E. Cummings Lower Drug Costs Now Act, that would mandate that the Secretary of Health and Human Services (HHS) identify 250 brand name drugs that lack competition in the marketplace and that account for the greatest cost to Medicare and the U.S. health system and then negotiate directly with drug

---

[20] https://www.rand.org/news/press/2021/01/28.html.

[21] *https://www.commonwealthfund.org/sites/default/files/documents/media_files_publications_issue_brief_2017_oct_sarnak_paying_for_rx_ib_v2.pdf.*

[22] *https://www.kff.org/health-reform/report/kaiser-health-tracking-poll-late-april-2017-the-future-of-the-aca-and-health-care-the-budget/.*

[23] *https://pubmed.ncbi.nlm.nih.gov/29620830/.*

manufacturers to establish a maximum fair price for a bare minimum of 25 of those drugs. *In a 2019 estimate by the Congressional Budget Office,*[24] *projections indicated that $456 billion in savings over 10 years would be realized by enacting the provision in H.R. 3 to allow Medicare to directly negotiate prescription drug prices with manufacturers.*

Last November, the House passed H.R. 5376, the Build Back Better Act (BBBA), that includes a provision to allow Medicare to directly negotiate the price of some drugs provided in Medicare Part D. We remain concerned that the House-passed BBBA does not include this more robust provision of price negotiation in H.R. 3. We believe that giving HHS the authority to negotiate drug prices with manufacturers is one of the most effective ways to lower the cost of prescription drugs and we urge lawmakers to include that provision of H.R. 3 or similar legislation in the final bill.

The House-passed BBBA allows HHS to negotiate the price of 10 of the most expensive drugs by 2025 and goes up to 20 drugs by 2028 on drugs that are beyond their period of exclusivity. The bill applies an excise tax on drug manufacturers for raising prices faster than the rate of inflation, reduces out-of-pocket expenses for customers and ensures patients pay no more than $35 a month for insulin products. *While ACP reaffirms its support for a full repeal of the noninterference clause, ACP is also supportive of an interim approach, such as allowing the Secretary of HHS to negotiate for a limited set of high-cost or sole-source drugs.*

Impose Caps on Out-of-Pocket Spending in Medicare Part D

American consumers must pay less at the pharmacy counter. The Medicare Part D benefit structure leaves millions of patients exposed to extreme out-of-pocket spending, while failing to create the proper incentives to direct patients towards drugs that cost less.

ACP was pleased to support a provision in legislation that Senators Wyden and Grassley introduced in the last Congress, the Prescription Drug Pricing Reduction Act of 2019, which would cap annual out-of-pocket spending for Medicare Part D beneficiaries who reach the catastrophic phase of coverage. In addition, ACP sup- ports adoption of a cap on out-of-pocket drug costs to protect Medicare beneficiaries from excessive exposure to these costs, which is too often the case today. Although we are supportive of these

[24] https://www.cbo.gov/system/files/2019-12/hr3_complete.pdf.

policies, we urge the Committee to consider the full gamut of likely ramifications from such changes, particularly when programmatic changes of this magnitude are being put forward.

One potential result, for example, is that such a cap on beneficiary out-of-pocket costs is likely to be offset at least in part by higher premiums, unless accompanied by other measures that address the underlying reason for high out-of-pocket costs, like excessive pricing. Notable among these is the application of any cap brought about by Part D reforms should be on a quarterly as opposed to an annual basis. This will help beneficiaries better afford their medications at the time they have to pay out-of-pocket for them—rather than at the end of a full calendar year—which could be many months after they have incurred the expense. Limiting beneficiary out-of-pocket expenses on a quarterly basis will make it much less likely they will forgo needed medications because they cannot afford them.

Increase Competition in the Marketplace to Lower the Cost of Prescription Drugs

The prescription drug market in the United States relies on competition to keep prices reasonable. Although many policies have been implemented to spur competition and decrease costs for patients, these policies may be outdated and should be redesigned and updated to achieve success in the current prescription drug market.

Improve Competition in Medicare Part D Low Income Subsidy Program

ACP supports the Medicare Part D low-income subsidy program (LIS) that assists seniors with fewer resources in paying for their prescription drugs. We also support modifications to this program to encourage the use of lower-cost generic or biosimilar drugs by eliminating cost sharing for generic drugs for LIS enrollees. Twelve million Medicare Part D beneficiaries are enrolled in the LIS program. Although use of low-cost generic drugs by Part D beneficiaries is relatively high and continues to increase as more generics become available, the generic drug use rate is lower among LIS enrollees than among other Medicare beneficiaries.

Despite the current rate of generic drug dispensing among low-income subsidy (LIS) enrollees and non-LIS enrollees, additional savings are possible for Medicare and its beneficiaries. The Centers for Medicare and Medicaid Services (CMS)[25] estimates that Medicare could have saved nearly $9 billion if available equivalent generics were used instead of brand-name drugs and could have passed on $3 billion in savings to the Part D program and its beneficiaries. Reducing or eliminating cost sharing for LIS enrollees would not require legislative action because it would not increase cost sharing, would reduce overall out-of-pocket costs for LIS enrollees, and would encourage use of generics among them. Reducing or eliminating cost sharing or copayments for generic drugs could also reduce Medicare spending[26] on reinsurance payments because a majority of enrollees who reach the catastrophic phase of coverage are in the LIS program. In addition to traditional generic drugs, biosimilar cost sharing should also ensure that LIS enrollees have an incentive to choose lower-cost alternatives to brand name biologic drugs. Biosimilars have the potential to save[27] $54 billion in direct spending on biologic drugs between 2017 and 2026.

Prohibit Gaming of the Patent System

ACP supports robust oversight and enforcement of restrictions on product-hopping, evergreening, and pay-for-delay practices to increase marketability and availability of competitor products and we urge the Congress to adopt policies that will prohibit drug companies from gaming the patent system through these practices.

There are several ways in which pharmaceutical manufacturers use the existing patent system for their benefit. Companies may apply for multiple patents on a single drug, creating what has been referred to as a patent thicket,[28] a "dense web of overlapping intellectual property rights that a company must hack its way through in order to actually commercialize new technology." In an egregious example, the parent company of the biologic

---

25 https://aspe.hhs.gov/sites/default/files/private/pdf/259326/DP-Multisource-Brands-in-Part-D.pdf.

26 https://aspe.hhs.gov/sites/default/files/private/pdf/259326/DP-Multisource-Brands-in-Part-D.pdf.

27 https://pubmed.ncbi.nlm.nih.gov/30083415/.

28 https://www.journals.uchicago.edu/doi/pdfplus/10.1086/ipe.1.25056143.

drug Humira[29] has filed 247 patent applications and has been granted more than 100, extending patent protection for the drug into the 2030s.

End the Practice of Product Hopping or Evergreening by Pharmaceutical Companies

Companies use product hopping or evergreening to prevent generic competition from entering the market by making small adjustments with minimal if any real therapeutic value to a drug that grant the company longer patent protection, or they remove the drug from market, forcing patients to switch to a reformulated version of the same drug. Applications for these types of modifications often occur toward the end of a product's patent life, when the drug is facing potential generic competition, in order to maximize the potential monopoly extension.

ACP Opposes Anti-competitive Pay-for-Delay Arrangements

ACP opposes anticompetitive pay-for-delay arrangements that curtail access to lower-cost alternative drugs. ACP believes applicable federal agencies should be empowered through guidance, congressional action, or additional resource support to address anticompetitive behaviors and gaming. Pay-for-delay, also known as "reverse payment settlement," is a patent settlement strategy in which a patent holder pays a generic manufacturer to keep a potential generic drug off the market for a certain period. The number of pay-for-delay agreements[30] increased from 3 in 2005 to 19 in 2009, after court decisions upheld the legality of such agreements, which prohibit generic drugs from entering the market on average nearly 17 months longer than agreements without compensation. In 2013, the Supreme Court ruled that although pay-for-delay agreements are not presumptively illegal, the FTC cannot be prevented from initiating legal action in regard to such agreements.[31]

Senators Klobuchar and Grassley have introduced legislation S. 1428, The Preserve Access to Affordable Generics and Biosimilars Act, which would

---

29 https://heatinformatics.com/sites/default/files/images-videosFileContent/i-mak.enbrel. Report-REVISED-2020-10-06.pdf.

30 https://www.ftc.gov/news-events/topics/competition-enforcement/pay-delay.

31 https://www.scotusblog.com/case-files/cases/federal-trade-commission-v-watson-pharmaceuticals-inc/.

prohibit brand name drug companies from compensating generic drug companies to delay the entry of a generic drug into the market. ACP calls for robust oversight and enforcement of pay-for delay agreement in order to limit anti-competitive behaviors that keep lower cost alternative off the market, and we appreciate that Senators have introduced legislation with the intent to address these harmful tactics.

Reduce Pharmaceutical Companies Market or Data Exclusivity Periods from 12 to 7 years

Pharmaceutical companies also claim that long exclusivity periods are needed to support innovation and allow a return on their investment and promote future innovation. Marketing exclusivity is granted by the FDA upon approval, during which a competitor, typically a generic drug, is prohibited from being marketed. Data exclusivity prohibits a competitor company from using the data collected by an originator company to gain approval of their drug. In the case of biosimilars, the high cost of developing and conducting trials undermines the potential cost-savings to the manufacturer if they are required to collect new data. *ACP opposes extending market or data exclusivity periods beyond the current exclusivities granted to small-molecule, generic, orphan, and biologic drugs and we support reducing the period of data and market exclusivity for biologic drugs from 12 years to 7 years.* Reducing the exclusivity period from 12 to 7 years, combined with provisions to prevent product hopping or evergreening[32] of biologic drugs, could get biosimilar or interchangeable drugs to market faster and save the federal government nearly $7 billion over 10 years. The Federal Trade Commission (FTC)[33] also supports a reduction in biologic exclusivity, noting that 12 years is unnecessary to promote innovation because biologic drug manufacturers are likely to earn substantial revenue even after the introduction of biosimilars.

---

[32] https://obamawhitehouse.archives.gov/omb/budget/.

[33] https://www.ftc.gov/sites/default/files/documents/reports/emerging-health-care-issues-follow-biologic-drug-competition-federal-trade-commission-report/p083901biologicsreport.pdf.

Eliminate Tax Deductions for Direct-to-Consumer Pharmaceutical Advertising

A study[34] of the period from 1997 to 2016 showed that direct-to-consumer (DTC) advertising for prescription drugs experienced rapid spending growth, from $2.1 billion (11.9 percent) of total spending in 1997 to $9.6 billion (32.0 percent) of total spending in 2016. Another study[35] showed that one third of the growth in drug spending is attributable to an increase in advertising. A review of available data showed that DTC advertising was associated with increases in prescribing of the advertised drug[36] and drug spending.[37] Although a complete ban on DTC advertising is unlikely given that many courts have ruled that it is allowed under the First Amendment, steps can be taken to limit the influence it may have on prescription drug expenditures.

Under current law, drug manufacturers may deduct the cost of advertising expenses from federal taxes. Eliminating the tax deduction only for prescription drug product claim ads does not run afoul of free speech concerns about banning DTC advertising. Further, a study of physicians by the FDA showed that although the physicians believed that DTC advertising prompted patients to ask questions and be more aware of possible treatments, they believed that such ads did not convey risks and benefits equally well.

We urge Congress to approve legislation, S. 141, the End Taxpayer Subsidies for Drug Ads Act, which would prohibit a tax deduction for expenses for DTC advertising of prescription drugs, thus eliminating the deduction that pharmaceutical companies use to pay for drug advertising.

Increase Transparency in the Marketplace

ACP policy supports transparency in the pricing, cost, and comparative value of all pharmaceutical products. For decades, pharmaceutical manufacturers have claimed that drug pricing is based on research and development cost and innovation and is well regulated by market forces. The spike in prices and increase in price for drugs already on the market have made many stakeholders wary, especially because many of these new therapies treat

---

34 https://pubmed.ncbi.nlm.nih.gov/30620375/.

35 https://www.nber.org/system/files/working_papers/w21714/w21714.pdf.

36 https://pubmed.ncbi.nlm.nih.gov/16076787/.

37 https://www.gao.gov/assets/gao-07-54.pdf.

small populations and there are few data to support that overall health care costs are reduced.

We support additional measures to improve transparency in the price of prescription drugs so that drug manufacturers disclose additional information concerning the reasons why drug prices may rise beyond the rate of inflation. Pharmaceutical companies should disclose actual material and production costs to regulators, and research and development costs contributing to a drug's pricing, including those drugs which were previously licensed by another company. Rigorous price transparency standards should be instituted for drugs developed from taxpayer-funded basic research.

We urge Congress to approve the FAIR Drug Pricing Act (S. 898), which would promote pricing transparency by requiring manufacturers to notify the Department of Health and Human Services (HHS) and provide a justification report 30 days before they increase the price of certain drugs.

Increase Transparency for Pharmacy Benefit Managers and Insurers

Pharmacy benefit managers[38] (PBMs) are for-profit companies that act as intermediaries for health insurers, self-insured employers, union health plans, Medicare Part D prescription drug benefit plans, and government purchasers in the selection, purchase, and distribution of pharmaceutical products for more than half the U.S. population. The ACP believes increased transparency[39] is needed on the part of PBMs and health plans to provide greater understanding of drug prices, help patients make informed decisions, and support a more sustainable health care system.

The continued lack of transparency from PBMs and insurers can hinder how patients, physicians, and others view the drug supply chain and can make it difficult to identify whether a particular entity is inappropriately driving up drug prices. This lack of transparency can also prevent viable policy solutions from being identified and further delay reforms that would help to rein in spending on prescription drugs. Although there have been many calls for transparency on the part of pharmaceutical companies and greater support for transparency in health care generally, all stakeholders must commit to improving transparency as the health care community works toward creating an innovative but sustainable prescription drug market.

---

[38] https://www.healthaffairs.org/do/10.1377/hpb20171409.000178/full/.

[39] https://www.acpjournals.org/doi/pdf/10.7326/M19-0035.

We provide the following recommendations to improve transparency in the prescription drug marketplace:

- Banning gag clauses that prevent pharmacists from informing patients when lower-cost alternatives are available, such as paying cash for a prescription instead of going through one's insurance coverage, is a reasonable step that has garnered bipartisan support.
- ACP supports the availability of accurate, understandable, and actionable information on the price of prescription medication. ACP urges health plans to make this information available to physicians and patients at the point of prescribing to facilitate informed decision making about clinically appropriate and cost-conscious care.
- ACP believes health plans, PBMs, and pharmaceutical manufacturers should report the amount paid for prescription drugs, aggregate number of rebates, and nonproprietary pricing information to the Department of Health and Human Services and make it publicly available. Any disclosure mandate should be structured in a way that deidentifies negotiated rebates with specific companies and protects confidential information that could be considered trade secrets or could have the effect of increasing prices.

Implement Reforms Concerning Step Therapy Practices

PBMs have developed a series of price management tactics to curb the rising cost of prescription drugs. Among these, step therapy policies, commonly called "failfirst"[40] policies, require patients to be initiated on lower-priced medications[41] before being approved for originally prescribed medications. Carriers can also change coverage in an attempt to force patients off their current therapies for cost reasons, a practice known as nonmedical drug switching.[42]

Evidence concerning the effectiveness of these tactics is mixed. Some studies[43] have found they can successfully drive cost savings without

---

[40] https://www.rheumatologyadvisor.com/home/topics/practice-management/acr-releases- new - step-thrapy-and-drug-pricing-position-statements/.

[41] https://www.healthaffairs.org/doi/10.1377/hlthaff.2014.0516.

[42] https://pubmed.ncbi.nlm.nih.gov/31081414/.

[43] https://acpo365-my.sharepoint.com/personal/glyons_acponline_org/Documents/ACP%20 Files/Motheral%20BR.%20Pharmaceutical%20step-therapy%20interventions:

negatively impacting patient care. Others[44] have found overall health spending actually increased due to an uptick in hospitalizations and other services resulting from new symptoms or complications. Meanwhile, these policies have drawn scrutiny for restricting patient access to effective treatments, putting patient health and safety in jeopardy by subjecting patients to potential adverse effects, interfering with the patient— physician relationship, and absorbing practice resources with burdensome approvals and documentation requirements.

In 2020, ACP released a position paper, that details our policies concerning Mitigating the Negative Impact of Step Therapy Practices and Non-Medical Switching of Prescription Drugs.[45] We provide the following recommendations to the Senate Finance Committee as it considers policies to reform the practice of step therapy and medication and medication switching:

- All step therapy and medication switching policies should aim to minimize care disruption, harm, side effects, and risks to the patient.
- All step therapy and nonmedical drug switching policies be designed with patients at the center, taking into account unique needs and preferences.
- All step therapy and nonmedical drug switching protocols be designed with input from frontline physicians and community pharmacists; feature transparent, minimally burdensome processes that consider the expertise of a patient's physician; and include a timely appeals process.
- Data concerning the effectiveness and potential adverse consequences of step therapy and nonmedical drug switching programs should be made transparent to the public and studied by policymakers. Alternative strategies to address the rising cost of prescription drugs that do not inhibit patient access to medications should be explored.

We also urge the Congress to approve The Safe Step Act (S. 464 and H.R. 2163), which would ensure patient access to appropriate treatments based on clinical decision-making and medical necessity, not arbitrary step therapy

---

%20a%20critical%20review%20of%20the%20literature.%20J%20Manag%20Care%20Pharm.

44 https://www.healthaffairs.org/doi/10.1377/hlthaff.2014.0516.

45 https://www.acponline.org/acp_policy/policies/step_therapy_nonmedical_switching_prescription_drugs_policy_2020.pdf.

protocols. This legislation would require insurers to implement a clear and transparent process to request an exception to a step therapy policy.

Conclusion

We appreciate the sustained effort of the Senate Finance Committee to lower the price of prescription drugs for our patients, but we urge you to act on our recommendations as soon as possible to ensure our patients can afford drugs prescribed by their physician. Should you have any questions regarding this statement, please do not hesitate to contact Brian Buckley our Senior Associate for Legislative Affairs at bbuckley@acponline.org.

American Consumer Institute

Center for Citizen Research
1701 Pennsylvania Avenue, NW, Suite 200
Washington, DC 20006
(703) 282–9400

Statement of Steve Pociask, President/CEO Strangling Generic Drugs is the Wrong Path to Lower Prices

Lowering drug prices is a public policy objective that everyone can agree on. About 18 million patients can't afford their prescribed medications, according to a recent poll,[46] including nearly 1 in 5 members of the poorest households. Unfortunately, Congress' plan to control pharmaceutical prices consists of half-baked proposals[47] that would do serious harm to consumers.

The legislation's central feature is an elaborate set of price controls—simply put, government-imposed ceilings on what drug makers can charge for their products. Although price controls are a tempting remedy to make medicines more affordable, their historical record is dismal. From 3rd-century

46 https://www.usnews.com/news/health-news/articles/2021-09-22/18-million-americans-cant-pay-for-needed-meds.

47 https://www.wsj.com/articles/a-toxic-drug-price-deal-11636415735?mod=opinion_lead_pos1.

Rome to modern-day Venezuela, artificial constraints on prices invariably lead[48] to shortages in the short-run and decreased innovation in the long-run as private companies abandon the market or rein in their investment.

A study[49] from the National Bureau of Economic Research, for example, estimated that cutting pharmaceutical prices by 40–45 percent by government fiat—roughly the reduction being proposed for some drugs—would cause pharmaceutical makers to significantly cut back on research and development, resulting in a 50–60 percent decrease in the number of compounds getting to human trials. That means fewer cutting-edge treatment options for patients.

Innovation in the brand-name pharmaceutical industry wouldn't be the only casualty of Congress' plan. The market for generic and biosimilar drugs—low-cost copies of a brand-name product—would be significantly disrupted, too. Makers of generics and biosimilars tend to compete against the costliest brand-name drugs, hoping to attract customers by undercutting their rival's price. As more manufacturers enter the market and competition intensifies, prices fall rapidly.

For example, products with a single generic maker are about 35 percent cheaper[50] than those with no generic competition, and prices drop by 95 percent when six or more generics are offered, according to FDA data. That explains why 92 percent of generic prescriptions in the U.S. are filled for $20 or less,[51] delivering more than $315 billion[52] in consumer savings every year.

But by forcing down the price of brand-name drugs, Congress' plan would weaken the enticement for generic and biosimilar competitors to enter the market. Though not as costly as developing a novel drug, creating generic or biosimilar medicines can be expensive. A 2013 paper[53] estimated that it takes 7 to 8 years to develop a biosimilar, at a cost of up to $250 million. Investors will be less likely to view the expense as worthwhile if the government can intervene to impose arbitrary caps[54] on drug prices. The result will be fewer generics and less competition for brandname products, undermining the price

---

48 https://www.wsj.com/articles/a-toxic-drug-price-deal-11636415735?mod=opinion_lead_pos1.

49 https://www.nber.org/system/files/working_papers/w11114/w11114.pdf.

50 https://www.fda.gov/about-fda/center-drug-evaluation-and-research-cder/generic-competition-and-drug-prices.

51 https://accessiblemeds.org/sites/default/files/2020-09/AAM-2020-Generics-Biosimilars-Access-Savings-Report-US-Web.pdf.

52 https://accessiblemeds.org/sites/default/files/2020-09/AAM-2020-Generics-Biosimilars-Access-Savings-Report-US-Web.pdf.

53 https://www.ncbi.nlm.nih.gov/pmc/articles/PMC4031732/.

54 https://www.statnews.com/2021/11/06/hurried-bills-congress-shouldnt-undermine-vast-savings-generic-biosimilar-drugs/.

reductions that Congress hopes to achieve. Lawmakers should be seeking to make it easier for generics and biosimilars to thrive, not more difficult.

Another provision of the bill punishes certain drug makers for raising their prices faster than inflation. Though matching pharmaceutical price increases with consumers' cost of living is intuitively appealing, this measure could easily backfire. Generic manufacturers generally price their products just above production cost, counting on the volume of sales—not revenue per unit—to turn a profit. While consumers benefit from rock-bottom prices, the viability of this pricing strategy hinges on drug makers' ability to modify the price as underlying production costs fluctuate. Given the complexity of the global pharmaceutical supply chain, it's impossible to foresee when the price of a raw input—potentially located in a foreign country—may spike, forcing the drug maker to rapidly increase its sale price in order to stay afloat. If penalized for doing so by an inflation cap, the manufacturer would curtail its production or withdraw from the market. Why would a generic drug manufacture enter the market and take this risk?

The design of the inflation penalty is especially problematic, since it is based on the percentage that a price increase exceeds inflation. That means a generic drug maker may face a penalty for increasing its price by a penny from $0.25 to $0.26 (a 4-percent increase), but a brand-name drug manufacturer could increase its price by 20 cents from $10.00 to $10.20 (a 2 percent increase) may avoid the penalty. Once again, this tilts the playing field against lower-cost medicines.

There are better ways to tackle drug costs. Accelerating FDA reviews[55] of generics and biosimilars promises to lower prices and expand consumer choice without disrupting competition. Reining in the excessive power[56] of pharmacy benefit managers (PBMs), which often exploit their position as middlemen in pharmaceutical transactions to extract exorbitant profits, should also be a priority for Congress.

Millions of patients need relief from spiraling pharmaceutical prices. Lawmakers should be focusing on real solutions, not miracle-cures that do more harm than good.

Steve Pociask is president and CEO of the American Consumer Institute, a nonprofit education and research organization. For more information on the

55 https://www.wsj.com/articles/fda-unveils-effort-to-get-biosimilar-drugs-on-the-market-faster-1531937491.

56 https://www.realclearhealth.com/articles/2016/07/21/the_middlemen_in_higher_drug_prices_109971.html.

Institute, visit www.TheAmericanConsumer.Org or follow us on Twitter @ConsumerPal.

American Diabetes Association

2451 Crystal Drive, Suite 900
Arlington, VA 22202

Statement of Lisa Murdock, Chief Advocacy Officer

Thank you, Chairman Wyden, Ranking Member Crapo and distinguished members of the Finance Committee, for providing the American Diabetes Association (ADA) the opportunity to submit written comments regarding the rising cost of prescription drugs in Medicare. We appreciate you considering this important topic at this critical time.

The ADA is the nation's leading voluntary health organization fighting to bend the curve on the diabetes epidemic and help people living with diabetes thrive. For 80 years the ADA has been driving discovery and research to treat, manage and prevent diabetes, while working relentlessly for a cure. We help people with diabetes thrive by fighting for their rights and developing programs, advocacy and education designed to improve their quality of life.

As you are no doubt aware, the increasing cost of prescription drugs has created an outsized burden on the diabetes community, which has grown to 37 million— more than one in 10—Americans. For people with diabetes, many of whom rely on insulin and other expensive medications to manage their condition, this financial barrier can mean the difference between life and death. The price of insulin has roughly tripled in the past decade, increasing from less than $100 for an average vial in 2009 to nearly $300 for the same vial today, even though today's insulin is nearly the exact same product as it was 10 years ago.[57] With these facts in mind, it should be little surprise that Americans spend more treating diabetes than any other chronic condition; that people with diabetes in the U.S. spend two and a half times more on health

[57] Rachel Gillett and Shayanne Gal, "One Chart Reveals How the Cost of Insulin Has Sky-rocketed in the US, Even Though Nothing About It Has Changed," *Business Insider,* September 18, 2019, *https://www.businessinsider.com/insulin-price-increased-last-decade-chart-2019-9.*

care than those who do not have diabetes; and that one in four insulin-dependent Americans report rationing their insulin supply due to the cost of the drug and financial difficulty.[58]

During the pandemic and consequent economic downturn, the diabetes community faced a disproportionate health burden of COVID–19. Americans with diabetes and other related underlying health conditions were hospitalized with COVID–19 six times as often and died of COVID–19 12 times as often as those who did not have diabetes.[59] One in 10 coronavirus patients with diabetes died within one week of hospital admission.[60] And Americans with diabetes accounted for 40 percent of COVID– 19 fatalities nationwide, despite making up just 10 percent of the U.S. population.[61] While we are still learning about the relationship between COVID–19 and diabetes, we know that unmanaged diabetes—whether a lack of medication use or missing doses—is a key factor in COVID–19 severity and complications, and an important indicator of whether someone with diabetes and COVID–19 is likely to have a longer hospitalization.[62]

---

58 American Diabetes Association, "Economic Costs of Diabetes in the U.S. in 2017," *Diabetes Care* 41, no. 5 (2018): 917–928, *https://care.diabetesjournals.org/content/41/5/917;* Sarah Stark Casagrande and Catherine C. Cowie, "Health Insurance Coverage Among People With and Without Diabetes in the U.S. Adult Population," *Diabetes Care* 35, no. 11 (2012): 2243–2249, *https://care.diabetes journals.org/content/35/11/2243;* Centers for Medicare and Medicaid Services, "National Health Expenditure Data—Historical," NHE Tables, December 16, 2020, *https:// www.cms.gov/research-statistics-data-and-systems/statistics-trends-and-reports/national healthexpenddata/nationalhealthaccountshistorical;* Darby Herkert et al., "Cost-Related Insulin Underuse Among Patients with Diabetes," *JAMA Internal Medicine* 179, no. 1 (2019): 112–114, *https://jamanetwork.com/journals/jamainternalmedicine/ article-abstract/2717499.*

59 Erin K. Stokes et al., "Coronavirus Disease 2019 Case Surveillance—United States, January 22–May 30, 2020," Morbidity and Mortality Weekly Report (MMWR), Centers for Disease Control and Prevention, June 15, 2020, *https://www.cdc.gov/mmwr/volumes/69/ wr/mm6924e2. htm?s_cid=mm6924e2_w#T1_down.*

60 Karena Yan, "1 in 10 People with COVID and Diabetes Die Within Seven Days of Hospital Admission," diatribe Learn, June 22, 2020, *https://diatribe.org/1-10-people-covid-and-diabetes- die-within-seven-days-hospital-admission.*

61 Jonathan M. Wortham et al., "Characteristics of Persons Who Died with COVID–19—United States, February 12–May 18, 2020," Morbidity and Mortality Weekly Report (MMWR), Centers for Disease Control and Prevention, July 10, 2020, *https://www.cdc.gov/ mmwr/volumes/69/ wr/mm6928e1.htm;* American Diabetes Association, "Statistics About Diabetes," *https:// www.diabetes.org/resources/ statistics/ statistics-about-diabetes.*

62 Dr. Sudip Bajpeyi and Ali Mossayebi, "Unmanaged Diabetes as a Poor Prognostic Factor in the Severity of Infection and Recovery Time of Hospitalized COVID–19 Patients," American Dia- betes Association, June 25, 2020, *https://www.diabetes.org/newsroom/ press-releases/2021/unmanaged-diabetes-associated-with-greater-COVID-19-severity.*

Beyond facing a heightened risk for the worst of the virus's health effects, Americans with diabetes have also experienced magnified financial challenges in the pandemic's wake. ADA surveys during the pandemic suggest that people with diabetes suffered pandemic-driven unemployment at a rate 50 percent higher than the national rate.[63] One-third of Americans with diabetes reported that they lost income due to COVID–19, and one in four reported needing to dip into their savings, take out a loan or use their stimulus checks to afford diabetes medication or supplies since the start of the pandemic.[64] Nearly one in five people with diabetes reported being forced to choose between buying food and filling their prescriptions.[65]

These troubling trends, coupled with the increasing cost of insulin, makes action by Congress to reduce the cost of insulin specifically, and prescription drugs more broadly, urgent. When it comes to insulin, we can learn from Medicare to expand cost-saving benefits to people with diabetes on commercial health insurance plans. One-third of Medicare beneficiaries have diabetes, and more than 3.3 million seniors on Medicare use insulin. During the Trump administration, the Centers for Medicare and Medicaid Services (CMS) Innovation Center launched the Senior Savings Model, a 5-year program to offer seniors Medicare Part D plan options that cap the beneficiary's cost sharing for insulin at $35 a month, regardless of the beneficiary's coverage phase. The Biden administration continued the pilot program in 2022, and more than 500 Part D plans are participating in the model this year.[66]

This successful bipartisan approach to reducing out-of-pocket costs for patients who use insulin can be replicated across insurance plans, and Congress has already taken steps to do just that. Last year, the House of Representatives passed the Build Back Better Act, which included a $35 monthly co-pay cap on insulin for commercial health insurance plans, group health insurance plans covered by the Employee Retirement Income Security Act (ERISA) and Medicare. Meanwhile several Senate Republicans

---

63 American Diabetes Association and dQ&A, "Diabetes and COVID–19: New Data Quantifies Extraordinary Challenges Faced by Americans with Diabetes During Pandemic," July 29, 2020, *https://www.diabetes.org/sites/default/files/2020-07/7.29.2020_dQA-ADA%20Data% 20Release. pdf.*

64 *Ibid.*

65 American Diabetes Association and Diabetes Daily, "Effects of the COVID–19 Pandemic on People with Diabetes," December 23, 2020, *https://www.diabetes.org/sites/default/files/2020-12/ADA%20Thrivable%20Data% 20Deck.pdf.*

66 "Part D Senior Savings Model," U.S. Centers for Medicare and Medicaid Services, February 28, 2022, *https://innovation.cms.gov/innovation-models/part-d-savings-model.*

introduced the Lower Costs, More Cures Act, which would make the Senior Savings Model and the $35 insulin co-pay cap in Medicare permanent. In February, the Affordable Insulin Now Act—a stand-alone bill with the Build Back Better Act's insulin co-pay cap provisions—was introduced in the House and the Senate.

As a result of the ADA's leadership in advocating for state and federal caps on cost sharing for insulin, 20 states and the District of Columbia have already enacted co pay caps. Still, since these caps are limited to individuals covered by state-regulated insurance, more is needed to expand and deepen the impact of limits on cost-sharing. We know that co-pay caps can provide immediate, noticeable financial relief to patients. An analysis of California Senate Bill 473—which would cap out-of- pocket costs for insulin at $50 per month for state regulated plans—would offer patients currently paying above the cap a 55 percent reduction in cost sharing, from an average of $88 per prescription to $39 per prescription. The analysis estimated a 10 percent decrease in diabetes-related emergency room visits, which could reduce ER costs by more than $2 million in the cap's first year should the state enact it.[67]

The best way forward is to enact a national insulin co-pay cap right now so Americans with diabetes can benefit from reduced costs regardless of the type of insurance they have. By contrast, policies that simply shift funds among industry players in the health care supply chain are less valuable unless patients themselves are realizing direct savings—at the pharmacy counter, in their premiums and in the cost of deductibles. Practical approaches like a monthly co-pay cap that put patients first should be a key goal of any effort to make drugs more affordable.

Given that people with diabetes typically require more than one medication to manage their diabetes and other co-morbidities—indeed, the U.S. diabetes community accounts for $1 of every $4 spent on health care, including prescription drugs, in America—we hope to see Congress take additional steps this year to make prescription medication and supplies for people with diabetes more affordable.[68] Among our priorities are:

- Increasing transparency throughout the pharmaceutical supply chain, including efforts to shed light on pricing practices, improve

---

[67] "Analysis of California Senate Bill 473 Insulin Cost Sharing," California Health Benefits Review Program, April 19, 2021, *http://analyses.chbrp.com/document/view.php? id=1566.*

[68] "Cost Effectiveness of Diabetes Interventions," National Center for Chronic Disease Prevention and Health Promotion, Centers for Disease Control and Prevention, March 7, 2022, *https:// www.cdc.gov/chronicdisease/programs-impact/pop/diabetes.htm.*

accountability in the pharmacy benefit manager (PBM) market, and ensure that rebates are benefiting patients and not artificially increasing prices or limiting patient options;

- Speeding competitive generic drug and biosimilar alternatives to market by, among other things, addressing loopholes in our patent system that allow manufacturers to stave off competition;
- Cracking down on insurance practices that push patients to choose between quality and affordability, including prior authorization and step therapy (or "fail first") policies that force patients to try the least expensive drug in a class first, even if their prescribing physician believes a different therapy is in the patient's best clinical interest; and
- Increasing oversight and regulation of specialty drug tiers used by insurers that shift the cost-sharing burden disproportionately onto patients with rare and/or chronic conditions who rely on these medications.

Thank you for the opportunity to submit this testimony for the record. The ADA looks forward to continuing to work with Congress to enact a national co-pay cap on insulin and identify other ways to reduce the cost of prescription drugs so that all Americans with diabetes can afford to stay safe and healthy.

American Federation of Teachers, AFL–CIO

555 New Jersey Ave., NW Washington, DC 20001
(202) 879–4400
https://www.aft.org/
March 21, 2022

The Honorable Ron Wyden
Chairman
U.S. Senate Committee on Finance
Dirksen Senate Office Bldg. Washington, DC 20510–6200
Re: Senate Committee on Finance Hearing, March 16, 2022
"Prescription Drug Price Inflation: An Urgent Need to Lower Drug Prices in Medicare"

Dear Chairman Wyden:

On behalf of the 1.7 million members of the American Federation of Teachers, including 200,000 nurses and other health professionals, I thank you for holding this important hearing on the affordability of pharmaceuticals and for your leadership on this critical issue.

No one should have to choose between feeding their families and paying for life-saving medication, but that is exactly what happens in American households because of the unjustified rising price tag of prescription drugs. I frequently hear stories from our members about patients who are skipping needed medications because they are forced to choose between their health needs and paying their mortgages or buying food.

AFT members and their families—from the bus driver living paycheck to paycheck, to the nurse who understands the lifeline that prescription drugs can be, to the retired teacher on a fixed income—are demanding that those in power in Washington, DC, take action to lower drug prices. It is devastating to hear retired educators and healthcare professionals, who have spent their lives helping people, talk about the struggles they face in taking care of their own health needs.

This hearing should serve as the first step toward passing legislation to reduce what patients pay for medicine. Legislation to address the medicine affordability crisis must include a mandate that the secretary of health and human services negotiate the price of a significant number of drugs covered by Medicare and ensure that prices don't rise faster than inflation. These price protections should be extended to all in need of medication.

As a union, we have worked hard to ensure that our members have access to high- quality, affordable healthcare, which is why we have fought for the Affordable Care Act, worked to end surprise medical billing, and demanded that healthcare workers have supportive work environments. We will continue to press for access to high- quality, affordable healthcare, and it is clear that comprehensive legislative action is needed to directly address the affordability of many pharmaceuticals.

Thank you again for your important leadership on this issue. Your work is crucial to ensuring that patients have access to the medicines they need.

Sincerely,
Randi Weingarten President

American Hospital Association

800 10th Street, NW Two CityCenter, Suite 400
Washington, DC 20001–4956
(202) 638–1100

On behalf of our nearly 5,000 member hospitals, health systems and other health care organizations, our clinician partners—including more than 270,000 affiliated physicians, 2 million nurses and other caregivers—and the 43,000 health care leaders who belong to our professional membership groups, the American Hospital Association (AHA) writes to express support for addressing the high cost of drugs in Medicare.

The AHA is deeply committed to the availability of high-quality, efficient health care for all Americans. Hospitals and health systems, and the clinicians who work in them, rely on lifesaving drug therapies to care for their patients. In addition, researchers in U.S. academic medical centers generate much of the evidence used to develop new drugs. However, an unaffordable drug is not a lifesaving drug.

The AHA continues to work with its members to document the challenges hospitals and health systems face with high drug prices and develop policy solutions to protect access to critical therapies while encouraging and supporting much-needed innovation. We encourage Congress to consider policy recommendations in the following areas.

Increase Competition and Innovation

Competition for prescription drugs generally results in increased options for lower cost therapies, particularly through the introduction of one or more generic competitors. We encourage Congress to implement policies that would increase the introduction of generic alternatives and discourage anti-competitive tactics while maintaining incentives for the development of innovative new therapies.

- Deny patents for "evergreened" products. Some drug manufacturers attempt to minimize or eliminate competition through product "evergreening." A manufacturer attempts to "evergreen" a product when it applies for patent and market exclusivity protections for a "new" product that is essentially the same as the original product, such as extended release formulations or combination therapies that simply combine two existing drugs into one pill. What generally happens is that, while the older version of the drug is no longer patent-protected and, therefore, generic alternatives may be offered, drug manufacturers promote the newer version as the "latest and greatest." Without important information on the comparative value of the newer drug, many providers and consumers switch to the brand-only "evergreened" product after intense marketing by the manufacturer that suggests that the newer version is superior. Patents and market exclusivity rights for products that are simply modifications of existing products should be denied unless the new product offers significant improvements in clinical effectiveness, cost savings, access or safety.

- Limit orphan drug incentives to true orphan drugs. Drug manufacturers receive a number of incentives to develop drugs for rare diseases. These incentives, which include waived FDA fees, tax credits and longer market exclusivity periods, are intended to spur innovation of therapies for which the manufacturer may otherwise not recoup their investment due to low volume. These incentives have contributed to the development of innovative, life-saving drugs where no therapies previously existed. However, in some instances, manufacturers have received orphan drug status for drugs that they subsequently marketed for other, non-rare indications. In these instances, manufacturers are receiving the incentives for drugs that are broadly used. For example, Humira (adalimumab), Procrit (epoetin alfa) and Prolia (denosumab) all are approved for orphan drug status; however, since receiving the designation, the drugs also have been marketed for a number of other, non-rare indications. Further, each of these drugs were among the top 10 highest-spend drugs for hospitals and health systems, and each had substantial price increases of at least 15% from 2015–2017.[69]

Congress should require FDA to collect information on other intended indications for a drug when evaluating eligibility for orphan drug status. FDA also should be required to do a post-market review at regular intervals throughout the market exclusivity period to determine whether the drug should

[69] AHA/FAH Drug Survey 2019.

retain its status as an orphan drug. In instances where the manufacturer is promoting the drug for other indications that do not meet the orphan drug status requirements, FDA should levy penalties, such as requiring that the manufacturer pay the government the value of the tax breaks and waived fees and potentially reducing the market exclusivity period.

Increase Drug Pricing Transparency

Payers, providers and the public have little information about how drugs are priced. This gap in information challenges payers' abilities to make decisions regarding coverage and pricing of drugs, and often results in mid-year cost increases that providers are unprepared to manage. Policies should be implemented to provide greater parity between drug manufacturers and other sectors of the health care system, including hospitals, which already disclose a considerable amount of information on pricing, input costs and utilization.

Increased disclosure requirements related to drug pricing, research and development should be included at the time of application for drug approval. There is very little evidence of what it actually costs to develop a new drug and how those costs factor into the pricing of a drug. Other components of the health care system are held to a much higher transparency standard. For example, hospitals provide detailed data to the Centers for Medicare and Medicaid Services (CMS) via the annual Medicare cost report, which includes information on facility characteristics, utilization, costs and charges, and financial data. Given the significant taxpayer investment in drugs—both through funded research and purchasing through public programs like Medicare and Medicaid—there should be greater transparency parity between drug manufacturers and other health care providers.

Drug manufacturers should be required to submit as part of the drug approval process information on anticipated product pricing for both a single unit and a course of treatment; anticipated public spending on the product (e.g., from government purchasers including Medicare, Medicaid and TRICARE, among others); and information on how the product was priced, including anticipated portion of the product price that will contribute to current or future marketing and research and development costs. In addition, drug manufacturers should be required to provide information on the research that contributed to the development of the drug and specify all entities that conducted research that contributed to the development of the drug, the amount spent on that research and the funding source.

Increased transparency into drug pricing could be used to hold drug manufacturers accountable for fairly pricing products, help calculate the value of a drug, and support future policymaking.

Improve Access Through Inflation-Based Rebates for Medicare Drugs

The Medicaid program consistently achieves better pricing on drugs than the Medicare program. The primary driver behind the lower net unit costs are mandated, additional rebates that kick in when the average manufacturer price (AMP) for a drug increases faster than inflation. A similar inflation cap should be implemented on the price of drugs under the Medicare program. Under Medicare Part B, such a cap could be operationalized through a manufacturer rebate to Medicare when the average sales price (ASP) for a drug increases faster than a specified inflation benchmark. A similar cap could be placed on increases in the prices of Part D drugs.

This policy would protect the program and beneficiaries from dramatic increases in the Medicare payment rate for drugs, notable past increases included examples like 533% (Miacalcin, used for treating bone disease), 638% (Neostigmine, used in anesthesia) and 1,261% (Vasopressin, used to treat diabetes and bleeding in a critical care environment). This policy also could potentially generate savings for drugs with price growth above the inflation benchmark. According to a 2019 report, the Congressional Budget Office estimated that an inflationary rebate requirement would reduce direct spending by about $35 billion over 10 years.[70]

Better Align Incentives by Testing Changes to the Federally-Funded Part D Reinsurance Program

Under the Part D prescription drug program, the federal government covers 80% of the costs for enrollees who cross the out-of-pocket threshold. Insurers and beneficiaries share the responsibility for the remaining 20%, at 15% and 5%, respectively. These reinsurance payments are substantial: in 2013, the federal government's portion totaled nearly $20 billion for approximately 2

---

[70] https://www.cbo.gov/system/files/2019-12/hr3_complete.pdf.

million Medicare beneficiaries.[71] This program shields Part D plan sponsors from high costs and may create disincentives for plan sponsors to aggressively negotiate drug prices with manufacturers and manage enrollees' care.

Congress should require CMS to design a pilot project to test a new Part D payment model that either reduces or eliminates reinsurance payments while making appropriate adjustments to the direct subsidy rate. While CMMI has recently taken action in an attempt to modernize the Part D program through rewards and incentives, medication management programs and changes to the Low-Income Subsidy, congressional action would require CMS to test whether shifting more of the financial risk to insurers leads to appropriate reductions in program spending due to stronger negotiations with drug manufacturers or improved care management. This alternative is consistent with a Medicare Payment Advisory Commission recommendation on improvements to the Part D program.

Protect the 340B Drug Pricing Program

The 340B program is a critical program that helps eligible providers to care for the patients and communities they serve. The program requires pharmaceutical companies participating in Medicaid to sell certain outpatient drugs at discounted prices to health care organizations that care for high numbers of uninsured and lowincome patients or care for specific populations, such as children or patients with cancer or AIDS. 340B hospitals use the savings they receive on the discounted drugs to stretch scarce federal resources and provide more affordable and effective care, just as Congress intended. In fact, 340B hospitals reinvest their 340B savings in programs that are critical for the communities and patients they serve, which can include enhancing patient services and access to care, as well as providing free or reduced priced prescription drugs to vulnerable patient populations. In 2018 alone, 340B hospitals provided $68 billion in community benefits. Despite the 340B program's proven track record for 30 years, pharmaceutical manufacturers have repeatedly attempted to scale back or significantly reduce its benefits to hospitals and the patients they serve.

Since July 2020, several of the largest drug manufacturers have engaged in unprecedented and unlawful actions to limit the scope of the 340B program by denying 340B pricing through contract pharmacies and demanding

---

[71] MedPAC, "Chapter 6: Sharing risk in Medicare Part D," June 2015.

superfluous, detailed reporting of 340B drug claims distributed through hospitals' contract pharmacies. These drug companies have knowingly violated the statute and ignored calls by both the Biden and Trump Administrations to end these harmful actions.

The Health Resources and Services Administration (HRSA) has long authorized 340B covered entities to contract with community pharmacies to dispense drugs to eligible patients in order to expand the reach of the program and ensure access to prescribed medications for their patients. The use of outside pharmacies is especially important for hospitals that are located in and/or serve rural communities, as many of these hospitals do not operate in-house pharmacies, so they must rely on contracting with outside pharmacies to ensure their patients have access to their medications. More than 80% of rural 340B hospitals use contract pharmacies to ensure their patients receive outpatient drugs, as well as other essential services. These contract pharmacy arrangements have also proven especially important during the COVID–19 pandemic when patients have relied more heavily on alternative pharmacy channels such as mail order, online and small localized retail pharmacies. Hospitals have increasingly contracted with such pharmacies to ensure that their patients are able to access their prescribed medications and are not lost to follow- up. For these reasons, it is imperative that these pernicious actions by pharmaceutical companies be stopped immediately and restore access to 340B pricing for hospitals with contract pharmacy arrangements.

The 340B program is now more crucial than ever as 340B hospitals continue to be on the front lines of the COVID–19 public health emergency, despite incurring historic financial and operational challenges. Among these challenges is the high cost of pharmaceuticals. As of January 2022, hospital drug expenses are 22% higher on an absolute basis and 65% higher on a per patient basis compared to pre-pandemic levels in January 2020.

The fact remains that pharmaceutical companies continue to raise the prices of their products and enjoy double-digit profit margins, while 340B hospitals continue to care for the nation's most vulnerable patients and communities and operate on razor-thin margins. It is imperative for Congress to continue its bipartisan support of the program and ensure that eligible hospitals and their patients can continue to benefit from the 340B program.

Conclusion

Thank you for your attention to the ever increasing cost of prescription drugs and consideration of our comments on behalf of hospitals and health systems. We look forward to working with Congress to lower the cost of drugs to protect access to critical therapies.

American Pharmacy Cooperative, Inc.

5601 Shirley Park Drive Bessemer, Alabama 35022

The Honorable Ron Wyden, The Honorable Mike Crapo, and members of the Committee:

Thank you for the opportunity to submit a statement for the record in connection with this Committee's March 16, 2022, hearing on prescription drug price inflation in Medicare. American Pharmacy Cooperative ("APCI"), consisting of more than 1,700 community pharmacies across thirty states, is appreciative of this Committee's attention to rising prescription drug prices for America's seniors and watched the hearing with great interest.

As you are likely aware, anticompetitive and predatory practices by pharmacy benefits managers ("PBMs") wreak havoc on independent community pharmacies across the country including but not limited to misaligned reimbursements based on opaque, trade secreted methodologies, retroactive DIR fees, restrictive narrow networks, and beneficiary steering of patients away from community pharmacies to PBM owned or affiliated pharmacies.

However, PBMs, on behalf of their client (and often affiliated) prescription drug plans ("PDPs"), also engage in practices that directly raise the costs of prescription drugs for senior beneficiaries in Medicare Part D and addressing those practices should figure centrally in any efforts to rein in rising drug costs.

In that regard, the 3 Axis Advisors report released earlier this month entitled: Deserving of Better: How American Seniors are Paying for Misaligned Incentives within Medicare Part D, illustrates the role PDP/PBM imposed DIR fees play in inflating medication costs at the drug counter in Medicare Part D.

More specifically, the report found, amongst other things, one large PDP/PBM in- creased prices at the counter 51% over a 30-month period on generic drugs.[72] While this would appear problematic in and of itself, during the same period the national average drug acquisition cost ("NADAC") saw 8.7% deflation over the same 30-month period for the same mix of generic drugs.[73] This represents an astounding *59% gap between drug costs at the counter for beneficiaries and NADAC.*

Equally concerning, the report also uncovered a 591.9% increase in retroactive DIR fees applied to community pharmacies during the same 30-month period.[74] The trend is unmistakable, despite acquisition costs for pharmacies deflating, costs rose for beneficiaries at an alarming rate while PBMs recouped more money via retroactive DIR fees.

3 Axis Advisors also uncovered that in addition to the 59% spread between costs at the counter and NADAC, and the rise in retroactive DIR fees, the same plan was recouping beneficiary cost shares collected by pharmacies via retroactive DIR fees thus charging beneficiaries cost shares that exceed the amount the pharmacies were reimbursed (this practice is referred to as a clawback).[75] More specifically, the report's single plan analysis found that during the first 6 months of 2021:

- A mean beneficiary clawback of $10.71;
- More than 27% of claims had a clawback; and
- Beneficiary clawbacks were in excess of $2.21 million.[76]

Put another way, beneficiaries under this plan were charged by their PDP/PBM $2.21 million more for prescription drugs than the pharmacies were reimbursed. This particular plan seems to be escalating the use of cost

[72] 3 Axis Advisors (2021). Deserving of Better: How American Seniors are Paying for Mis-aligned Incentives within Medicare Part D (hereinafter referred to as "3 Axis report"). Available online at *https://static1.squarespace.com/static/5c326d5596e76f58ee234632/t/622631f0c98dae49c09a3d86/1646670321833/3AxisAdvisors_Medicare_DIR_Report_Final_0322.pdf.*

[73] *Id.;* NADAC is administered by CMS and is used today in most Medicaid fee for service programs with pharmacies being reimbursed at the average acquisition cost for a drug plus a professional dispensing fee based on pharmacies' average cost to dispense a prescription drug.

[74] *Id.*

[75] *Id.*

[76] *Id.*

share clawbacks with the average value of the clawback increasing by 1,648% from 2019 to 2021.[77]

In light of the foregoing, the report's findings that moving away from PDP/PBM pricing games and towards a transparent drug pricing reimbursement model would yield significant savings should come as no surprise. However, the potential savings found was eye opening. Specially, the report found an estimated *$18.7 billion in potential savings across Part D* in 2021 alone by moving from the current PDP/ PBM negotiated price model to a transparent model in which pharmacies are reimbursed based upon NADAC plus an average dispensing fee of $10.[78]

Conclusion

The 3 Axis Advisors' report findings bear repeating:

- Report's single plan analysis found 51% increase in prices at counter for generic medications in a 30-month period while NADAC saw 8.7% deflation during the same period all while DIR fees increased 591%.
- Report's single plan analysis also uncovered a PDP/PBM charging beneficiaries cost shares that exceed the amounts the pharmacy is reimbursed after DIR fees are assessed with the average beneficiary clawback increasing 1,648% from 2019 to 2021.
- Report found potential savings via a move to NADAC of $18.7 billion plan wide in 2021 alone.

In light of the foregoing, APCI believes that a move to a NADAC based reimbursement model should figure centrally in any efforts to lower drug costs for Part D beneficiaries. Not only would it save beneficiaries and taxpayers money, it would strip PDPs/PBMs of their ability to manipulate drug prices for their own selfish gain.

It is APCI's sincere hope the 3 Axis report's findings is a catalyst to beginning conversations regarding a move to a transparent NADAC based model with this Committee along with exploring additional actions that can lower drug prices and protect patients, taxpayers, and community pharmacies.

---

[77] *Id.*
[78] *Id.*

Should you have any questions or APCI can provide anything additional, please contact the undersigned at gregr@apcinet.com.

Thank you again for your leadership and attention to this important issue.

Sincerely,
Greg Reybold, Esq.
Director of Healthcare Policy and General Counsel

Association for Accessible Medicines

601 New Jersey Ave., NW, Suite 850 Washington, DC 20001
202–249–7100
info@accessiblemeds.org
accessiblemeds.org

The Association for Accessible Medicines (AAM) and its Biosimilars Council are the nation's leading trade association for the manufacturers and distributors of FDA-approved generic and biosimilar medicines. AAM's members provide more than 52,000 jobs at nearly 150 facilities in the United States and manufacture more than 60 billion doses of medicines every year.[79] AAM appreciates the opportunity to submit this statement for the record for the Senate Finance Committee's hearing on "Prescription Drug Price Inflation: An Urgent Need to Lower Drug Prices in Medicare."

America's patients rightfully expect Congress to address the ever-increasing prices of brand-name prescription drugs. High launch prices on new brand biologics and annual price increases on existing brand-name drugs, combined with an increasing trend of anti-competitive tactics designed to delay or prevent competition from more affordable biosimilars and generics, are pushing access to medicines out of reach for too many patients. These dynamics are compounded by flawed policies that reward health plans for the use of high-cost, high-rebate brand drugs and that allow plans to raise the out-of-pocket costs for generics, even as the prices for those generics are falling. As a result, Medicare's seniors are missing out on billions of dollars in savings from biosimilar and generic drugs each year.

[79] AAM, "A Blueprint for Enhancing the Security of the U.S. Pharmaceutical Supply Chain," October 2021 (https://accessiblemeds.org/blueprint).

However, the untested approach in the House-passed Build Back Better Act (H.R. 5376) does not address these challenges and could in fact harm future savings from generic and biosimilar medicines. The Build Back Better Act's approach to direct negotiations in Medicare and inflation-based penalties, as passed by the House, would alter the incentive for generic and biosimilar manufacturers to develop new medicines. In contrast, the bipartisan Prescription Drug Pricing Reduction Act of 2019 ("Grassley-Wyden") would effectively tackle the high cost of brand-name prescription drugs without disrupting the ability of generic and biosimilar manufacturers to compete.

In light of the proven track record of savings from generic and biosimilar competition, addressing the existing barriers to competition would produce more immediate results and be more successful in lowering the cost of prescription drugs for patients for years to come. AAM estimates seniors could save as much as $74 billion over the next 10 years, with additional savings for taxpayers and the federal government of more than $66 billion, by maximizing patient access to generic and biosimilar medicines already approved by FDA.[80]

Specifically, AAM recommends the Senate Finance Committee advance the following reforms:

- Address the biosimilar rebate trap and increase patient access to biosimilar medicines;
- Ensure that patients have access to lower-cost generics at launch;
- Modernize the Part D benefit to encourage more generic and biosimilar adoption;
- Ensure that patient out-of-pocket costs reflect the low cost of generics; and

[80] HHS, "Savings Available Under Full Generic Substitution of Multiple Source Brand Drugs in Medicare Part D," January 2018 *(https://aspe.hhs.gov/sites/default/files/private/pdf/259326/DP-Multisource-Brands-in-Part-D.pdf);* FDA, Remarks from FDA Commissioner Scott Gottlieb, M.D., FDA's Biosimilars Action Plan, September 2018 *(https://www.fda.gov/news-events/press-announcements/remarks-fda-commissioner-scott-gottlieb-md-prepared-delivery-brookings-institution-release-fdas);* Avalere, "Effect of Potential Policy Change to Part D Generic Tiers on Patient Cost Sharing and Part D Plan Costs," February 2019 *(https://avalere.com/in- sights/effect-of-potential-policy-change-to-part-d-generic-tiering-on-patient-cost-sharing-and-part-d-plan-costs);* AAM, Modeling the Budget and Premium Impacts of Updating Medicare Part D to Increase Generic & Biosimilar Adoption, October 2019; Milliman Research Report, "Five Year Analysis of the Drug Pricing Lab's Production Plus Profit Pricing (P-Quad) Proposal for Biologic Drugs," March 2021 *(https://www.drugpricinglab.org/wp-content/uploads/2021/03/MSK-Bio-logic-P-quad-Whitepaper_2021.03.08.pdf).*

- Eliminate the penalty on generics in Medicaid.

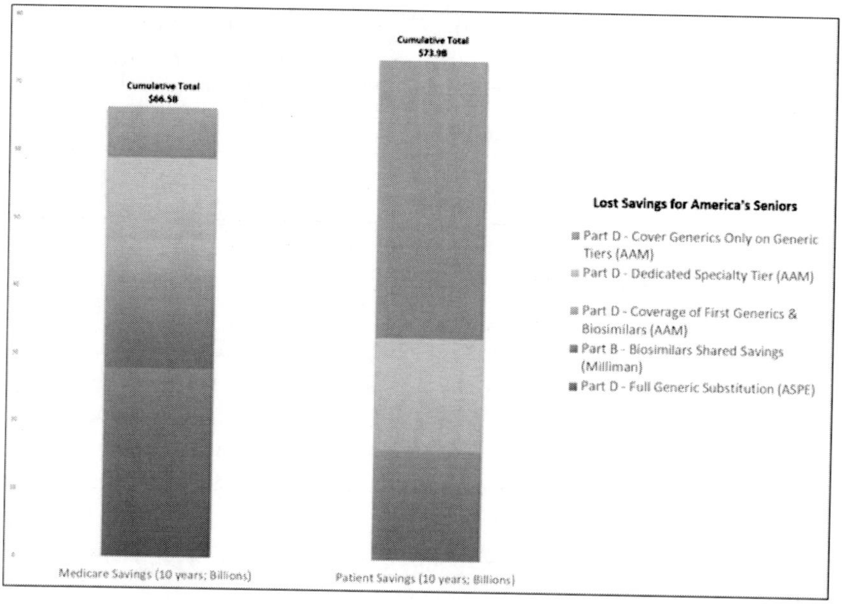

Together, these policies could save patients and taxpayers billions in 2022 and more in future years through increased competition, lower out-of-pocket costs and reduced spending on prescription drugs.[81]

Generic and Biosimilar Medicines Drive Savings, Brand-Name Drugs Increase Costs

The generic and biosimilar markets are fundamentally different than the brandname and biologic markets. While brand-name drugs operate in a market where there is no direct price competition from generics and biosimilars due to government-awarded exclusivities and patent protections, generic and biosimilar medicines compete within a multi-competitor model with drug prices decreasing as more competitors enter the market. Not surprisingly, these differences lead to dramatically different results for patients.

Generic and biosimilar medicines are successful in lowering the cost of prescription drugs. Experience shows drug prices decline rapidly when

[81] AAM, "Prescription for Savings," January 2021 *(https://accessiblemeds.org/Rx4Savings)*.

generics enter the market. According to FDA, prices fall by an average of 39% for the first generic and by nearly 80% when four or more generics enter the market.[82] Evidence with the biosimilars market shows average cost savings of 45%.[83] Importantly, biosimilar com- petition also results in lower brand biologic prices—by about 25% on average.[84]

Competition from generic and biosimilar medicines leads to significant savings for patients and the health care system. Over the last 10 years, generics and bio- similars provided more than $2 trillion in savings—including $469 billion from new generics and more than $12 billion from biosimilars. In addition to the cost savings provided, patient access to life-savings treatments is broadened as the price of medicine falls. A recent analysis of Medicare Part D from the Congressional Budget Office (CBO) notes, "the number of standardized prescriptions dispensed for generic drugs more than doubled from 2009 through 2018."[85] And the independent consulting firm IQVIA found that biosimilar competition has provided for new access to care—more than 10 million additional days of patient therapy beyond what would have been expected.

Independent research from MedPAC, CBO, AARP and HHS's ASPE examining trends in the prices of prescriptions drugs reach the same undeniable conclusion: generic prices continue to decrease, while brand-name drugs continue to rise.

- MedPAC: "Generic drug prices in Part D declined by an average of 13.7% from 2006–2018 and experienced an 11% decline from 2018–2019."[86]
- CBO: "In Medicare Part D, the average price of a generic prescription was $22 in 2009 and gradually fell to $17 in 2018."[87]

---

[82] FDA, "New Evidence Linking Greater Competition and Lower Generic Drug Prices," December 2019 *(https://www.fda.gov/about-fda/center-drug-evaluation-and-research-cder/generic-competition-and-drug-prices#:~:text=New%20Evidence%20 Linking%20Greater%20Generic,differ ent%20sources%20for%20wholesale%20prices).*

[83] AAM, Analysis of Average Sales Price Files, January 2022.

[84] *Ibid.*

[85] CBO, "Prescription Drugs: Spending, Use, and Prices," January 2022 *(https://www.cbo.gov/publication/57050).*

[86] MedPAC, "March 2021 Report to the Congress: Medicare Payment Policy," March 2021*(https://www.medpac.gov/wp-content/uploads/2021/10/mar21_medpac _report_ch13_sec.pdf).*

[87] Ibid., CBO.

- AARP: "Between 2016 and 2017, retail prices for 390 widely used generic prescription drugs decreased by an average of 9.3 percent."[88]
- ASPE: "Our review of the evidence strongly supports the conclusion that generic drug prices are not an important part of the drug cost problem facing the nation."[89]

Notably, recent analysis from MedPAC and CBO shows the increases in the prices of brand-name drugs are significant enough to completely offset the increased use of lower-cost generic medicines. CBO found, "Despite increases in the use of lower- cost generic drugs over the 2009–2018 period, the average price of a prescription drug did not fall significantly, because of increases in the prices of brand-name drugs."[90]

Patients savings, however, often goes unrealized. HHS found "incompletely aligned incentives for generic substitution leave significant savings uncaptured."[91] Seniors and the Medicare Part D program would have saved $3 billion in 2016 if generics had been dispensed rather than the brand-name drug.[92] In 2018, FDA reported that patients could have saved "more than $4.5 billion in 2017" if they had the ability to purchase FDA-approved biosimilars.[93] AAM's Biosimilars Council conducted simi- lar analysis and found patients had unrealized savings of more than $10 billion from the lack of access to lower-cost biosimilar medicines through 2018.[94]

Moreover, updated analysis from Avalere shows generic drugs are increasingly being placed on higher formulary tiers for seniors with Medicare Part D coverage. From 2011 to 2022, the number of generic drugs on the lowest cost-sharing tier declined from 71% to 14%.[95] Generic drugs are now

---

[88] AARP, "Trends in Retail Prices of Generic Prescription Drugs Widely Used by Older Americans: 2017 Year-End Update," April 2019 *(https://www.aarp.org/content/dam/aarp/ppi/2019/04/trends-in-retail-prices-of-generic-prescription-drugs-widely-used-by-older-americans.pdf)*.

[89] ASPE, "Understanding Recent Trends in Generic Drug Prices," January 2016 *(https://aspe.hhs.gov/reports/understanding-recent-trends-generic-drug-prices)*.

[90] *Ibid.*, CBO.

[91] *Ibid.*, HHS 2018.

[92] *Ibid.*

[93] *Ibid.*, FDA 2018.

[94] Biosimilars Council, "Failure to Launch: Patent Abuse Blocks Access to Biosimilars for America's Patients," June 2019 *(https://accessiblemeds.org/resources/reports/white-paper-part-1-failure-launch-patent-abuse-blocks-access-biosimilars-americas)*.

[95] *Ibid.*, Avalere 2019; Avalere, "57% of Generic Drugs Are Not on 2022 Part D Generic Tiers," January 2022 *(https://avalere.com/insights/57-of-generic-drugs-are-not-on-2022-part-d-generic- tiers)*.

placed on non-generic tiers 57% of the time.[96] As a result, patients are now paying more, even sometimes paying the full cost of the drug, even as generic prices have continued to fall. Avalere estimated seniors would save more than $4 billion a year if generic medicines were placed only on generic formulary tiers.[97]

Figure 4.

Average Price of a Prescription Drug Obtained Through Medicare Part D and Medicaid

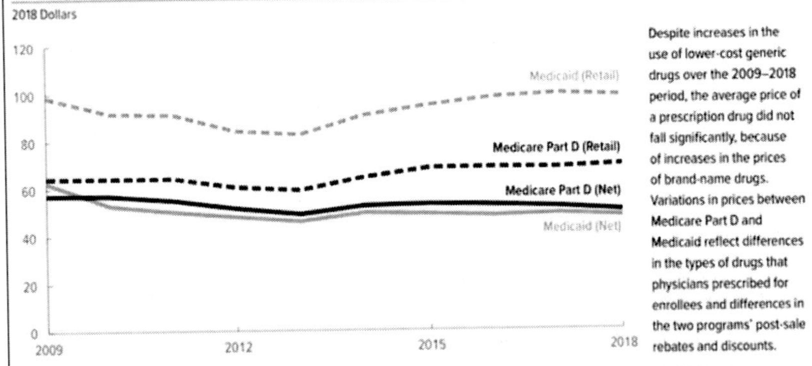

Data source: Congressional Budget Office, using administrative data for Medicare Part D and Medicaid. See www.cbo.gov/publication/57050#data.

The Generic and Biosimilar Markets Are Designed and Function Differently than the Brand Drug Markets.

The pharmaceutical industry in the United States is predicated on a balance between innovation and access. Brand-name drug companies are rewarded for inventing and developing new treatments and cures. In return for the innovation, current law provides brand-name drug companies with 12 years of exclusivity for biologics and 20 years, from filing, for each patent. There is also regulatory exclusivity provided to incentivize pediatric and orphan drug development. During the period of patent and marketing exclusivity, brand-name drugs are priced and sold free from competition from generics and biosimilars, and discounts or rebates may be negotiated with pharmacy benefit managers (PBM) for formulary placement.

Developers of generic and biosimilar medicines are provided with the opportunity to begin marketing the same or highly similar medicine with the same clinical benefit for patients if the developer can address the patents and exclusivity. As noted earlier, the introduction of competition into the market

[96] *Ibid,* Avalere 2022.
[97] *Ibid,* Avalere 2019.

significantly reduces the price of medicine, and patients benefit from greater, more affordable access to FDA- approved drugs. Thus, generic and biosimilar medicines consequently play an integral role in patient health.

Once medicines are approved and launched, brand-name drug companies maximize revenue through price rather than volume and negotiate discounts or rebates with other stakeholders in the supply chain. In contrast, generic drug manufacturers compete solely on the basis of price and the ability to supply. As a result, brand- name drug companies retain 76% of all revenue, while other stakeholders in the supply chain capture 24%.[98]20 For generic drug manufacturers, the economic reality is different.

Generic drug manufacturers retain 36%, while other stakeholders capture 64% of all revenue.[99]21

In the brand-name drug market, brand-name drug companies use their leverage in the supply chain to negotiate formulary placement through rebate agreements with PBMs and health insurers. There is little room for wholesalers and pharmacies to capture large margins due to their relative lack of negotiating power. And pharmacy reimbursement for brand-name drugs is tied to the reported price and there is generally only one product available.

For the generic drug market, wholesalers, through collaborative purchasing agreements with pharmacies across the country, and group purchasing organizations exert leverage through their purchasing power and the robust competition among multiple generic manufacturers who are making identical products. More than 90% of all generic drug sales are controlled by three consolidated wholesaler-pharmacy groups.[100]22 This results in significant downward pressure on price, which can result in sustainability challenges for generic manufacturers and can leave generic drugs vulnerable to drug shortages.

---

[98] USC Schaeffer, "The Flow of Money Through the Pharmaceutical Distribution System," June 2017 (https://healthpolicy.usc.edu/research/flow-of-money-through-the-pharmaceutical-distribution-system/).

[99] *Ibid.*

[100] Adam Fein, "The 2018–19 Economic Report on Pharmaceutical Wholesalers and Specialty Distributors," October 2018 *(https://www.drugchannels.net/2018/10/new-201819-economic-report-on.html).*

Build Back Better's Proposed Reforms Harm Generic and Biosimilar Development

The House-passed Build Back Better Act (H.R. 5376) threatens to reduce seniors' access to generics and biosimilars, potentially dampening competition for years to come, with its approach to direct negotiations in Medicare and inflation-based rebate penalties. In contrast, the bipartisan Prescription Drug Pricing Reduction Act of 2019 ("Grassley-Wyden") would effectively tackle the high cost of brand-name prescription drugs without disrupting the ability of generic and biosimilar manufactur- ers to compete.

Direct Medicare Negotiations

The Build Back Better Act's direct Medicare negotiations would alter the careful balance struck between innovation and access enacted as part of the Hatch-Waxman Amendments in 1984 and the Biologics Price Competition and Innovation Act (BPCIA) in 2010. The negotiations framework severely erodes the incentives for biosimilar and generic development, keeping drug prices high for some seniors, while forgoing additional cost savings.

Biosimilars are complex products that can require 8 to 10 years to develop, at a cost of $100 to $250 million.[101]23 After years of high-risk investment, the biosimilar industry is poised to deliver tremendous savings to the U.S. health care system, improving access for patients and lowering prescription drug costs. New biosimilars are expected to launch for a range of treatments for patients with diabetes, arthritis, macular degeneration, oncology and more. As shown below, 42 biosimilars are on track to launch in the coming years.[102]24 However, the negotiation framework in the Build Back Better Act threatens this progress and could undermine biosimilar competition, resulting in fewer options for care and higher costs for patients.

---

[101] AAM, "The Evidence Is Clear: Biosimilar Competition Will Achieve More Savings for Patients Than Build Back Better's Negotiations," December 2021 *(https://accessiblemeds.org/re-sources/blog/competition-biosimilars-will-achieve-more-savings-bbb-negotiation).*

[102] Cardinal Health, "2022 Biosimilars Report," February 2022 *(https://www.cardinalhealth.com/content/dam/corp/web/documents/Report/cardinal-health-2022-biosimilars-report.pdf).*

Figure 43. **New and upcoming biosimilars launches**

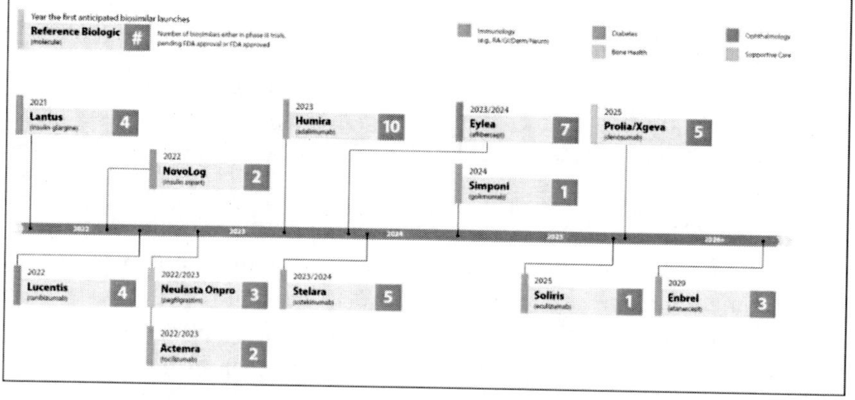

Under the Build Back Better proposal, HHS would have the authority to negotiate prices with manufacturers for 100 drugs or more by 2030, a number of them ref- erence biologics that could be subject to biosimilar competition. IQVIA estimates biosimilars will deliver more than $130 billion in savings by 2024. That is greater savings for patients than the Build Back Better proposal and it starts right now. And as more biosimilars and interchangeable biologics become available, there is the potential for much larger savings as providers and payers take advantage of the op- portunities to improve access and reduce costs for patients with these products.

The House-passed version of the Build Back Better Act, however, would put these savings in jeopardy. The aggressive use of non-innovative patents by brand-name pharmaceutical companies delays entry for biosimilars past the point of the negotiation window. As a result, it takes biosimilars many years to launch, and AAM would welcome further efforts by Congress to address patent abuse and accelerate timelines for biosimilar competition. But rather than addressing the core problem of patent abuse, the Build Back Better framework imposes price controls that could actually reduce biosimilar competition and reward brand manufacturers.[103] While Build Back Better's reforms may reduce the cost of some brand-name drugs for Medicare, it would do so at the expense of biosimilar development for all patients. This would harm long-term savings available through competition, and it would directly

[103] AAM, "Medicare Negotiations Serve as a Catalyst to a Perpetual Monopoly," November 2021 (https://accessiblemeds.org/resources/blog/medicare-negotiations-serve-catalyst-perpetual- monopoly).

result in higher prices for employers and private market payers who are counting on biosimilar competition.[104]

The cumulative result is that the uncertainty associated with developing and bring- ing a biosimilar to market would skyrocket, and the potential market opportunity for lower-cost competitors would be cut by at least 60%. At the time biosimilar developers decide on whether to commit to a $100–$250 million investment, manufac- turers will have no way to know whether a reference product will be selected for negotiation or what the negotiated price might be. The resulting uncertainty created by the Build Back Better Act's negotiation framework therefore threatens the future of an industry that has already demonstrated its promise by helping cut by 50% the spending growth rate in oncology treatments. While the approach in the Build Back Better Act may result in savings on faster timelines than biosimilars are able to launch, the dampening effect on competition may result in few options for patients and additional downstream savings never materializing. The proposal can and must be adjusted to avoid harming the incentives to develop generic and biosimilar medicines for seniors, children and other patients should Congress advance them further.

Inflation-Based Rebates

In addition, the House-passed Build Back Better Act would apply inflation-based rebate penalties to generics. This is misguided and would limit patients' access to low- cost medicines. The proposal is based on a policy designed for the brand drug market. Under the policy, drugs face a penalty when a product's average price rises faster than inflation (less than 2% in recent years). But while FDA-approved generics function the same way as innovative drugs for patient health, their market functions very differently, and any policies should be tailored to the market. The Prescription Drug Pricing Reduction Act ("Grassley-Wyden") recognized those differences and thus did not include generic and biosimilar medicines in its inflation-based rebate penalties.

Inexpensive products are particularly sensitive to percentage-based triggers for an inflation-based penalty. For instance, a change of one penny in the average price of a generic costing 20 cents per pill would likely trigger the

---

104 AAM, "Proposed BBB Negotiation Framework Discourages Biosimilar Competition, Imposes Higher Costs on Commercially Insured Patients and Their Employers," December 2021 *(https:// accessiblemeds.org/resources/blog/proposed-bbb-negotiation-framework-discourages-biosimilar- competition-imposes-higher).*

penalty. And unlike brand drugs, generics compete based on lower list prices and can experience volatile swings in their Average Manufacturer Price (AMP) even when they do not raise their price. This can occur when a generic keeps its prices unchanged but experiences changes in the quantity purchased as other manufacturers compete for business. The result is that a generic may keep its price level but see its AMP increase because of changes in customer purchasing patterns.

This is not merely hypothetical. Generic manufacturers are already struggling with the impact of this policy as applied in the Medicaid market. A survey of AAM members determined that 40 to 100% of total penalties assessed under the Medicaid policy were attributable to changes in customer purchasing behavior, meaning that the majority of instances where companies incurred the Medicaid inflation penalty were not associated with a true increase in the drug's list price. Moreover, half of the respondents indicated the penalty was applied to products that were recently or currently on the FDA shortage list.

The proposed policy, which applies to generic drugs sold in Medicare Part D and the commercial market, creates an additional barrier to a sustainable market for vulnerable products. It undermines the ability of low-cost generics to stay on the market and can serve as a barrier to reentering a market—even to prevent a drug shortage.

In the updated Build Back Better text released on December 11th, the Senate Finance Committee narrowed the applicability of the inflation-based rebate penalty on generics in Medicare Part D. The penalty would apply only to single-source generics with a total cost greater than $100 per beneficiary per year and provides the HHS Secretary with discretion to exempt products due to shortages or supply chain disruptions. This is a material improvement to the House-passed Build Back Better Act.

AAM strongly recommends aligning the current inflation-based penalty under Medicaid with the Build Back Better's definition should this policy move forward. While generic medicines are not a contributing factor to the drug pricing problem and should therefore be exempt from any inflation-based penalties, Congress should at a minimum align the policies to minimize the operational costs associated with compliance. Generic manufacturers already operate on relatively low margins and onerous requirements and penalties serve only to threaten the sustainability of the market.

Building a Better Prescription Drug Market Rests on More Generic, Biosimilar Competition and Access

Increasing competition and patient access to generic and biosimilar medicines must be at the center of any reform to the prescription drug market. AAM's recommended reforms build on the progress made in recent years to increase patient access to lower-cost medicines, but it is without question that much more can and should be done to achieve the full potential of generic and biosimilar competition. Modernizing the Medicare program is an important place to start.

Medicare modernization is integral to both lower drugs costs for patients and make the federal health programs more sustainable for future generations. Generic and biosimilar medicines face significant barriers to use and adoption in Medicare because of policy choices that unintentionally incentivize plans to prioritize formulary placement of high-cost brand drugs. These challenges are the result of the design of the Part D Coverage Gap Program, which rewards plans for preferring a high-cost brand drug, and the Part D drug rebate sharing formula, which allows plans to benefit from covering high-rebate brand drugs—even when it results in higher costs for Medicare and patients.

To this end, AAM recommends the Senate Finance Committee advance the following reforms:

- Address the biosimilar rebate trap and increase patient access to biosimilar medicines.

The manner by which drug rebates can be used by high-cost brand-name drugs to block generic or biosimilar competition has been well documented. Rebate traps are of particular concern in the Medicare program because of the manner in which rebates are shared with CMS. Specifically, plans retain all rebates until the catastrophic phase of the benefit, at which point plans retain 20% of the rebates—even though plans are liable for only 15% of the costs. This means that the value of high rebates on brand drugs, combined with the impacts of beneficiary cost-sharing differences and Part D subsidies and program design, may drive plans to give equivalent or preferential tier placement to higher-cost brand drugs because the rebates are more valuable to the plan—even if the brand drugs have a higher net price or result in higher costs to patients and taxpayers.

As generics seek to compete and biosimilars are poised to enter the Part D market, the rebate sharing formula continues to be a major concern. This practice undermines efforts to reduce patient out-of-pocket spending by further inhibiting access to lower-cost generic products, forcing additional costs onto America's seniors. Congress has a number of options available to address this issue, such as revising the rebate sharing formula such that plans are permitted to keep only the portion of rebates for which they are financially liable or even requiring rebate pass-through before a patient enters the catastrophic phase of the benefit. Moreover, we encourage Congress to ensure that Medicare policies encourage true price competition and do not create perverse financial incentives favoring high-cost brand-name medicines.

In addition, AAM supports the following policies to help increase biosimilar adoption, generating savings for patients and the federal government:

- Modest increase to Medicare Part B reimbursement (ASP+8%). This policy was included in the Prescription Drug Pricing Reduction Act ("Grassley- Wyden"), introduced as The BIOSIM Act (H.R. 2815) by Representatives Kurt Schrader (D–OR) and Adam Kinzinger (R–IL), and included in The Lower Drug Costs Now Act (H.R. 3).[105]27
- Establish a Medicare shared-savings demonstration program. Bipartisan leg- islation has been introduced in the Senate and House as the Increasing Access to Biosimilars Act (S. 1427/H.R. 2869) by Senators John Cornyn (R–TX) and Michael Bennet (D–CO) and Representatives Tony Cardenas (D–CA) and Angie Craig (D–MN).[106]28 Estimates prepared by Milliman suggest that this demonstration program could save up to $3.2 billion for patients and as much as $12.5 billion for the federal government over the next 10 years.[107]

---

[105] AAM Letter of Support for BIOSIM Act *(http://biosimilarscouncil.org/wp-content/uploads/2021/04/AAM-BC-Letter-of-Support-BIOSIM-Act-04-22-21.pdf);* Rep. Kurt Schrader, "Schrader Introduces Bipartisan Bill to Make Biosimilar Drugs More Affordable to Patients," September 2019 *(https://schrader.house.gov/newsroom/ documentsingle.aspx?DocumentID =392607).*

[106] AAM Letter of Support for Increasing Access to Biosimilars Act *(https:// biosimilars.staging. wpengine.com/wp-content/uploads/2021/04/AAM-BC-Letter-of-Support-for- Increasing-Access-to-Biosimilars-Act-04-28-21.pdf);* Sen. John Cornyn, "Cornyn, Bennet Introduce Bill to Address High Cost of Prescription Drugs for Seniors," July 2020 *(https:// www.cornyn.senate.gov/content/news/cornyn-bennet-introduce-bill-address-high-cost-prescrip- tion-drugs-seniors);* Rep. Tony Cardenas, "Cardenas, Hudson, Craig, Fitzpatrick Introduce the Increasing Access to Biosimilars Act," March 2020 *(https://cardenas.house.gov/media-center/ press-releases/c-rdenas-hudson-craig-fitzpatrick-introduce-increasing-access).*

[107] *Ibid.,* Milliman.

- Reduce cost sharing for patients in Medicare Part B. This policy was introduced in the 116th Congress as the ACCESS Act (H.R. 4597) by Representative Scott Peters (D–CA).[108]
- Allow biosimilars to qualify for mid-year formulary changes. We encourage CMS to align the regulation surrounding mid-year formulary changes and notice requirements to make biosimilars consistent with those of small-molecule drugs. This would provide plan sponsors with another lever to use to encourage beneficiary use of the lower-cost biosimilar option.
- Ensure that plan utilization management strategies do not prohibit the use of biosimilars. Specifically, we encourage CMS to clarify that utilization management tools are based on the molecule, not the product. This would make it easier for a patient currently receiving biologic therapy to switch to a lower-cost biosimilar without once again being subject to step therapy requirements that they have already navigated.
- Reduce cost sharing for seniors in Medicare and for low-income beneficiaries.

Generic and biosimilar medicines can provide significant savings for patients only if they are covered on the appropriate Medicare Part D formulary tier. Ensuring coverage of newly available generic and biosimilar medicines, reducing patient cost sharing through proper formulary tier coverage and creating a new specialty tier for biosimilars can significantly encourage generic and biosimilar adoption. To this end, AAM recommends three distinct policy solutions:

- Ensure Medicare Part D plans cover new generic medicines, particularly first generics, at launch;
- Create a separate specialty tier to allow for differentiation among specialty brands and more affordable generics and biosimilars; and,
- Reduce cost sharing for seniors by providing for placement of all generic medicines on formulary tiers designated as generic and separate from highpriced brand-name drugs.

---

108 Rep. Scott Peters, "Reps. Peters, King, Cardenas Introduce Bipartisan Bill to Make Cost-Effective Biosimilars More Accessible," October 2019 *(https://scottpeters.house.gov/media-center/press-releases/reps-peters-king-brindisi-introduce-bipartisan-bill-to-make-cost-0).*

First generics—drugs approved by FDA as the first competitor to a brand—benefit patients and the health care system. First generics represent new competition and lower prices beginning, on average, 40% lower than brand drugs. But Medicare prescription drug formularies are covering only 21% of the first generics launched in 2020. Commercial health plan formularies, by contrast, covered 66% of first generics.[109] This is not a one-time statistical blip. It is the continuation of a trend whereby Medicare drug plans are significantly slower to cover first generics, delay- ing seniors' access to lower-cost competition. Even when Medicare drug plans do cover first generics, these plans tend to place them on brand drug tiers with higher patient cost sharing, rather than on low copay generic tiers.

In addition, seniors are not realizing the full value of lower-cost generics. As noted earlier, generic drugs have increasingly been moved to brand tiers with higher copays—even when the cost of the generic drug has declined. Not only has this caused significant increases in out-of-pocket costs for beneficiaries, but it even means that patients may be responsible for the full cost of the drug. A recent analysis found that in cases where the generic is covered on Tier 3, nearly 45% of Medicare Part D beneficiaries paid the full cost of their generic at least once while in the initial coverage limit of their benefit.[110] In other words, their generic drug cost less than the plan's required copayment, causing the patient to pay the full price of the product at the pharmacy.

Should one or more of these policies be enacted in the next few months, seniors could select these new coverage options during open enrollment beginning October 2022 with coverage effective in January 2023. A combination of these policies would ensure that patients have access to safe, affordable generic and biosimilar medicines, as well as ensure a viable and competitive prescription drug market for years to come.

In doing so, accelerating coverage of newly launched generics could lower premiums by $2.5 billion and federal health spending by $7.3 billion.[111] Creating a new specialty tier for specialty generics and biosimilars would

[109] AAM, "New Generics Are Less Available in Medicare Than Commercial Plans," July 2021 (https://accessiblemeds.org/sites/default/files/2021-07/AAM-New-Generics-Are-Less-Available-in-Medicare-2021.pdf).

[110] Avalere, "Some Part D Beneficiaries May Pay Full Price for Certain Generic Drugs," July 2021 (https://avalere.com/insights/some-part-d-beneficiaries-may-pay-full-price-for-certain-generic-drugs).

[111] AAM, "White Paper: Access Denied: Why New Generics Are Not Reaching America's Seniors," October 2019 (https://accessiblemeds.org/sites/default/files/2019-09/AAM-White-Paper-Access-Denied-First-Generics-web_0.pdf).

likely have a negligible impact on premiums, while reducing federal health spending (savings up to $11 billion) depending on how it is implemented. And while ensuring generic medicines are on generic cost-sharing tiers (Tiers I and II) may nominally increase premiums, it would save seniors as much as $4 billion per year in lower out-of-pocket costs.[112]

The bipartisan Ensuring Access to Lower-Cost Medicines Act (H.R. 2846) was introduced by Rep. David McKinley (R–WV) and Rep. Ann Kuster (D–NH).[113] Similar policies were offered as an amendment by Sen. Robert Menendez (D–NJ), Sen. James Lankford (R–OK), Sen. Ben Cardin (D–MD) and Sen. Steve Daines (R–MT) in the 116th Congress during the Senate Finance Committee's markup of the Prescription Drug Pricing Reduction Act ("Grassley-Wyden").

Another option to consider is reducing cost sharing for low-income Medicare beneficiaries (LIS). LIS beneficiaries typically utilize more expensive brand-name drugs even when lower-cost biosimilar and generic medicines are available. In 2018, HHS estimated the Part D program and its beneficiaries could have saved $2.8 billion with full generic substitution in 2016.[114] Reducing the out-of-pocket costs for low- income seniors through policies designed to encourage the greater use of generic medicines could save up to $18 billion over 10 years, according to CBO.[115] We encourage Congress to support legislation to this end.

- Modernize the Part D benefit to encourage more generic and biosimilar adoption.

The Medicare Part D benefit should be updated to incentivize the use of lower-price, high-quality medicines by eliminating the perverse incentives that favor high-cost brand-name drugs. AAM recommends that such efforts:

---

[112] Avalere, "Medicare Part D Generic Drug Tiering Request for Comment: Implications for Patient Out-of-Pocket Spending and Part D Plan Costs," February 2019 *(https://avalere.com/wp-content/uploads/2019/02/20190228-White-Paper-Part-D-Generic-Tiering.pdf).*

[113] Rep. Annie Kuster, "Kuster, McKinley Introduce Bipartisan Legislation to Help Save Seniors Billions in Drug Costs," April 2021 *(https://kuster.house.gov/news/documentsingle.aspx?DocumentID=3535#:~:text=Act%20last%20Congress.-,The%20Ensuring%20Access%20to%20Lower%2DCost%20Medicines%20for%20Seniors%20Act,charged%20the%20higher%20brand%20rate.).*

[114] *Ibid.*, HHS 2018.

[115] CBO, "Proposals for Health Care Programs—CBO's Estimate of the President's Fiscal Year 2017 Budget" [Line 59], March 2016 *(https://www.cbo.gov/system/files/2020-03/56243-2016- 03-29-health-programs.pdf).*

- Incentivize the use of lower-cost biosimilars and generics by decreasing plan liability for these products; and
- Align plan incentives for using low-cost products by decreasing government reinsurance and increasing plan liability in the catastrophic phase.

The House-passed Build Back Better Act sets plan liability in the catastrophic phase of the Part D benefit at 60% for all prescription drugs. The Prescription Drug Pricing Reduction Act ("Grassley-Wyden") differentiates between brand-name (66%) and generics (60%). AAM recommends setting plan liability at 50% for generics and 50% for biosimilars to encourage greater adoption of these lower-cost medicines.

- Eliminate the penalty on generics in Medicaid.

Manufacturers of affordable generic medicines are now paying millions of dollars in penalties on prescription drugs that have not been subject to a price increase. These unpredictable, onerous penalties—totaling $1.6 billion over 10 years—make it challenging to continue production of low-margin generics and threaten patient access to life-saving medicine. Repealing the Medicaid Generics Penalty alleviates the harmful and unintended consequences of this policy on patients.

We strongly encourage Congress to advance the Protecting Access to Affordable Medicines Act (H.R. 2868) introduced by Representative G.K. Butterfield (D–NC) and Billy Long (R–MO). This proposal would exempt the lowest-cost generics, those with a price of less than $1 per unit, and would help address the misguided application of the Medicaid rebate on generic medicines, thus reducing the risk of drug shortages and benefiting patients through sustainable access to low-cost generics.[116]

---

[116] AAM Letter of Support for the Protecting Access to Affordable Medicines Act (2021); Rep. G.K. Butterfield, "Congressman Butterfield Introduces Bipartisan Bill to Fix Medicaid Penalty for Low-Cost Generics," October 2020 *(https://butterfield.house.gov/media-center/press-releases/congressman-butterfield-introduces-bipartisan-bill-to-fix-medicaid#:~:text=Federal%20Agency%20Help-,Congressman%20Butterfield%20Introduces%20Bipartisan%20Bill%20to,Penalty.%20for%20Low-Cost%20Generics&text=This%20will%20help%20ensure%20that,to%20quality%20and%20affordable%20medications.).*

Conclusion

Congress is right to try to meet the expectations of a nation concerned about the high prices of brand-name drugs. But policies to reform drug pricing should be focused on ensuring that Americans have access to more affordable medicines by eliminating barriers and improving incentives for competition. The House-passed Build Back Better Act offers an untested approach that, in our estimation, would harm the development of generic and biosimilar medicines. The Senate Finance Committee has an opportunity to advance policies that will yield more immediate and lasting results in lowering the cost of prescription drugs for patients. We welcome the opportunity to work together toward that shared goal.

March 16, 2022

Association of Community Cancer Centers

1801 Research Boulevard, Suite 400
Rockville, MD 20850
T: 301–984–9496
F: 301–770–1949
www.accc-cancer.org

The Honorable Ron Wyden
Chairman
U.S. Senate, Committee on Finance
221 Dirksen Senate Office Building
Washington, DC 20510

The Honorable Mike Crapo
Ranking Member
U.S. Senate
Committee on Finance
239 Dirksen Senate Office Building
Washington, DC 20510
RE: "Prescription Drug Price Inflation: An Urgent Need to Lower Drug Prices in Medicare"

Dear Senators Wyden and Crapo,

On behalf our member cancer programs and practices, the Association of Commu- nity Cancer Centers (ACCC) would like to thank the Senate Finance Committee for holding this hearing on "Prescription Drug Price Inflation: An Urgent Need to Lower Drug Prices in Medicare". In considering legislation to reduce out-of-pocket prescription drug costs for Medicare beneficiaries, it is important for the Committee to consider the cancer care provider perspective, and we appreciate the opportunity to submit the following statement for the record.

ACCC is the leading education and advocacy organization for our nation's cancer care community, representing a network of 28,000 multidisciplinary practitioners from 2,100 hospitals and practices nationwide. The diversity of our membership uniquely positions ACCC to effectively engage with policymakers about the need for reforms to reduce out-of-pocket costs for prescription drugs and drugs administered in both academic and community-based oncology practices, clinics, and hospitals.

ACCC supports the goal of reducing the cost of prescription drugs for Medicare beneficiaries. However, we are concerned that the "maximum fair price" standard proposed for achieving cost savings in the Build Back Better Act (BBBA) would neg- atively impact reimbursement for providers that administer drugs covered under Medicare Part B. We also fear this legislation would threaten the financial viability of cancer programs and practices across the country and reduce Medicare bene- ficiary access to crucial medications and treatments. We therefore request that the Committee pursue legislative solutions that hold providers harmless in the drug pricing negotiation between the federal government and drug manufacturers.

The current level of reimbursement for Medicare Part B drugs affords cancer care providers the necessary capital to fund crucial elements of a comprehensive cancer care program. This not only includes the cost of overhead, but the ability to invest in new and innovative technologies, patient care coordination and supportive care services, and adequate staffing structures for care delivery. By reducing reimburse- ment for Medicare Part B drugs, we believe that the drug pricing provisions of the BBBA would limit the ability of cancer programs to provide quality care to the di- verse communities they serve.

Moreover, we are concerned that reductions in drug reimbursement outlined in the BBBA may worsen the financial challenges that many community cancer programs are already experiencing. Oncology programs and practices in smaller communities, rural areas, and areas of high Medicare penetration stand to be most severely affected by these reimbursement cuts. These community providers may be faced with the difficult decision to reduce available treatment options and services or even close their doors as a result. This would create new access issues for Medicare beneficiaries, with a disproportionate effect on the poor, vulnerable, and people of color.

ACCC believes that the most effective treatment options should be available to patients at the lowest cost, and any proposed changes in reimbursement for drugs should promote health equity while maintaining the ability of cancer programs to provide necessary support services for potentially disadvantaged populations. Therefore, we are troubled by the drug pricing provisions of the BBBA because of their potential to exacerbate existing inequities in cancer care delivery.

For these reasons, we encourage the Committee to refine the drug pricing provisions of the BBBA to remove providers from the middle of proposed drug pricing negotiations between the federal government and drug manufacturers. The proposal to establish a new negotiated price would severely impact reimbursement for providers that administer the selected Part B drugs, with the largest and most immediate impact on providers that treat predominantly Medicare beneficiaries. This change in pricing structure would also impact commercial reimbursement in a way that unfairly penalizes providers.

As the voice of our nation's cancer care community, we strongly urge the Committee to consider the impacts of drug price negotiation on cancer care providers and their ability to provide high quality, equitable care to the patients they serve. If you have any questions, please contact Matt Devino at mdevino@accc-cancer.org or (301) 263– 3510.

Respectfully,
Krista Nelson, MSW, LCSW, OSW–C, FAOSW President

Center for Fiscal Equity

14448 Parkvale Road, Suite 6
Rockville, MD 20853 fiscalequitycenter@yahoo.com

Statement of Michael Bindner

Chairman Wyden and Ranking Member Crapo, thank you for the opportunity to address this issue.

These concerns have been with us for decades. They still demand attention. PhARMA and AARP have put so much money into advertising on both sides that something must either be done, or loudly ignored. The advertisements on both sides have, to date, provided more heat than light - which was to be expected. Let us try to move to the facts so that we might find solutions.

The decision to not allow Medicare Part D to follow the Department of Veterans Af- fairs and negotiate down drug prices helped end the balanced budget that President Bush inherited from President Clinton.

This bill also pushed Bruce Bartlett out of the Republican Party and prompted the writing of the book that sealed the deal. The passage of that legislation was fishy, from leaving the vote open unto the wee hours of the night to future hiring of the law's author by big PhARMA.

While the Affordable Care Act helped ameliorate the worst feature of Part D, the coverage gap in the middle, it did not eliminate it. Perhaps competition will allow that gap to be filled.

PhARMA relies, in part, on claims that negotiation will lead to cost shifting. The dirty little secret in this debate is that single-payer solutions in the rest of the OECD have already resulted in cost shifting, where the rest of the world shifts its cost to the United States. Most people with insurance don't notice this. Single payer healthcare, either through a public option or Medicare for All, will further bury this. For now, allowing drug price negotiation will give drug companies leverage to renegotiate their deals with the rest of the world.

PhARMA also relies on the claims that new cures for pandemics and subsidizing the development of orphan drugs and new therapies requires the right to charge the most the market can bear. This ignores the fact that most basic research comes through government grants and contracts, not drug company profits. The latter fund commercial, not scientific, development.

In comments to Ways and Means, House Budget and this Committee in 2019 and 2020, we discussed how to fund orphan drugs and new treatments so that no one remains untreated due to insurance coverage.

A main problem with high-cost drugs, especially orphan drugs, is the high development costs and the cost of small batch manufacturing. This could drive the need to raise drug prices for mature drugs in order to subsidize the orphans, although some hikes are undertaken because no one can stop them. The solution for this is for NIH and the FDA to own the rights to orphan drugs and to contract out research and development costs as it does basic research, as well as testing and production.

PhARMA would still make reasonable profit, but the government would eat the risk and sometimes reap the rewards. NIH/FDA might even break even in the long term, especially if large volume drugs which were developed with government grants must pay back a share of basic research costs and the attached profits, as well as regulatory cost.

Universal coverage, starting with a public option under the Affordable Care Act, with eventual evolution to some type of single-payer system is inevitable. Unless we start building negotiation into the system now, we will give the drug companies a reason to oppose reform later.

A public option will only pass if pre-existing condition reforms are abolished with public option enrollment being automatic upon rejection. The public option must be subsidized, replacing Medicaid for the disabled and those not requiring long-term nursing care. Long-term care should be removed from states and replaced with a new federal Medicare Part E.

The profit motive, with the need to constantly increase profits to attract Wall Street investment or keep stock prices growing will lead to an ever increasing number of people who will be considered uninsurable, thus relying on the public option.

Most healthcare systems will provide services to both comprehensive insurance beneficiaries, the retired, the disabled and those with the public option. In other words, Medicare for All is our future, with the only exception being firms abandoning the system and providing their own doctors while making arrangements with local hospitals and specialists—essentially creating local HMOs.

The major issue here is funding, although more efficiency will reduce prices. Costs are already minimized by the for-profit and by governmental medical care (which often uses for profit networks). To repeat, with a shout THE ISSUE IS PRICE, NOT COST!

Attachments are included on Universal Coverage and our updated Tax Reform Plans discuss these issues in further detail. The latter finds the money to both pay for healthcare and an expanded child tax credit without expanding the "welfare state" bureaucracy so many love to hate.

Thank you again for the opportunity to add our comments to the debate. Please contact us if we can be of any assistance or contribute direct testimony.

Attachment One—Hearing on "Pathways to Universal Health Coverage," June 12, 2019

There are three methods to get to single-payer: a public option, Medicare for All and single-payer with an option for cooperative employers.

The first to set up a public option and end protections for pre-existing conditions and mandates. The public option would then cover all families who are rejected for either pre-existing conditions or the inability to pay. In essence, this is an expansion of Medicaid to everyone with a pre-existing condition. As such, it would be funded through increased taxation, which will be addressed below. A variation is the expan- sion of the Uniformed Public Health Service to treat such individuals and their families.

The public option is inherently unstable over the long term. The profit motive will ultimately make the exclusion pool grow until private insurance would no longer be justified, leading-again to Single Payer if the race to cut customers leads to no one left in private insurance who is actually sick. This eventually becomes Medicare for All, but with easier passage and sudden adoption as private health plans are either banned or become bankrupt. Single-payer would then be what occurs when.

The second option is Medicare for All, which I described in an attachment to June 18th and 19th's comments and previously in hearings held May 8, 2019 (Finance) and May 8, 2018 (Ways and Means). Medicare for All is essentially Medicaid for All without the smell of welfare and with providers reimbursed at Medicare levels, with the difference funded by tax revenue.

Medicare for All is a really good slogan, at least to mobilize the base. One would think it would attract the support of even the Tea Partiers who held up signs saying, "don't let the government touch my Medicare!" Alas, it has not. This has been a conversation on the left and it has not gotten beyond shouting slogans either. We need to decide what we want and whether it really is Medicare for All. If we want to go to any doctor we wish, pay nothing and have no premiums, then that is not Medicare.

There are essentially two Medicares, a high option and a low one. One option has Part A at no cost (funded by the Hospital Insurance Payroll Tax and part of Obamacare's high unearned income tax as well as the general fund), Medicare Part B, with a 20% copay and a $135 per month premium and Medicare Part D, which has both premiums and copays and is run through private providers. Parts A and B also are contracted out to insurance companies for case management. Much of this is now managed care, as is Medicare Advantage (Part C).

Medicaid lingers in the background and the foreground. It covers the disabled in their first two years (and probably while they are seeking disability and unable to work). It covers non-workers and the working poor (who are too poor for Obamacare) and it covers seniors and the disabled who are confined to a long-term care facility and who have run out their assets. It also has the long-term portion which should be federalized, but for the poor, it takes the form of an HMO, but with no premiums and zero copays.

Obamacare has premiums with income-based supports (one of those facts the Republicans hate) and copays. It may have a high option, like the Federal Employee Health Benefits Program (which also covers Congress) on which it is modeled, a standard option that puts you into an HMO. The HMO drug copays for Obamacare are higher than for Medicare Part C, but the office visit prices are exactly the same.

What does it mean, then, to want Medicare for All? If it means we want everyone who can afford it to get Medicare Advantage Coverage, we already have that. It is Obamacare. The reality is that Senator Sanders wants to reduce Medicare copays and premiums to Medicaid levels and then slowly reduce eligibility levels until ev- eryone is covered. Of course, this will still likely give us HMO coverage for everyone except the very rich, unless he adds a high-option PPO or reimbursable plan.

Either Medicare for All or a real single payer would require a very large payroll tax (and would eliminate the HI tax) or an employer paid subtraction value-added tax (so it would not appear on receipts nor would it be zero rated at the border, since there would be no evading it), which we discuss below, because the Health Care Reform debate is ultimately a tax reform debate. Too much money is at stake for it to be otherwise, although we may do just as well to call Obamacare Medicare for All and leave it alone.

The third option is an exclusion for employers, especially employee-owned and cooperative firms, who provide medical care directly to their employees without third party insurance, with the employer making HMO-like arrangements with local hospitals and medical practices for inpatient and specialist care.

Employer-based taxes, such as a subtraction VAT or payroll tax, will provide an incentive to avoid these taxes by providing such care. Employers who fund catastrophic care or operate nursing care facilities would get an even higher benefit, with the proviso that any care so provided be superior to the care available through Medicaid or Medicare for All. Making employers responsible for most costs and for all cost savings allows them to use some market power to get lower rates.

This proposal is probably the most promising way to arrest health care costs from their current upward spiral—as employers who would be financially responsible for this care through taxes would have a real incentive to limit spending in a way that individual taxpayers simply do not have the means or incentive to exercise. The employee ownership must ultimately expand to most of the economy as an alternative to capitalism, which is also unstable as income concentration becomes obvious to all.

Attachment Two—Tax Reform, Center for Fiscal Equity, December 7, 2021 Individual Payroll Taxes. Employee Payroll Tax of 7.2% for Old-Age and Survivors

Insurance. Funds now collected as a matching premium to a consumption tax based contribution credited at an equal dollar rate for all workers qualified within a quarter. An employer-paid subtraction value-added tax would be used if offsets to private accounts are included. Without such accounts, the invoice value-added tax would collect these funds. No payroll tax would be collected from employees if all contributions are credited on an equal dollar basis. If employee taxes are retained, the ceiling would be lowered to $100,000 to reduce benefits paid to wealthier individuals and a $16,000 floor should be established so that Earned Income Tax Credits are no longer needed. Subsidies for single workers should be abandoned in favor of radically higher minimum wages. If a $10 minimum wage is passed, the employee contribution floor would increase to $20,000.

Wage Surtaxes. Individual income taxes on salaries, which exclude business taxes, above an individual standard deduction of $100,000 per year, will range from 7.2% to 57.6%. This tax will fund net interest on the debt (which will no longer be rolled over into new borrowing), redemption of the Social Security Trust Fund, strategic, sea and non-continental U.S. military deployments, veterans' health benefits as the result of battlefield injuries, including mental health and addiction and eventual debt reduction.

Our proposed brackets have been increased from $85,000 to $100,000 because this is the income level at the top of the 80% of tax paying households who earn the bottom third of adjusted gross income. Earners above this level are considered middle class. Likewise, the top 1% of income earners are at the $500,000 level, which will be used as the start of the highest rate.

Asset Value-Added Tax (A–VAT). A replacement for capital gains taxes, dividend taxes, and the estate tax. It will apply to asset sales, dividend distributions, exercised options, rental income, inherited and gifted assets and the profits from short sales. Tax payments for option exercises, IPOs, inherited, gifted and donated assets will be marked to market, with prior tax payments for that asset eliminated so that the seller gets no benefit from them. In this perspective, it is the owner's increase in value that is taxed. As with any sale of liquid or real assets, sales to a qualified broad-based Employee Stock Ownership Plan will be tax free. These taxes will fund the same spending items as income or S–VAT surtaxes.

This tax will end Tax Gap issues owed by high income individuals. A 26% rate is between the GOP 23.8% rate (including ACA–SM surtax) and the Democratic 28.8% rate as proposed in the Build Back Better Act. It's time to quit playing football with tax rates to attract side bets. A single rate also stops gaming forms of ownership. Lower rates are not as regressive as they seem. Only the wealthy have capital gains in any significant amount. The de facto rate for everyone else is zero. For now, however, a 28.8% rate is assumed if reform is enacted by a Democratic majority in both Houses.

Subtraction Value-Added Tax (S–VAT). These are employer paid Net Business Receipts Taxes. S–VAT is a vehicle for tax benefits, including

- Health insurance or direct care, including veterans' health care for non- battlefield injuries and long-term care.
- Employer-paid educational costs in lieu of taxes are provided as either employee-directed contributions to the public or private unionized school of their choice or direct tuition payments for employee children or for workers (including ESL and remedial skills). Wages will be paid to students to meet opportunity costs.
- Most importantly, a refundable child tax credit at median income levels (with inflation adjustments) distributed with pay.

Subsistence-level benefits force the poor into servile labor. Wages and benefits must be high enough to provide justice and human dignity. This allows the ending of state administered subsidy programs and discourages abortions, and as such enactment must be scored as a must pass in voting rankings by pro-life organizations (and feminist organizations as well). To assure child subsidies are distributed, S– VAT will not be border adjustable.

The S–VAT is also used for personal accounts in Social Security, provided that these accounts are insured through an insurance fund for all such accounts, that accounts go toward employee ownership rather than for a subsidy for the investment industry. Both employers and employees must consent to a shift to these accounts, which will occur if corporate democracy in existing ESOPs is given a thorough test. So far it has not. S–VAT funded retirement accounts will be equal-dollar credited for every worker. They also have the advantage of drawing on both payroll and profit, making it less regressive.

A multi-tier S–VAT could replace income surtaxes in the same range. Some will use corporations to avoid these taxes, but that corporation would then pay all invoice and subtraction VAT payments (which would distribute tax benefits. Distributions from such corporations will be considered salary, not dividends.

Invoice Value-Added Tax (I–VAT). Border adjustable taxes will appear on purchase invoices. The rate varies according to what is being financed. If Medicare for All does not contain offsets for employers who fund their own medical personnel or for personal retirement accounts, both of which would otherwise be funded by an S–VAT, then they would be funded by the I–VAT to take advantage of border adjustability. I–VAT also forces everyone, from the working poor to the beneficiaries of inherited wealth, to pay taxes and share in the cost of government. Enactment of both the A–VAT and I–VAT ends the need for capital gains and inheritance taxes (apart from any initial payout). This tax would take care of the low-income Tax Gap.

I–VAT will fund domestic discretionary spending, equal dollar employer OASI contributions, and non-nuclear, non-deployed military spending, possibly on a regional basis. Regional I–VAT would both require a constitutional amendment to change the requirement that all excises be national and to discourage unnecessary spending, especially when allocated for electoral reasons rather than program needs. The latter could also be funded by the asset VAT (decreasing the rate by from 19.5% to 13%).

As part of enactment, gross wages will be reduced to take into account the shift to S–VAT and I–VAT, however net income will be increased by the same percentage as the I–VAT. Adoption of S–VAT and I–VAT will replace pass-through and propri- etary business and corporate income taxes.

Carbon Added Tax (C–AT). A Carbon tax with receipt visibility, which allows comparison shopping based on carbon content, even if it means a more expensive item with lower carbon is purchased. C–AT would also replace fuel taxes. It will fund transportation costs, including mass transit, and research into alternative fuels (including fusion). This tax would not be border adjustable unless it is in other nations, however in this case the imposition of this tax at the border will be noted, with the U.S. tax applied to the overseas base.

Tax Reform Summary

This plan can be summarized as a list of specific actions:

1) Increase the standard deduction to workers making salaried income of $35,000 and over, shifting business filing to a separate tax on employers and eliminating all credits and deductions—starting at 7.2%, going up to 28.8%, in $50,000 brackets.
2) Shift special rate taxes on capital income and gains from the income tax to an asset VAT. Expand the exclusion for sales to an ESOP to cooperatives and include sales of common and preferred stock. Mark option exercise and the first sale after inheritance, gift or donation to market.
3) Employers distribute the child tax credit with wages as an offset to their quar- terly tax filing (ending annual filings).
4) Employers collect and pay lower tier income taxes, starting at $100,000 at 7.2%, with an increase to 14.4% for all salary payments over $150,000 going up 7.2% for every $50,000 up to $250,000.
5) Shift payment of HI, DI, SM (ACA) payroll taxes to employers, remove caps on employer payroll taxes and credit them to workers on an equal dollar basis.
6) Employer paid taxes could as easily be called a subtraction VAT, abolishing cor- porate income taxes. These should not be zero rated at the border.
7) Expand current state/federal intergovernmental subtraction VAT to a full GST with limited exclusions (food would be taxed) and add a federal portion, which would also be collected by the states. Make these taxes zero rated at the border. Rate should be 19.5% and replace employer OASI contributions. Credit workers on an equal dollar basis.
8) Change employee OASI of 7.2% from $18,000 ($20,000 for $10 minimum wage) to $100,000 income are optional taxes for Old Age and Survivors Insurance.

Chronic Care Policy Alliance

1001 K Street, Sixth Floor Sacramento, CA 95814

Statement of Tom McCoy

Chronic Care Policy Alliance (CCPA) is a network of organizations dedicated to ensuring people living with chronic disease have access to quality, affordable healthcare. That is why as the Senate Finance Committee explores prescription drug prices, CCPA urges the Committee to focus on the costs borne by patients while recognizing the immense value prescription drugs bring to improving patient outcomes by improving their well-being, their quality of life, and even their lifespan.

The development of new treatments and reasonable access to them is critical to the continued improvement of the lives of patients with chronic conditions. New treatments can change a debilitating or fatal disease into a manageable condition. Therefore, any reforms need to ensure they do not impede current and future development and exploration of cures and treatments.

Patients depend on treatments and recognize the need to foster the development of these treatments—and Congress has been a strong partner in building the regulatory framework that has led to astounding new treatments in recent years. Under- cutting the system that has produced these treatments, including innovative vaccines and treatments for COVID-19 in record time, is a misguided endeavor.

Furthermore, as the Committee considers prescription drug policies, it should keep a patient-centered focus and ensure any changes to prescription drug policies benefit patients. Any savings to the federal government created by policy changes should be used to directly reduce consumers' cost.

As Congress considers potentially sweeping reforms to prescription drug policies, whether those proposed in the Build Back Better Act or other legislation, it is important that Congress evaluate our health system holistically to determine both opportunities for reform as well as the impact each reform will ultimately have on patients. Focusing on costs without focusing on patients could easily create unintended consequences and bring harm to patients.1 Instead, Congress should focus on specific policies that directly reduce patient costs, such as ensuring prescription drug rebates that are passed directly benefit patients.

We look forward to working with you on future policy reforms that protect patients and guarantee access to quality, affordable healthcare.

ERISA Industry Committee

701 8th Street, NW, Suite 610
Washington, DC 20001
Main 202.789.1400
http://www.eric.org/

Chairman Wyden, Ranking Member Crapo, and Members of the Committee, thank you for the opportunity to submit a statement for the record on behalf of The ERISA Industry Committee (ERIC) for the hearing entitled "Prescription Drug Price Inflation: An Urgent Need to Lower Drug Prices in Medicare."

ERIC is a national nonprofit organization exclusively representing the largest employers in the United States in their capacity as sponsors of employee benefit plans for their nationwide workforces. ERIC's member companies voluntarily provide benefits that cover millions of active and retired workers and their families across the country. With member companies that are leaders in every sector of the economy and with stores, factories, offices, warehouses, and other operations in every state, ERIC is the voice of large employer plan sponsors on federal, state, and local public policies impacting their ability to sponsor benefit plans and to lawfully operate under ERISA's protection from a patchwork of different and conflicting state and local laws, in addition to federal law.

You are likely to engage with an ERIC member company when you drive a car or fill it with gas, use a cell phone or a computer, watch TV, dine out or at home, enjoy a beverage, fly on an airplane, visit a bank or hotel, benefit from our national defense, receive or send a package, go shopping, or use cosmetics.

ERIC member companies provide comprehensive health benefits (including drug coverage) and pay the vast majority of these costs incurred by plan beneficiaries— as such, they have a significant stake in, and deep commitment to, efforts to curb the unsustainable rising costs of prescription drugs. Brand prescription drug costs have increased by nine percent annually for the past decade, and much of the burden is falling on the employers who, on average, pay 75 percent of the cost of care for 181 million American employees and family members. Additionally, drug costs represent the fastest-growing component of health care costs for employers and plan beneficiaries.[117] We strongly believe that healthy, functioning, competitive markets can drive lower prices and improve value. But we also recognize that markets sometimes fail or don't even exist, and in those cases, government involvement is needed.

Employer-sponsored health coverage is popular and valued by employees across the country. But to be a sustainable benefit, health coverage needs to be high quality and affordable. As you consider policies to lower prescription drug costs in Medicare, we urge the Committee to ensure that these policy changes do not result in shifting costs onto the millions of employees, families, and retirees who receive their health care benefits from their employers. ERIC urges Congress to ensure that measures such as negotiating prescription drug costs and inflation caps in the Medicare program do not make matters worse for private sector payors, and to adopt robust safeguards to ensure that employers and consumers do not experience cost-shifting increases due to changes in how the Medicare program pays for drugs. An internal analysis by the American Health Policy Institute (AHPI) finds that if drugmakers seek to make up for lost revenue due to Medicare price caps, employer-sponsored insurance premiums would increase by up to 3.7 percent per year above their current cost trends. In just the first five years, if Medicare negotiation is implemented, employers, employees, and their families would face more than $125 billion in increased drug costs.[118] Employees and their families who receive their health benefits from their employer are already experiencing high drug costs and spend on average $4,571 per year.[119] These cost increases are unsustainable for working Americans.

Conclusion

ERIC and its member companies are committed to advancing policies that will lower costs and improve the quality of health care. We look forward to working with you as you develop Medicare prescription drug policy to ensure it does not adversely affect employer-sponsored coverage for American workers, their families, and retirees.

---

117 https://chroniccarealliance.org/letter-to-congress-please-oppose-harmful-policy-change-to-medicare-part-d/.

118 https://www.pbgh.org/wp-content/uploads/2021/09/Employer-Group-Letter-on-Drug-Pricing-to-Hon.-Ron-Wyden.pdf.

119 Black, Michelle. Value Penguin. February 28, 2022. https://www.valuepenguin.com/pharmaceutical-spending-study.

Fresenius Kabi USA, LLC

Three Corporate Drive Lake Zurich, IL 60047 T 847–550–2300
T 888–391–6300
https://www.fresenius-kabi.com/us

U.S. Senate Committee on Finance
Dirksen Senate Office Bldg.
Washington, DC 20510–6200

RE: Fresenius Kabi Statement for the Record Senate Finance Committee Hearing on "Prescription Drug Price Inflation: An Urgent Need to Lower Drug Prices in Medicare" March 16, 2022.

Thank you for the opportunity to provide comment in response the committee's hearing, entitled "Prescription Drug Price Inflation: An Urgent Need to Lower Drug Prices in Medicare."

Fresenius Kabi is a generic and biosimilar manufacturer that employs more than 4,000 people in the United States with key domestic manufacturing, research and development, and distribution centers in Illinois, Nevada, North and South Carolina, New York, Pennsylvania, and Wisconsin. Fresenius Kabi specializes in bringing affordable medicines to patients with critical and chronic conditions.

Access to complex generic and biosimilar medicines represents a critical lifeline to millions of Americans. In 1984, Congress created a competitive pharmaceutical market with the passage of the Hatch-Waxman Amendments. The law has successfully delivered decades of savings for patients and the U.S. health care system. Generic medicines account for 90% of all prescriptions filled and just 18% of total Medicare drug spending, and more than nine out of ten generic prescriptions are filled for $20.00 or less.

Conversely, biologics represent approximately 10% of prescriptions filled but more than 80% of Medicare drug spending. In the coming years, biosimilars are poised to deliver tremendous savings to patients and the U.S. health care system with treatments for diabetes, arthritis, macular degeneration, cancer and more, but cannot deliver those savings in the current environment. Like Hatch-Waxman, the Biologics Price Competition and Innovation Act of 2009 (BPCIA) created an expedited pathway for biosimilars, but it did not account for the market distortions we see today. In 2022, this design is necessary but not sufficient to introduce the competitive forces needed to address the root causes of high-cost biologics, including patent policies and the extreme leverage of payers, which are more likely to protect branded biologics and disadvantage biosimilars.

Although price-setting seems to be an attractive route to pursue for Congress, it will not yield the results needed to sustain a healthy market, that includes innovation, in the long term because high list prices are a mere symptom of a deeper problem. By addressing the root causes of the problem, Congress can enjoy the success of cultivating the most robust and competitive market in the world, much like the success of the U.S. generics market.

Medicare direct negotiation does not address the root causes of the pricing problem, which is protracted brand monopolies due to patent misuse by branded drug companies and misaligned incentives due to rebating tactics in Medicare Part D. The current proposal allows government price setting in year 13 for biologics, instead of rebalancing the patent system to give biosimilar makers the ability to introduce competition after the product patent has expired, a similar time frame to the BBB proposal depending on the quality and quantity of the innovation in question. As written, the proposal does not address the root causes of the problem and will only reduce costs of some brand-name drugs for Medicare in the short term. Because it severely erodes the incentives for future development of biosimilars and complex generic medicines it will yield less savings for patients and the Medicare program over time.

Instead, we urge Congress to take on the anti-competitive tactics used by brand pharmaceutical companies to delay competition on their most profitable drugs. By addressing patent quality in the biologics market and ending the sophisticated life cycle management strategies, such as patent thickets and product hopping, designed to render the biosimilar irrelevant upon launch, Congress can gain a more robust result through competition, while still maintaining the U.S. as the innovation leader of the world.

Secondarily, delayed competition, resulting from the proliferation of low-quality patents, exacerbates the second root cause of high drug prices, which is the misaligned incentives in Medicare Part D. This imbalance allows rebates and list prices to grow unchecked and may force eventual biosimilar entrants to fight for market share in an environment where rebates perversely incentivize the prescribing of more expensive drugs. This practice undermines efforts to reduce patient out-of-pocket spending by further inhibiting access to lower-cost generic and biosimilar products.

Illustrative Example: Medicare Direct Negotiation (BBBA)

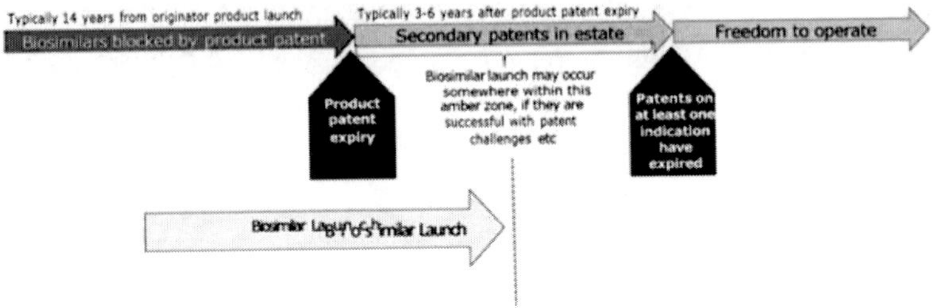

- Under the current proposal, biosimilar makers would not be able to launch in time to stop price setting as the compound patent would not have expired by year 13
- Price setting in this manner would replace the biosimilars market and not achieve the same price erosion as competition would in the long-term
- A market-based solution that includes strong patents that live or die on their merits and are not shielded from scrutiny by secondary continuation patents, would incentivize biosimilar challenges and achieve the result that Congress wants, without risking the loss of innovation.

We urge Congress to tackle the root causes of high drug prices by directly addressing patent quality and misaligned Medicare Part D incentives, which keep competition on the costliest drugs at bay, or at a disadvantage of leverage. We welcome the opportunity to discuss BBB's approach and the implications for development of lifesaving and affordable generics and biosimilars. Ensuring America's seniors can access lower-cost medicines is a goal we share.

Should you have any questions or would like to learn more about Fresenius Kabi, please do not hesitate to be in touch.

Regards,
Sarah D'Orsie
Vice President of Government Affairs and Policy

Health Equity Collaborative

1001 Connecticut Avenue, NW, Suite 730
Washington, DC 20036
www.healthequitycollaborative.org

The Health Equity Collaborative appreciates the opportunity to submit a statement for the record on the Senate Finance Committee's hearing titled "Prescription Drug Price Inflation: An Urgent Need to Lower Drug Prices in Medicare". Confronting the rising cost of healthcare remains a top priority of the Health Equity Collaborative. Average insurance premiums, which total $21,342 per family of four, and other expenses like out-of-network specialists and prescription drugs have reached record levels. We believe every sector of the healthcare industry needs to be held accountable and do their part in lowering the high insurance and prescription drug costs for underserved and diverse communities.

We applaud the House's passage of The Build Back Better Act for its historic investment in public health initiatives and subsequent focus from both Chambers to remedy the social inequities surrounding rising health care costs. However, it's critical to highlight the lack of provisions examining the role that Pharmacy Benefit Man- agers (PBMs) play in driving up prescription drug costs.

Despite wielding significant power to control costs, PBMs have directly benefitted from lack of oversight in the rebate market all the while maintaining a vested interest in keeping higher, not lower drug prices. These rebates are not shared directly with patients, and these middlemen collect as much as half the spending on brand name medicines. Discounts do not directly help vulnerable populations because they are not applied directly to consumer out of pocket costs. Rebates have skyrocketed from $102 billion in 2014 to $187 billion in 2020. Consumers deserve more transparency at the Pharmacy counter.

At this critical moment, congressional action is needed to identify and reform any perceived misaligned incentives or anti-competitive practices in the healthcare supply chain. This includes PBMs. In January 2021, the U.S. Senate Finance Committee released an investigative report on pricing schemes focused on insulin, finding that "PBM's formularies of covered drugs can affect patient's out-of-pocket spending for up to 50% of their co-pay." Increasing scrutiny and legislative regulations on PBMs would create immense cost savings.

The 116th Congress's "C–THRU Act" would enforce transparency on rebates, discounts, and other accrued payments, including their impact on Medicare Part D. This would ensure that Medicare enrollees receive a fair share of rebate savings by requiring cost sharing for Part D enrollees to be based off the negotiated price of the drug. Another policy solution, the Drug Price Transparency Act of 2021, would limit which type of prescription drug rebates are exempt from federal anti-kickback laws. This would narrow the range of possible pricing schemes PBMs could use. Middlemen do not deserve to profit while health care costs skyrocket beyond the reach of most Americans, including those in vulnerable populations.

There is no health equity without health justice, and there will be no long-term solutions unless we dismantle structural barriers that preclude people from accessing affordable medicines. While certainly not exhaustive, ensuring greater transparency and accountability within the pharmaceutical supply chain is one step towards improving the health of our nation's patients of color and creating a more equitable healthcare system.

Healthcare Leadership Council

750 9th Street, NW, Suite 500
Washington, DC 20001
202–452–8700
March 16, 2022

The Honorable Ron Wyden
Chairman
U.S. Senate
Committee on Finance
Washington, DC 20510

The Honorable Mike Crapo
Ranking Member
U.S. Senate
Committee on Finance
Washington, DC 20510

Dear Chairman Wyden and Ranking Member Crapo:

Thank you for holding a hearing on "Prescription Drug Price Inflation: An Urgent Need to Lower Drug Prices in Medicare." The Healthcare Leadership Council (HLC) appreciates the opportunity to share its thoughts with you on this important issue.

HLC is a coalition of chief executives from all disciplines within American healthcare. It is the exclusive forum for the nation's healthcare leaders to jointly develop policies, plans, and programs to achieve their vision of a 21st century healthcare system that makes affordable high-quality care accessible to all Americans. Members of HLC hospitals, academic health centers, health plans, pharmaceutical companies, medical device manufacturers, laboratories, biotech firms, health product distributors, post-acute care providers, home care providers, and information technology companies'advocate for measures to increase the quality and efficiency of healthcare through a patient- centered approach.

Competition and Innovation

The U.S. healthcare system has seen an increase in the cost of prescription drugs which has adversely affected patients, providers, payers, and other healthcare stakeholders. Increases in drug prices are often due to the lack of competition in the prescription drug marketplace. As a diverse coalition of healthcare stakeholders across the U.S. healthcare system, we believe innovation is essential to increasing market competition to deliver affordable, cutting-edge drug therapies to the public. HLC believes policies that encourage competitive markets and support innovation will lower drug costs and improve access to treatment. HLC supports a continuation of streamlining the Food and Drug Administration's (FDA) responsibilities and processes, which would include decreasing the backlog of generic drug approvals at the FDA and broadening FDA authority to accelerate review and approval for new generic drugs. Addressing barriers to and encouraging the entry of new generic drugs into the market will create more competition and help to lower drug prices.

Importation

HLC has provided an informed perspective on this issue throughout the sustained period in which we have seen pressure to allow wholesale importation of prescription drugs from outside U.S. borders. Our position is shaped by a membership that includes both pharmaceutical manufacturers and healthcare payers and providers, but also the healthcare product distributors that would be charged with facilitating movement of these imported drugs into the United States.

We have found that the promised cost savings from importation cannot be realized. When shipping, relabeling, storage, liability coverage, and other costs are factored into the economics of importation, the cost differential between obtaining medicines from the United States and those countries that employ government price controls are largely erased. Further, as multiple Canadian authorities have pointed out, Canada is frequently faced with drug shortage challenges and simply does not have the capacity to meet its own citizens' needs, as well as demand from the United States, so importation from Canada is not feasible.

In Republican and Democratic presidential administrations, U.S. Department of Health and Human Services Secretaries and FDA Commissioners have consistently attested that wholesale drug importation cannot be implemented without unacceptable risks to the American public. Today, those risks are more acute than ever before. Policymakers should consider the following when making decisions regarding drug importation:

- We have a substance use disorder crisis in this country, much of it fueled by the proliferation of lethal fentanyl that is originating in other countries and finding its way here through our ports and via the international mail service. Law enforcement authorities have said their resources are being stretched to the breaking point by the influx of illegal drugs. Government authorized whole- sale drug importation will only make law enforcement's task more difficult.
- It is a fallacy that drugs coming in from Canada can be assumed safe. Today, according to the National Association of Boards of Pharmacy, there are over 35,000 online drug sellers, many of them based in Canada. More than 95 percent of these operations are in violation of applicable laws. There is no way for the FDA to guarantee that prescription drugs imported to the United States from Canada did not originate in another country where they could have been counterfeited or adulterated.
- We are in a global counterfeit drug crisis. The World Health Organization has estimated that one in every 10 pharmaceutical products in low- and middle-income countries is falsified or substandard. Americans have benefited from a closed drug supply system in which manufacturing and distribution of prescription medications is approved and overseen by the FDA. Opening our borders to imported pharmaceuticals will only place Americans at

greater danger from those of ill intent who see the United States as a lucrative market.

Price Controls

We also believe policymakers must consider the ramifications for future medical innovation should other governments' price controls be imported into the United States economy. Today, we are the world's leading developer of new treatments and therapies. Americans are living healthier, longer lives because of an environment that encourages investment in pharmaceutical research and development. Even if wholesale importation were workable, the tradeoff in reduced research and development resources and investment would be unacceptable.

In fact, a recent Congressional Budget Office report estimated the number of drugs that will be introduced in the U.S. market under price controls over the next 30 years would be reduced by one over the 2022–2031 period, four over the subsequent decade, and five over the decade after that.[120] This is not a practical approach to reduce prescription drug costs, especially as it comes at the expense of a patient losing out on a potential lifesaving drug. In addition, the list price of drugs in 2021 rose less than the Consumer Price Index (CPI) and the net price of drugs dropped by 1.2 percent. As such, allowing the government to set the price for drugs in an environment where the list price of drugs is increasing less than the CPI is simply not needed.

As a diverse coalition of healthcare stakeholders across the U.S. healthcare system, we believe there are numerous policy actions that can have an impact on drug affordability without endangering the health and safety of the American people. They include FDA reforms to bring generic medications to the market at a faster pace; modernization of federal fraud and abuse laws to enable pro-patient, value focused collaboration among payers, providers, and manufacturers; and creating a cap on out-of-pocket drug costs in Medicare.

HLC members from all health sectors agree that treatment affordability and accessibility must continue to be health policy priorities. Opening our borders, however, to drugs of unverifiable origin at a time of increased global drug counterfeiting and trafficking of illicit substances is not an acceptable

[120] U.S. House of Representatives, Committee on Oversight and Reform. Drug Pricing Investigation: Majority Staff Report. December 2021.

solution to achieve this goal. Al- lowing the importation of prescription drugs will create more problems than it solves. It is clear that both the "Prescription Drug Price Relief Act" and "Affordable and Safe Prescription Drug Reimportation Act" would have a devastating effect on the innovation taking place to develop new treatments and cures for diabetes, heart disease, Alzheimer's, cancer, and many other health conditions. Investors will not devote dollars to the development of therapies that will be subject, directly, or indirectly, to harsh government price controls. It's right to pursue greater affordability; but not with a tradeoff that includes a diminished ability to fight disease. Government can take steps to address patient out-of-pocket costs and can also use trade negotiations to ensure other countries pay more of their fair share toward drug development; but we shouldn't sacrifice our current level of medical innovation.

Medicare Part D Improvements and Maximum Out-of-Pocket Cap

The Medicare Part D prescription drug program has successfully provided comprehensive, affordable drug coverage to seniors since 2006. We agree, however, that there are modifications and changes to the program that would improve incentives for all stakeholders, provide real financial protection for sicker beneficiaries, and reduce taxpayer costs. We support the concept of an out-of-pocket cap within Medicare Part D that does not negatively impact beneficiaries by significant premium increases or access restrictions.

In the current Medicare Part D program, beneficiaries are only responsible for five percent of drug costs above the catastrophic threshold. However, five percent of a $100,000 drug can be burdensome for seniors. Annual out-of-pocket expenses for these patients are significant. Beneficiary spending exceeds more than $3,000 on average, and one in 10 beneficiaries spends at least $5,200 for out-of-pocket prescription drug costs. HLC supports an out-of-pocket cap that provides all seniors with certainty and financial relief. We believe that any changes to the Medicare Part D program should be patient-centered and address beneficiaries' affordability issues.

HLC believes that establishing an out-of-pocket cap is a meaningful way to help seniors afford the lifesaving prescription drugs they need, especially those who are not eligible for supplemental help. The cost associated with an out-of-pocket cap needs to be shared among stakeholders, including, but not limited to health plans, pharmaceutical manufacturers, and the federal government.

Thank you for the opportunity to comment on "Prescription Drug Price Inflation: An Urgent Need to Lower Drug Prices in Medicare." HLC looks forward to continuing to collaborate with you on this important issue. If you have any questions, please do not hesitate to contact Debbie Witchey at (202) 449–3435 or dwitchey@hlc.org.

Sincerely,
Mary R. Grealy President

Jack Kemp Foundation

2012 Wyoming Avenue, NW, #301
Washington DC 20009

Statement of Ike Brannon, Ph.D., Senior Fellow the BBB's Threat to Biosimilar Drug Development

In 2019, longtime pharmaceutical industry critic Peter Bach took to The Wall Street Journal to declare that the U.S. should throw in the towel on copycat versions of the nation's highest priced specialty drugs in favor of government price controls. The recommendation was rightly maligned by those who recognize the undeniable role drug competition plays in driving down medicine costs for patients and taxpayers alike.

Yet 2 years later Congressional Democrats, perhaps unwittingly, appear poised to incarnate the Bach proposal.

Democrats have included a number of provisions intended to reduce drug prices in the Build Back Better bill, which is currently being debated in the U.S. Senate after having passed the House of Representatives on Friday. But the fact that the current bill's provisions that call for Medicare to essentially regulate prices and limit any future price increases would come at a high cost.

For starters, it would completely upend our country's wildly successful decades-long model of allowing new drugs to enjoy short periods of exclusivity, followed by a period of robust competition from generics and— for large molecule biologic drugs— biosimilars.

The inevitable outcome of such a price regulatory regime would be the likely evisceration of the market for biosimilar drugs, leaving us with less drug development, less competition, and reduced progress in the market for biologic drugs.

Biologics—complex drugs that are made via the use of living cells—comprise the fastest-growing class of medicine in the United States. In the last decade nearly all the blockbuster drugs that have been introduced have been biologics.

Biologics have also proven to be very expensive to develop and manufacture. Unlike classic small-molecule medicines, biologic drugs are created within living systems and are highly sensitive, which means that manufacturers must control the nature of starting materials and employ hundreds of process controls to guarantee quality. The cost of researching, developing, and producing these drugs contributes to their high prices.

One way the U.S. has tried to reduce the price of biologic drugs has been to encourage the introduction of biosimilar drugs. Biosimilars are akin to generics in that they are near-replicas of the original biologics, but creating the therapeutic equivalent of a biologic is a far more complex task than making a generic equivalent of a small-molecule drug: Biosimilar manufacturers are not granted access to the DNA used in reference products, and must invest in research and development to create close facsimiles of the originals. So while biosimilars are touted as lower-cost versions of their reference products, they nevertheless require significant investment as well.

However, the U.S. has been slow to approve biosimilar drugs, which has dampened their effect on drug prices. For instance, the EU approved its first biosimilar drug in 2006, but the first U.S. drug—Zarxio—did not reach the market until 2015. Today, the EU has approved 69 biosimilar drugs and the U.S. has just 31, many of which have been approved only recently and have yet to come to market.

No one would claim that the sizable difference in approvals between the U.S. and EU has to do with a lax EU regulatory state, given its famously sclerotic and cautious bureaucracy and its unquestioning embrace of the precautionary principle: It is clear that something is amiss in the U.S. biosimilar market. Part of it has to do with the fact that the current system has allowed drug companies to delay biosimilar competition via the courts and what some construe as a form of patent abuse, but the FDA's lengthy and complex process to approve biosimilar drugs is a bigger problem.

A more vigorous FDA, combined with legislation that removed most of the legal barriers and patent abuse that stymie biosimilar competition, would make it easier for biosimilar drugs to enter the market. This would go a long way towards constraining the prices of new drugs in a way that wouldn't have an untoward effect on development.

Instead, many Democrats see the bureaucratic and legalistic barriers as an immutable fact of life rather than a problem to be fixed, and embrace government price-setting instead.

As such, the current drug provisions in Build Back Better would basically end the decades-old model of encouraging competition via generics and go towards a centrally regulated market—more so than even Europe.

Orrin Hatch, my former employer in the U.S. Senate, recently came out of retirement to issue a statement decrying the notion of price controls and the possible demise of the Hatch-Waxman Act, the legislation that created the market for generic drugs and later biosimilars.

Current members of Congress should heed Senator Hatch's caution. Even a feint towards such a command-and-control drug market would cause biosimilar investment to plummet: it may be difficult to fully revive such investment later if pharmaceutical companies fear that such a draconian step would remain a possibility with the next administration.

The more practical and less damaging way to help reduce price pressures for prescription drugs would be to fix the pipeline for biosimilars and let competition drive down prices—just as generics have done.

Ike Brannon is a former senior economist for the United States Treasury and the Senate Finance Committee.

National Association of Chain Drug Stores

1776 Wilson Blvd., Suite 200
Arlington, VA 22209
703–549–3001
www.nacds.org

U.S. Senate
Committee on Finance
Dirksen Senate Office Building Washington, DC 20510

Re: Statement for the Record — "Prescription Drug Price Inflation: An Urgent Need to Lower Drug Prices in Medicare"

Dear Chairman Wyden, Ranking Member Crapo, and Members of the Senate Finance Committee:

The National Association of Chain Drugs Stores (NACDS)[121] thanks the Senate Finance Committee for the opportunity to submit this statement for the record following the Committee's hearing titled, "Prescription Drug Price Inflation: An Urgent Need to Lower Drug Prices in Medicare."

In the Medicare Part D program, drug costs—and corresponding patient out-of-pocket costs—are on the rise. As Medicare beneficiaries' trusted access points to needed medications, pharmacies know firsthand the dire consequences associated with increasing drug costs and out-of-pocket spending. For instance, higher out-of-pocket costs have been repeatedly connected to patients not taking their medication as prescribed, otherwise known as medication nonadherence, which has serious downstream impacts on worsening health and higher medical spending. In fact, a literature review of 160 studies illustrated that an increase in patient share of medication costs is directly associated with a significant decrease in medication adherence.[122] For example, higher out-of-pocket costs for medication have been associated with patients bypassing getting their medication filled because they cannot afford the co-pay, or otherwise results in patients inappropriately using their medication to make their supply last longer, such as cutting pills in half or skipping doses.[123]

For many chronic conditions, patients may not immediately feel the impact of skipping their medications, but in time, medication non-adherence leads to serious consequences in poorer health outcomes, increased morbidity and mortality, and higher downstream spending. When medications are not taken as prescribed, patients do not receive the expected, optimal benefit. For costly chronic conditions, such as diabetes, heart failure, hypertension, or cardiovascular disease, for example, non- adherence may lead to worsening of the condition and the need for more costly medications and treatments in the future; or worse, an emergency department visit for an avoidable heart attack or heart failure exacerbation. The negative impact of medication nonadherence has been well demonstrated across many other conditions as well.

---

[121] NACDS is located at 1776 Wilson Boulevard, Arlington, VA 22209.

[122] Eaddy MT, et al., "How Patient Cost-Sharing Trends Affect Adherence and Outcomes," Pharmacy and Therapeutics, January 2012, available at https://www.ncbi.nlm.nih.gov/pmc/articles/PMC3278192/.

[123] Kaiser Family Foundation, March 1, 2019, available at https://www.kff.org/health-costs/press-release/poll-nearly-1-in-4-americans-taking-prescription-drugs-say-its-difficult-to-afford- medicines-including-larger-shares-with-low-incomes/.

To combat high drug prices, out-of-pocket costs, and the associated negative impacts of both on Medicare Part D beneficiaries, NACDS urges the Committee to consider the following two policy solutions:

- Recommendation 1: Congress should implement standardized pharmacy quality measures to effectuate comprehensive pharmacy direct and indirect remuneration (DIR) reform that best serves Medicare patients and improves healthcare quality, equity, and reduces preventable spending.
- Recommendation 2: Congress should protect pharmacies' proprietary data collected through any mandatory reporting requirements of drug acquisition costs to promote competition and discourage the misuse of such information.

NACDS offers more background on these policies below.

- Recommendation 1: Congress should implement standardized pharmacy measures to effectuate comprehensive pharmacy DIR reform that best serves Medicare patients and improves healthcare quality, equity, and reduces preventable spending.

The Centers for Medicare and Medicaid Services (CMS) is currently considering a proposal to reduce prescription drug prices for Medicare Part D patients by adopting a revised definition of "negotiated price" for a covered Part D drug that would include all pharmacy price concessions (also known as "pharmacy direct and indirect remuneration" or "pharmacy DIR fees") at the point of sale. This proposal would bring transparency to pharmacy DIR fees, while also lowering beneficiaries' out-of- pocket costs by $21.3 billion over 10 years, or approximately 2 percent.[124] In comments submitted to CMS this month, *NACDS provides strong support for the Administration's work to bring transparency to pharmacy DIR and urges CMS to finalize the rule for contract year 2023.* NACDS' support is premised on the simple fact that the proposal will better align marketplace competition with the interests of Medicare patients, and lead to lower total healthcare costs, including lower out-of-pocket costs for beneficiaries.

Still, as retail pharmacies continue their commitment to serve Medicare patients, NACDS knows that successful DIR reform does not end with

[124] 87 Fed. Reg. 1842, 1849 (January 12, 2022).

transparency of pharmacy DIR fees. *In tandem with pharmacy DIR fee transparency, NACDS continues to advocate, as we have for the past eight years, that comprehensive pharmacy DIR reform must include the standardization of performance- based pharmacy price concessions and incentive payments that are currently based on arbitrary and inconsistent performance measures. We believe Congress can help accomplish this final step towards comprehensive pharmacy DIR reform to improve quality, equity and reduce preventable spending.*

In its current proposal, CMS acknowledges that performance-based pharmacy price concessions, net of all pharmacy incentive payments, increased, on average nearly 170 percent per year between 2012 and 2020 and now comprise the second largest category of DIR received by sponsors and PBMs, behind only manufacturer rebates.[125] CMS further acknowledged that performance-based incentive payments—payments paid to a pharmacy based on performance—have been extremely unlikely in recent years. NACDS concurs that this has been the experience of pharmacies.

NACDS highlights that since the proposed rule does not address the present regime of a lack of incentive payments paired with the prevalence of price concessions based on performance, it would still perpetuate significant, outstanding challenges that must be addressed to achieve comprehensive DIR reform and redirect incentives to emphasize better care for beneficiaries. Stated more precisely, pharmacy price concessions, including those based on performance, included in the negotiated price would remain contingent, variable, and without regard to beneficiary outcomes and care experience. Price concessions that are supposed to be performance-based could continue to be calculated lower and lower, without any regard to performance at all. Such a structure undermines CMS' goals to serve Part D beneficiaries in ways that improve healthcare quality, equity and minimize preventable spending. *Therefore, we urge Congress to consider legislation that would standardize pharmacy performance measures used to determine price concessions so that pharmacies can be fully apprised of performance expectations and opportunities* before signing a Part D contract, rather than after-the-fact, as is the current untenable situation. Implementing standardized pharmacy performance measures would also help to redirect and align incentives toward providing better care, equity, and experiences for beneficiaries.

---

[125] 87 Fed. Reg. at 1916.

Further, CMS' current requirement for the disclosure of performance measures to the agency is critically important as a first step in reforming DIR for the benefit of Medicare beneficiaries but is inadequate in effectuating comprehensive pharmacy DIR reform. Congress should implement clear rules and pharmacy measures needed to produce pharmacy incentives to improve performance based on quality and patient outcomes. These measures should be defined, transparent, consistent across plans, and used with time to adjust performance to ensure improvement. Additionally, these measures must be pharmacy-specific, proven, and based on achievable criteria that consider the drugs dispensed and the disease state(s) being managed. Doing so will help ensure fairness for both Part D plans and pharmacies, and benefit access to Medicare beneficiaries, while also promoting trust that is sorely lacking in the current process. Importantly, effective pharmacy- level performance measures should first recognize that there should be reimbursement for dispensing medications, separate from performance-based quality measures.

The development of pharmacy-level quality measures is already underway. Several pharmacy quality measures have been developed, tested, and endorsed by the Pharmacy Quality Alliance (PQA) over the last two years for the purpose of evaluating the quality of pharmacies and assessing pharmacist-provided care and pharmacy- based services. To date, PQA has endorsed five pharmacy quality measures, primarily focused on medication adherence.[126],[127] Additional measures are in development, including measures focused on patient health outcomes for some of the most common, costly conditions including high blood pressure and diabetes (A1c), among others.[128]

Implementing standardized pharmacy performance measures would not only help to provide pharmacies with clarity on their performance expectations and opportunities but would also help to redirect and align incentives toward providing better care, equity, and experiences for beneficiaries based on evidence-based, tested quality measures. Beyond this, implementing standardized pharmacy performance measures would help reduce the total cost of care by aligning incentives for pharmacies, plans, and PBMs to further improve medication adherence, patient health outcomes, and prevent downstream unnecessary spending in addition to undue harm and suf- fering for patients. To effectuate this meaningful, needed change for Medicare bene-

---

[126] Pharmacy Quality Alliance, available at https://www.pqaalliance.org/pqa-endorses-pharmacy-performance-measures-for-medication-adherence-and-specialty-turnaround-time.

[127] Pharmacy Quality Alliance, available at https://www.pqaalliance.org/pqa-endorses-pharmacy-performance-measures.

[128] Pharmacy Quality Alliance, available at https://www.pqaalliance.org/pharmacy-measures.

ficiaries, Congress must take the final step in comprehensive pharmacy DIR fee reform by implementing standardized pharmacy measures.

- Recommendation 2: Congress should protect pharmacies' proprietary data collected through any mandatory reporting requirements of drug acquisition costs to promote competition and discourage the misuse of such information.

Within the realm of prescription drug pricing, some policymakers have considered updates to the National Average Drug Acquisition Cost (NADAC) survey in the Medicaid program. For example, some policymakers have argued that pharmacy responses to the NADAC survey should be mandatory. As Congress considers changes to the NADAC survey, NACDS urges the Committee to ensure that any proprietary pharmacy data collected must remain confidential and not publicly disclosed. Congress should also abstain from policies that could utilize information collected through a mandatory NADAC reporting program to other federal programs like Medicare.

Public disclosure of this information could have a market-distorting effect that harms pharmacies' ability to negotiate effectively, which could ultimately harm Medicaid beneficiaries and the pharmacies that serve them. For example, such disclosure could result in higher acquisition costs for pharmacies. Given the widespread concerns with mandatory NADAC reporting, Congress should not consider policies that would permit proprietary information to likewise skew competition and the patient experience in Medicare.

Conclusion

In conclusion, NACDS urges the Committee to advance legislation that would require implementation of standardized pharmacy quality measures in the Part D program so that implementation can be aligned with proposed rulemaking to effectuate more holistic DIR reform for beneficiaries, as well as consider the impact of NADAC proposals to influence the overall cost of drugs. NACDS looks forward to working with the Committee on both of these important policies. For questions or further discussion, please contact NACDS' Christie Boutte, Senior Vice President, Reimbursement, Innovation & Advocacy, at cboutte@nacds.org or 703–837–4211.

National Breast Cancer Coalition

2001 L Street, NW, Suite 500, PMB #50111
Washington, DC 20036
P 202–296–7477
F 202–314–3458
https://www.stopbreastcancer.org/

Statement of Fran Visco, J.D., President

Thank you, Chairman Wyden, Ranking Member Crapo, and Members of the Senate Finance Committee, for the opportunity to submit a statement for the record of the hearing this Committee, held on March 16, 2022: "Prescription Drug Price Inflation an Urgent Need to Lower Drug Prices in Medicare."

My name is Fran Visco, and I am a breast cancer survivor, a wife, a mother, a lawyer, and President of the National Breast Cancer Coalition (NBCC). My statement represents the hundreds of member organizations and thousands of individual members of the Coalition. NBCC is a grassroots organization dedicated to ending breast cancer through action and advocacy. The Coalition's primary goals are to advocate for federal funding for breast cancer research and collaborate with the scientific community to implement new models of research, improve access to quality health care, treatments, and breast cancer clinical trials for women and men; and expand the influence of breast cancer advocates wherever breast cancer decisions are made.

Congress must help put an end to drug prices that create financial toxicity for patients, adversely disrupt the health-care system, and have little relation to value to human life. The U.S. spends more than double what other industrialized countries do per capita on prescription drugs, and 79% of Americans agree that the cost of prescription drugs is too high. It is not just a belief. It is reality. Medical debt is the largest source of personal debt in the U.S. Two-thirds of all personal bankruptcies are due to medical bills. About 115 million Americans under 65 report issues with medical bills and have skipped medical care due to cost.[129]

Because our mission is to end breast cancer, we focus specifically on oncology drugs, and the trends there are troubling. A JAMA study, published in July 2021, found that between 2009 and 2019, 74% of the 65 cancer drugs

[129] Breaking News: Medical Debt and Your Credit Report, Oncolink, March 23, 2022.

the group looked at increased in price faster than the rate of inflation. The median monthly treatment cost rose from $5,790 in 2009–2010 to $14,580 in 2018–2019.[130] In 2019, national out- of-pocket expenses in the U.S. for female breast cancer were $3.14 billion.[131] Most troubling is that there is generally no relationship between a drug's clinical effectiveness or reducing mortality and its price or subsequent price increases. We will not end breast cancer or any disease until everyone has access to affordable, effective interventions.

Affordable access to prescription drugs has been a priority for NBCC since its inception. From advocacy for access to quality care for all to drug pricing workshops to interactions with the FDA and public statements on specific drug pricing, NBCC has been a voice for value, evidence-based approaches, and affordable, accessible treatments. The government's ability to negotiate drug pricing is but one necessary reform to help save lives.

A recently published study found non-initiation (patient did not fill their prescription) for 30 percent of prescriptions written for anticancer drugs among many Medicare part D beneficiaries. Many Medicare Part D beneficiaries must pay a percentage of the price for high-priced drugs for each medication fill. Many beneficiaries typically pay hundreds or thousands of dollars for a single fill. The study's findings support current legislative efforts to increase the accessibility of high-price medications by reducing out-of-pocket expenses under Medicare Part D.[132]

The purpose of a healthcare system must be to do what is best for peoples' lives. The system must be designed to achieve that goal. At NBCC, we believe that value to patients should be the cornerstone of the conversation about drug pricing. Today, U.S. drug manufacturers enjoy monopolistic market power and set prices as high as possible. As a result, many of their drugs launch with huge price tags despite little added value or innovation.

Some recent examples of this in breast cancer include:

- TECENTRIQ - (atezolizumab) was approved via accelerated approval for first- line treatment of advanced or metastatic triple-negative breast cancer (TNBC) in 2020, using the surrogate endpoint of progression-free survival (PFS) as the primary endpoint. The list price of TECENTRIQ- is $13,860 per month.

---

130 July 1, 2021 Analysis of Launch and Post approval Cancer Drug Pricing, Clinical Benefit, and Policy Implications in the U.S. and Europe.

131 CDC, Annual Report to the Nation on the Status of Cancer, October, 2021.

132 Many Medicare Beneficiaries Do Not Fill High-Price Specialty Drug Prescriptions, Health Af- fairs, April 2022. https://doi.org/10.1377/hlthaff.2021.01742.

- On April 22, 2020, the FDA granted accelerated approval to sacituzumab govitecan-hziy (TRODELVY, Immunomedics, Inc.) for metastatic triple-negative breast cancer based on a single-arm trial (not a randomized trial). The approval was based on the surrogate endpoint of response rate. The list price of TRODELVY is $6,600 per month.

While drug price negotiation is critical to providing access to quality health care to all Americans, it is just a start. NBCC believes that the next conversation in drug pricing must be about value-based drug prices so that Americans have access to drugs that actually benefit them at prices they can afford.

To this end, NBCC adopted the following five principles for value-based drug pricing:[133]

Everyone Must Benefit from Drug Pricing Reform

Drug pricing reform must be comprehensive. New and existing drugs must be subject to pricing reform, and private and government-provided insurance coverage must be included.

Drug Prices Must Reflect Value to People's Lives

Health-care consumers generally and breast cancer advocates more specifically want drugs that significantly extend the length and/or quality of their lives. The reality is that most drugs coming to market today do neither of these but do carry significant financial costs.

NBCC urges reform that results in an evidence-based system where drugs are priced based on how well they improve people's lives. Value-based approaches to drug pricing can encourage drug makers to produce more of what people need, drugs that will enhance health and/or quality of life.

---

[133] Comprehensive Reform to Lower Prescription Drug Prices, Madeline Twomey, Center for American Progress, January 29, 2019; How Medicare Could Get Better Prices on Prescription Drugs, Kevin Outterson and Aaron S. Kesselheim, Health Affairs Vol. 28, 2009.

Independent and Fair Assessments Must Determine Value

Independent analyses should inform drug value assessments. Organizations conducting assessments must be independent, free of any conflicts of interest, and have a transparent and reviewable methodology.

The Process Must Include Educated Patient Advocates

Educated patient advocates who represent a constituency must have a meaningful seat at the table in determining value in all aspects of drug pricing policy, including evaluation and negotiation.

Patient advocates must be centered in the drug pricing discussion. Educated patient advocates can bring a truly comprehensive view to the table on what matters most to a healthcare system focused on "peoples" lives.

Reform Must Include Strong Enforcement Mechanisms

Drug price policies must include strong, meaningful, and effective enforcement mechanisms.

NBCC will continue to work with you on our shared goal to make certain that effective treatments are also affordable and accessible. The ability to negotiate drug prices under Medicare is a necessary step to that end.

Thank you again for the opportunity to submit testimony. We look forward to working with the Senate Finance Committee on this issue of critical importance to Amer- ican consumers.

National Community Pharmacists Association

100 Daingerfield Road
Alexandria, VA 22314
(703) 683–8200
www.ncpa.org

Chairman Wyden, Ranking Member Crapo, and Members of the Committee:

Thank you for conducting this hearing on prescription drug affordability and the need to lower costs for patients. In this statement, NCPA will offer support and suggestions on a number of policy considerations that would lower out of pocket costs for seniors, provide certainty for pharmacies, and protect taxpayers by bringing more transparency to Medicaid spending.

NCPA represents America's community pharmacists, including 19,400 independent community pharmacies. Almost half of all community pharmacies provide long-term care services and play a critical role in ensuring patients have immediate access to medications in both community and long-term care (LTC) settings. Together, our members represent a $67 billion healthcare marketplace, employ 215,000 individuals, and provide an expanding set of healthcare services to millions of patients every day. Our members are small business owners who are among America's most accessible healthcare providers.

Our pharmacies and the patients they serve have long had concerns about pharmacy benefit managers (PBMs), their anticompetitive practices, and the role they play in ever-increasing drug costs. These concerns have been further exacerbated because of the COVID–19 pandemic's impact on small businesses. Independently owned pharmacies have served as lifelines as essential businesses during the pandemic, but PBM practices are causing these small businesses to struggle to remain viable and keep doors open to provide continued access and care. We appreciate the efforts of the Chairman and Ranking Member to discuss these practices and the impact on the drug prices on Medicare patients.

Pharmacy Direct and Indirect Remuneration (DIR) fee Reform

NCPA has long advocated for relief from Medicare Part D pharmacy DIR fees, a top priority. In January, the Centers for Medicare & Medicaid Services (CMS) released a proposed rule which would address many of the concerns NCPA has raised with the agency, this Committee, and the relevant Committees of jurisdiction in the House of Representatives. In the rule, CMS acknowledges pharmacy price concessions, also known as pharmacy DIR fees, have increased more than 107,400 percent over a 10-year period.[134]

---

[134] Proposed Rule: Medicare Program; Contract Year 2023 Policy and Technical Changes to the Medicare Advantage and Medicare Prescription Drug Benefit Programs, *https://www.federalregister.gov/d/2022-00117/p-714.*

NCPA provided comments to CMS on the proposed rule, requesting the agency to resolve or clarify the several issues summarized below to have a positive impact on patients, the Medicare program, and community pharmacies.[135]

NCPA requested CMS provide the following to maximize the benefit for patients and community pharmacies:

- CMS must ensure transparency of pharmacy reimbursement at the point of sale and ensure the lowest possible reimbursement equals the amount paid on a pharmacy remittance advice, paid within the CMS prompt pay rules of 14 calendar days. Transparency to pharmacies and patients is critical. Therefore, CMS needs to:
    - Clarify that the definition of "other stakeholders" includes the dispensing pharmacy;
    - Verify the lowest possible reimbursement will be visible to pharmacies at the point of sale on the paid claim response;
    - Provide clear guidance that any post-point-of-sale adjustments must be positive incentive payments for pharmacy performance only;
    - Specify that the coordination-of-benefits requirements do not apply to pharmacy incentive payments;
    - Confirm that all pharmacy price concessions must be attributable at the claim level even if not computed or assessed at the time of dispensing the Medicare Part D drug;
    - Address how CMS guidance would apply if plan sponsors or PBMs were to begin restructuring pharmacy fees on a basis other than claim-level fees;
    - Require that pharmacy administrative service fees are properly reported by Medicare Part D plans, as plans are currently incentivized not to report these fees at all; and
    - Clearly provide a workable and inclusive definition of pharmacy price concession that addresses any fee paid by a pharmacy or deducted from payments to a pharmacy, or any other

[135] NCPA offers these comments on the proposed rule without commenting on CMS' statutory authority to modify the definition of "negotiated prices." NCPA is presently the lead plaintiff in a lawsuit challenging CMS' existing regulatory definition of "negotiated prices," *see NCPA v. Becerra,* No. 1:21–cv–131 (D.D.C.), and nothing in this letter should be construed as a waiver of the arguments that NCPA and the other plaintiffs have made in the litigation challenging the existing regulatory definition.

remuneration received directly or indirectly by the Medicare Part D sponsor or its intermediary contracting organization.

- CMS must close the coverage gap loophole. The proposed rule creates a loophole that would treat patients differently depending on their phase in the Medicare Part D benefit, would permit PBMs to continue to play games with pharmacy price concessions for pharmacies and inflate prescription costs for the most vulnerable patients, and would add needless administrative expenses by forcing the use of two systems, one within the coverage gap and the other outside of it.
- CMS must require standardized pharmacy performance measures for incentive payments. There is currently an inequitable application of metrics for community pharmacies. Even pharmacies that earn high performance ratings are nevertheless punished by pharmacy DIR fees based on arbitrary PBM measures.
- CMS must enforce existing network adequacy and contract provision requirements. Maintaining adequate access for patients to prescription drugs is predicated on the participation of pharmacies in Medicare Part D plan networks.
- CMS must address NCPA's concerns and recommendations when pro- mulgating the final rule for small business pharmacies to remain viable participants in the Medicare Part D program. An "Actuarial Memorandum of the Model and Assumptions in Analyzing the 2023 Proposed Rule Regarding Pharmacy Price Concessions at Point of Sale" was prepared for Avalere Health on behalf of NCPA.[136] NCPA commissioned this memorandum because CMS failed to adequately test the assumptions that this proposal could result in a "modest" potential indirect positive effect on pharmacy payment, and CMS did not consider this proposal's impact on small business pharmacies. The memorandum reveals that CMS miscalculated the positive impact on pharmacy. If plans lower net reimbursement by 2 percent because of this rule, a reasonable assumption based on PBMs' long history of reduced pharmacy reimbursement in the Medicare Part D program, the average pharmacy would face a 2 percent reduction in reimbursement.[137]

---

[136] See discussion at p. 14 and Appendix attached of NCPA comment letter at, https://ncpa.org/sites/default/files/2022-03/ncpa-comment-cms-part-d-proposed-rule.pdf.

[137] Actuarial Memorandum of the Model and Assumptions in Analyzing the 2023 Proposed Rule Regarding Pharmacy Price Concessions at Point of Sale, prepared for Avalere Health and com- missioned by NCPA, p. 9 and Table 7 (Appendix to comment letter).

We are grateful that Congress included some version of pharmacy DIR fee reform in every drug pricing package over the last legislative cycle (Grassley-Wyden, H.R. 3, H.R. 19, and S. 3129), which has helped to get us to the point where CMS is moving forward with rulemaking to apply all pharmacy price concessions at the point of sale. However, if this rule is finalized, it may be necessary to have additional statutory authority and clarity that would allow CMS to move forward to address other issues, such as standardized quality metrics. We hope that Congress will work with us to standardize pharmacy quality metrics for pharmacy incentive payments this year, so that comprehensive pharmacy DIR fee reform can be implemented in 2023.

Conclusion

In conclusion, prescription drug prices continue to grow at an alarming rate. There are many factors in the pharmaceutical supply chain and delivery system that may contribute to this growth, including pharmacy benefit manager "middlemen." NCPA stands ready to work with Congress and the administration to implement policies that will lower drug prices at the pharmacy counter for our patients.

National Council on Disability

1331 F Street, NW, Suite 850
Washington, DC 20004
202–272–2004 Voice
202–272–2022 Fax
https://ncd.gov/

Dear Chairman Wyden, Ranking Member Crapo, and Members of the Committee:

Thank you for the opportunity to submit this statement for the record. On behalf of the National Council on Disability (NCD), I write to raise concern about provisions in the House-passed Build Back Better Act (H.R. 5376) that would allow the Secretary of Health and Human Services (HHS) to negotiate prices for some high-cost drugs covered under Medicare Part B and Part D. NCD respectfully advises the committee to include a provision in the bill that prohibits HHS from relying on QALY-based cost effectiveness reports, whether from research entities that conduct such research, e.g., the Institute for Clinical and Economic Review (ICER), or reliance upon prices paid by foreign countries, where those countries utilize the QALY methodology to determine coverage for prescription medicines. This is in line with the Patient Protection and Affordable Care Act's prohibition on HHS' reliance on QALY-based cost effectiveness research in Medicare. Further, we advise including a provision that requires HHS to rely on value assessments made by the Patient-Centered Outcomes Research Institute, which conducts value assessments without the use of the QALY.

As an independent federal advisory body to the President, his Administration, Congress, and federal agencies, NCD unequivocally agrees that drug prices need to be lowered as high drug prices can themselves be a source of health inequity for millions of people with disabilities. However, our agency would like the Committee to be aware of the unintended and discriminatory implications that would negatively affect people with disabilities and chronic illnesses absent parameters governing the drug negotiation process. NCD is concerned that most of the proposed "applicable countries" identified in H.R. 5376 as countries to reference when determining the average international market price per unit for a particular drug or treatment use QALY-based cost-effectiveness to determine their national health system's coverage of prescription drugs and treatments.

Congress has previously determined that the QALY methodology is discriminatory in both design and its impact and restricts access to necessary prescription drugs. These concerns led Congress to prohibits its use by the Secretary of HHS in coverage determinations in Medicare under the 2010 Patient Protection and Affordable Care Act[138] as well as by the Patient-Centered Outcomes Research Institute.[139] In addition, HHS' regulation implementing Section 504 of the Rehabilitation Act of 1973 prohibits

---

[138] Patient Protection and Affordable Care Act, Pub. L. 111–148, title VI, § 6301(c), March 23, 2010 (codified as 42 U.S.C. 1320e–1(e)) (The Patient-Centered Outcomes Research Institute . . . shall not develop or employ a dollars-per-quality adjusted life year (or similar measure that discounts the value of a life because of an individual's disability) as a threshold to establish what type of health care is cost effective or recommended The Secretary shall not utilize such an adjusted life year (or such a similar measure) as a threshold to determine coverage, reimbursement, or incentive programs under subchapter XVIII).

[139] *Id.*

discrimination on the basis of disability in all programs or activities conducted by HHS.[140]

In January 2021, NCD raised similar concerns in response to the Centers for Medicare and Medicaid Services' (CMS) Most Favored Nation (MFN) Rule that was implemented in an attempt to control Medicare prescription drug costs. NCD determined that the MFN Rule, like the drug price negotiation provisions of H.R. 5376, was contrary to federal law by adopting foreign drug prices set in reliance on the QALY.[141] Furthermore, the MFN Rule explicitly acknowledged that a portion of the MFN Model's savings "is attributable to beneficiaries not accessing their drugs through the Medicare benefit, along with the associated lost utilization." CMS' "Extreme Disruption" possibility predicted that, for the potential $286.3 billion in Medicare savings, nearly half would be due to seniors foregoing necessary medicines and treatments. The MFN Model is a clear example of how value assessments like QALYs unintentionally result in limiting access to healthcare.

As the Committee discusses the best way to lower drug prices, for the reasons stated above, NCD reaffirms our advice to prohibit the use of QALY-based cost methodologies and reliance upon international pricing that uses those methodologies. We further reaffirm our advice to adhere to the Patient Protection and Affordable Care Act's prohibition on HHS' reliance on the QALY methodology in Medicare.

Most Respectfully,
Andre´s J. Gallegos Chairman

National Taxpayers Union

122 C Street, NW, Suite 650
Washington, DC 20001
Phone: (703) 683–5700
Fax: (703) 683–5722
https://www.ntu.org/

---

140 Enforcement of Nondiscrimination on the Basis of Handicap in Programs or Activities Conducted by the Department of Health and Human Services, 45 CFR Part 85 (1988).

141 https://ncd.gov/publications/2021/ncd-letter-cms-most-favored-nation-rule#_ftn6.

The Honorable Ron Wyden
Chair
U.S. Senate
Committee on Finance
219 Dirksen Senate Office Building
Washington, DC 20510

The Honorable Mike Crapo
Ranking Member
U.S. Senate
Committee on Finance
219 Dirksen Senate Office Building
Washington, DC 20510

Dear Chair Wyden, Ranking Member Crapo, and Members of the Committee:

On behalf of National Taxpayers Union (NTU), the nation's oldest taxpayer advocacy organization, I write in regard to your March 16th hearing, "Prescription Drug Price Inflation: An Urgent Need to Lower Drug Prices in Medicare."

NTU has conducted research and advocacy on prescription drug pricing policy, which significantly impacts American taxpayers, in Congress and the states for decades. We have long believed that prescription drug policy should focus on increasing market competition and providing targeted, fiscally responsible relief for patients facing high costs, rather than artificially setting prices or forcing private manufacturers into deeply imbalanced negotiations with the federal government. Unfortunately, several recent proposals in the House and Senate have leaned heavily into these price controls and faux "negotiations."[142]

We write once again to urge lawmakers to pursue narrow, targeted solutions for Americans facing high drug costs, rather than sweeping tax-and-mandate schemes that will ultimately push the cost bubble for researching, developing, manufacturing, and delivering prescription drugs on to other parts of the private health sector.

---

[142] For example, *see* Subtitle I of Title XIII (page 175) in: House Committee on Rules. "Build Back Better Act—Rules Committee Print 117–18 Section-By-Section." November 2021. Retrieved from: *https://rules.house.gov/sites/democrats.rules.house.gov/files/Section_by_Section_BBB_RC P117-18_.pdf#page=175.* (Accessed March 14, 2022.)

Below, we briefly review some of NTU's recent work on prescription drug policy, and share some recommendations that would offer more tangible and lasting cost relief for patients than federal price controls.

NTU's Recent Work on Prescription Drug Policy

In November 2021, NTU analyzed the broad outlines of a deal negotiated between moderate Democrats and liberals to include prescription drug pricing provisions in the FY 2022 reconciliation bill, formerly known as the Build Back Better Act (BBBA).[143]

We noted that the negotiated deal among Democratic lawmakers included three broad planks: (1) a requirement for Medicare to negotiate the prices of prescription drugs on a top-down basis, replacing private-sector negotiations between Part D plans and drug manufacturers, (2) inflation caps in Medicare Parts B and D that would require manufacturers to rebate Medicare when increasing the price of their drugs beyond a broad measure of consumer inflation, and (3) reform and redesign of the Part D prescription drug benefit for seniors.

Of the first plank, requiring Medicare negotiation, we argued that:

> . . . requiring Medicare to negotiate drug prices would upend private-sector negotiations happening every year in Part D. And by seeking hundreds of billions of dollars in the form of higher taxes or rebates, policymakers could undermine the resources necessary to develop new and improved prescription drugs for patients in America and around the world.[144]

Of the second plank, inflation caps in Medicare, we noted in July 2021 that:

> To peg the allowable price Medicare will pay for a prescription drug to a broad measure of price increases like the Consumer Price Index (CPI) is to effectively attempt to set the price of the drug. While there are obvious examples of abusive price increases that are clearly not tied to market

---

[143] Lautz, Andrew. "Analyzing the New Prescription Drug Pricing Proposal For Reconciliation." NTU, November 5, 2021. Retrieved from: *https://www.ntu.org/publications/detail/analyzing-the-new-prescription-drug-pricing-proposal-for-reconciliation.*

[144] *Ibid.*

conditions, such as Martin Shkreli increasing the price of malaria and HIV medicine from $13.50 to $750, manufacturers can and do weigh more than just CPI in setting the price of drugs. Private payers in Part D should be able to push back on what they deem to be excessive price increases in negotiations with manufacturers, and private payer negotiations also affect the price of drugs in Part B because Part B reimbursement is based on average sales price.[145]

NTU also led a coalition of taxpayer, consumer, and free-market advocates who wrote to Congress in December 2021, warning of the impacts these two planks in BBBA could have on generic drug competition:

We are also deeply concerned about the impact these two proposals could have on generic drug and biosimilar development. The top-down negotiation requirement is structured in such a way that it will undermine the carefully balanced policy that provides space for generic drug and biosimilar manufacturers to develop products that offer lower-cost alternatives to popular brand-name drugs.

The inflation caps are also as damaging to generic manufacturers as they are to others, if not more so. Applying a broad-based measure of consumer price growth to the growth of a medical product is clunky at best, and could severely undermine manufacturers' ability to account for the cost growth of developing, manufacturing, and distributing their products at worst.[146]

Generic drugs have helped push down the costs of brand-name products for decades since the passage of the landmark, bipartisan Hatch-Waxman Act in 1984, and even a co-author of that legislation, former Sen. Orrin Hatch (R–UT), has warned that provisions in BBBA could "undermine generic competition" and "jeopardize . . . biopharmaceutical innovation."[147]

---

[145] Lautz, Andrew. "Senate Finance Drug Pricing Framework Risks Similar Pitfalls of Price-Setting H.R. 3." NTU, July 7, 2021. Retrieved from: *https://www.ntu.org/publications/detail/senate-finance-drug-pricing-framework-risks-similar-pitfalls-of-price-setting-hr-3.*

[146] Lautz, Andrew. "NTU-Led Coalition Warns of BBB's Impact on Drug Competition." NTU, December 9, 2021. Retrieved from: *https://www.ntu.org/publications/detail/ntu-led-coalition- warns-of-bbbs-impact-on-drug-competition.*

[147] *See:* BioUtah." Hatch Warns of Dangers to Generic Drug Market." November 18, 2021. Retrieved from: *https://bioutah.org/hatch-warns-of-dangers-to-the-generic-drug-market/.* (Accessed November 30, 2021.)

NTU's Federal Policy Recommendations for Prescription Drug Cost Support

Fortunately, there are bipartisan proposals currently on the table in Congress that could reduce costs for patients who may be struggling in America—all without the harmful price controls or higher taxes that could undermine research and development in America's biopharmaceutical sector.

One major proposal that has long earned NTU's support is the third plank of BBBA's prescription drug section—Medicare Part D reform and redesign. Several versions of this redesign have transferred some of the risk in the Part D benefit from America's taxpayers to the private insurers offering plans in Part D, and have used the cost savings to propose setting the first ever out-of-pocket cap for Part D. This would protect seniors from paying above a certain amount per year in drug costs—anywhere from $2,000 per year to $3,100 per year[148] — and could save some of the seniors with the highest costs in the program thousands of dollars per year.

In February of last year, NTU also proposed several policy reforms that could increase competition in the prescription drug market, lower costs, or accomplish both aims:

- Ensure pharmaceutical manufacturers (and other American industries) can continue to fully and immediately recover their research and development (R&D) costs, rather than amortizing them over five years;
- Reduce, rather than increase, distortionary rebates in the Medicaid program;
- Make the elimination of price controls and the protection of intellectual property two primary goals of U.S. free trade agreements; and
- Reduce regulatory barriers to competition and patient barriers to accessing biosimilars.[149]

---

148 7 Lautz, Andrew. "Analyzing the New Prescription Drug Pricing Proposal for Reconciliation." NTU, November 5, 2021. Retrieved from: *https://www.ntu.org/publications/detail/analyzing-the-new-prescription-drug-pricing-proposal-for-reconciliation.*

149 Lautz, Andrew. "A Taxpayer- and Market-Oriented Path Forward for Federal Prescription Drug Policy." NTU, February 25, 2021. Retrieved from: *https://www.ntu.org/publications/de-tail/a-taxpayer-and-market-oriented-path-forward-for-federal-prescription-drug-policy.*

We believe all of these reforms would lead to more lasting and effective change for patients and taxpayers than price controls that could destroy parts of the private biopharmaceutical sector and undermine efforts to increase prescription drug competition. Thank you for your consideration of NTU's views as a taxpayer advocate. Should you wish to discuss NTU's reform recommendations at greater length, I am at your service.

Sincerely,
Andrew Lautz,
Director of Federal Policy

Pharmacy Checker

333 Mamaroneck Avenue White Plains,
NY 10605 Tel. (718) 554–3067
info@pharmacychecker.com
www.pharmacychecker.com

U.S. Senate Committee on Finance

Dirksen Senate Office Bldg. W
ashington, DC 20510–6200
March 25, 2022

Statement of Lucia Mueller and Gabriel Levitt

Thank you for the opportunity to comment.

The heart and soul of PharmacyChecker's mission is to help people find affordable and safe medicine. We vehemently support ending the ban on Medicare drug price negotiations, but we also believe safe importation of lower-cost medicines is critical now. PharmacyChecker's verifications of online pharmacies and drug price comparisons help alleviate the crisis of high drug prices for individual patients by publishing free, useful information on international pharmacy standards of practice and drug price comparisons of those mail order international pharmacies with U.S. discount pharmacy options.

Patients deserve a choice when it comes to their medications and should enjoy the commonsense systems and competition the Internet has fueled across all industry sectors. It is well known that tens of millions of Americans have chosen to buy more affordable prescription drugs from Canada and other countries. PharmacyChecker's main advocacy focus is online access to lower-cost and safe imported medications for Americans. This requires (1) rational policies applied to Internet safety so that patient-consumers can buy their prescription medication from international online pharmacies; and (2) federal policies that do not prevent patients from importing affordable medicines they need.

Sadly, the pharmaceutical industry spends considerable resources to convince Congress that prescription drugs from other countries are somehow dangerous or counterfeit. The January 2022 report published by PharmacyChecker.com, "Not Made in the USA: The Global Pharmaceutical Supply Chain and Prospects for Safe Drug Importation," brings transparency to this very issue by identifying countries of manufacture for the top 100 drugs by total expenditures in Medicare Part D in 2018, showing that most of the prescription drugs Americans get at local pharmacies are not made here.[150] Additionally, looking at wholesale and retail channels, "Not Made in the USA" discusses the vast domestic vs. international price discrepancies of these top 100 drugs. Below are the Key Findings and Policy Recommendations of that report relevant to the issue of high drug prices in America.

Dataset

The dataset of drugs for this report comes from the Medicare Part D Drug Spending Dashboard & Data.[151] The drugs chosen to determine their countries of origin were the top 100 drugs by total spending in 2018. Where there were generic drugs listed, we looked at the brand name product to assess the

150 Levitt, G. and Mueller, L. 2022. "Not Made in the USA: The Global Pharmaceutical Supply Chain and the Prospects for Safe Drug Importation," *https://www.pharmacychecker.com/research/not-made-in-the-usa/*.

151 Medicare Part D drug spending dashboard. (2020, December 22). Centers for Medicare and Medicaid Services, CMS, *https://www.cms.gov/Research-Statistics-Data-and-Systems/Statistics-Trends-and-Reports/Information-on-Prescription-Drugs/MedicarePartD*.

manufacturing origin of that drug.[152] Eighty-five of the 100 were single source drugs with no generic availability in 2018.

Key Findings

- A large majority of the top 100 drugs in Medicare Part D are made outside the U.S.:
  - 68% of finished drug formulations (FDFs)[153]
  - 78% of active pharmaceutical ingredients (APIs)[154]

These brand name products ranged from exceedingly expensive cancer, biologic, and specialty drugs to more widely prescribed maintenance medications.

- Almost all imported brand name drugs are made in countries with manufacturing safety practices equal or superior to those in the United States.

Similar to generic drugs, most brand FDFs and their APIs are foreign made. What differs is that most FDA-approved brand name drugs, including their APIs, are made in high-income countries with the strongest pharmaceutical regulations. Of the 100 Medicare Part D drugs assessed in our report, 32 were finished in the U.S.; 67 were finished in countries that have comparable to if not stronger systems of pharmaceutical manufacturing than the U.S.: the countries in the European Union, Canada, Japan, Singapore, Switzerland, and the United Kingdom. One drug, brand Neurontin (gabapentin), was formulated in India.

- Among drugs from the dataset that are accessible to patients for purchase online, average international mail order prices were 75.53% lower than average

---

[152] Spending on those generic products is captured in the source data.

[153] Finished Drug Formulation (FDF) is the term for the final drug product prescribed to a patient by a medical professional.

[154] Active Pharmaceutical Ingredients (APIs) are the key components of a medicine that produce the intended effects in the body. Since a large majority of prescription drugs sold in the U.S. are made with foreign APIs, tracking where they originate is an important public health issue.

U.S. pharmacy prices. Average prices available of drugs only shipped from Canadian dispensing pharmacies were 70.18% lower than average U.S. pharmacy retail prices.

Policy Recommendations for the Federal Government

- Through legislation, expressly allow importation of brand name drugs by companies, other than their manufacturers, from countries known to have similarly strong pharmaceutical regulations as the U.S., subject to rational regulatory safeguards.

Under current law, Section 804 of the FDCA, importation of commercial quantities of prescription drugs for re-sale without the authorization of the manufacturer is only permitted from Canada. Its relatively small size to the U.S., 38 million compared to 330 million, precludes long-term and meaningful parallel trade in pharmaceuticals with the United States. In contrast, the combined markets of Canada, Japan, the European Union, and the United Kingdom, have 667 million people— twice the U.S. population. If other high-income countries with strong pharmaceutical regulations are added, including Australia, Israel, New Zealand, Singapore, and Switzerland, the relevant market size is almost 700 million. Those regions and countries are also where most of our brand name drugs are manufactured. Section 804 must be amended to allow non-manufacturers importation from those countries, too.

The amendment to allow imports from this greater network of countries would be specific to brand name drugs manufactured in the listed countries.

Currently, Section 804 precludes the importation of biologics. The most expensive category of medical products on the market, biologics represent about 40% of all pharmaceutical expenditures,[155] but only about 2% of prescriptions written.[156] As previously mentioned, wholesale prices for biologics are on average almost three times higher in the U.S. than in the

---

[155] Aitken, M. (2020, March 9). Biologics market dynamics: setting the stage for biosimilars [PDF]. IQVIA Institute for Human Data Science, *https://www.ftc.gov/system/files/documents/public_events/1568297/aitken_-_biologics_market_dynamics_setting_the_stage_for_biosimilars_ slides.pdf.*

[156] Roy, A., and The Apothecary. (2019, March 8). Biologic medicines: the biggest driver of rising drug prices. *Forbes, https://www.forbes.com/sites/theapothecary/2019/03/08/biologic-medi-cines-the-biggest-driver-of-rising-drug-prices/?sh=6019fbed 18b0.*

OECD.[157] Thus, Section 804 must be amended to permit the importation of biologics.

Ostensibly, the preclusion of biologics in Section 804 was due to the greater challenges in safe distribution of what are referred to as "large molecule" pharmaceuticals that are produced with living organisms and therefore require special technology to ship under temperature controls. Today, U.S. pharmacy benefit managers, such as Optum,[158] are already actively importing biologics, albeit under the authorization and with the cooperation of the manufacturers. A federal rule should require wholesale importers of biologic drugs to meet or exceed manufacturer specifications for safe, international shipping. Optum's marketing materials provide a roadmap to develop the standard).[159]

The current federal rule allowing wholesale importation under Section 804, requires that the U.S. importer only imports from a wholesaler that received the products for import directly from the manufacturer. This rule makes it easier for drug manufacturers to use inventory management to prevent unwanted distribution of their products from lower to high priced markets. The rule should be revised to allow the U.S. importer to import from a secondary wholesaler, as long as that wholesaler received the products from the wholesaler that first received the products from the manufacturer. This revision would maintain a closed distribution channel while allowing for the development of a competitive marketplace in pharmaceutical trade, similar to the European Union.

- Remove barriers and provide guidance to assist individual patients who seek to import brand name drugs pursuant to a valid prescription.

The Secretary of Health and Human Services is already seeking new ideas on expanding personal drug importation to help patients access lower drug prices internationally.[160]

---

157 Mulcahy, A.W., Whaley, C.M., Gizaw, M., Schwam, D., Edenfield, N., and Becerra-Ornelas, A.U. (2021). International prescription drug price comparisons: Current empirical estimates and comparisons with previous studies. RAND Corporation, *https://www.rand.org/pubs/re- search_reports/RR2956.html.*

158 Six thoughts: Temperature-controlled shipping. (n.d.). Health Services Innovation Company | Optum, *https://www.optum.com/business/resources/library/cool-thoughts-shipping-sensitive- medications.html.*

159 *Ibid.*

160 Requests for proposals for insulin reimportation and personal prescription drug importation; Withdrawal (86 FR 36283). (2021, July 9). Food and Drug Administration,

Federal law allows personal importation of lower-cost medicines, subject to Section 804(J) of the Food, Drug and Cosmetic Act. A few million Americans each year already import lower-cost medicine for personal use. While they are not charged or prosecuted for illegal imports, individuals purchase medicine, often over the Internet within a grey marketplace, receiving conflicting messages from regulators, industry-sponsored and non-profit organizations on what they should and shouldn't do.

Organizations like PharmacyChecker and the Canadian International Pharmacy Association provide guidance to patients and healthcare providers for those who choose to import medicine for personal use. Those private sector solutions are helpful, but a publicly or non-profit funded effort is needed to bring greater awareness and stakeholder acceptance of safe personal drug importation.

To maximize the utility of personal drug importation as a safe and accepted channel for drug affordability, the following is proposed:

1) Create an HHS task force with a diverse set of stakeholders to review best practices in safe personal drug importation and create FDA recommendations to the public. As part of its mandate, the task force would identify all current programs and channels of personal drug importation, assessing their strengths and weaknesses.
2) Revise the FDA's public communications to include useful recommendations for patients who choose to import a lower cost medicine for personal use and clarify that the agency will not prevent the personal import of a brand name drug from licensed pharmacies in Australia, Canada, the European Union, Israel, Japan, New Zealand, Switzerland, Singapore, and the UK. www.federal register.gov/documents/2021/07/09/2021-14637/requests-for-proposals-for-insulin-reimportation-and-personal-prescription-drug-importation.

As a general model, the U.S. can look to Australia, in which personal importation is expressly legal and the government provides warnings and guidance.[161] As Australians do not face the same problems as Americans do

https:// www.federalregister.gov/documents/2021/07/09/2021-14637/requests-for-proposals-for-insulin- reimportation-and-personal-prescription-drug-importation.

161 Personal importation scheme. (2015, March 18). Australian Government Department of Health | Therapeutic Goods Administration (TGA), *https://www.tga.gov.au/personal-importa- tion-scheme.*

with drug affordability, Australians' necessity for personal importation is not as widespread. Thus, the FDA would need to create more robust warnings and guidelines for patients in the United States.

- Instead of reactionary, mercantilist policies to bring drug manufacturing home, pursue greater global collaboration and coordination towards an international agreement to better regulate and ensure the safe manufacture and high quality of APIs.[162]

APIs are made all over the world and shipped globally to different drug companies for the manufacture of FDFs. This global competition has meant much lower cost generic drugs worldwide, including in the U.S. For reasons of national security, whether due to geopolitical tensions with China or reliance on foreign supplies during the pandemic, there is a new rallying cry for greater autarky with pharmaceuticals. A more longstanding, and less politically charged issue is that, for over 20 years, the FDA has been criticized for its inability to keep up with federal requirements on inspections and oversight of global API manufacturers.

In terms of national security, the U.S. should identify the greatest vulnerabilities and create practical contingency plans involving alternative suppliers or ramping up domestic production. The FDA has reported to Congress on the extent of our vulnerabilities, and they are not as great as the rhetoric on this issue. China accounts for 13% of all FDA registered API manufacturers, a significant but not overwhelming figure. As a matter of national defense policy, we need to identify alternative suppliers for those pharmaceutical ingredients and appropriate special funding and production plans to ramp up domestic manufacturing of the most critical pharmaceuticals.

Outside the above-mentioned national security issues, we must accept the reality of global pharmaceutical manufacturing. To maximize safety and minimize cost, the U.S. should set clear goals for international harmonization on API standards, cGMP, and distribution. The European Medicines Agency is already leading this effort, with the FDA as a participant.[163] FDA's MRAs with all EU countries on drug manufacturing, finalized in 2019, occurred

---

162 Mayr, M. (2017, September 19). International cooperation for inspections of API manufacturers. The place of the Certification Procedure in the global regulatory environment. Prague [PDF]. European Medicines Agency, *https://www.edqm.eu/sites/default/files/20092017-m_mayr-international_cooperation_for_inspections_of_api_manufacturers.pdf.*

163 *Ibid.*

because the FDA knows that the future lies in globally accepted standards and even shared regulatory authority.

Efforts to harmonize API quality standards have been ongoing for 20 years through the International Council for Harmonisation of Technical Requirements for Pharmaceuticals for Human Use (ICH), the Pharmaceutical Inspection Co-operation Scheme, and the World Health Organization. The FDA publishes a questions-and- answers document for the regulated industry called "Q7 Good Manufacturing Practice Guidance for Active Pharmaceutical Ingredients" that is the product of those efforts.[164]

The next step is for the FDA to prioritize working with those international forums and counterpart national drug regulators to create a global regulatory approval scheme for API manufacturers. The goal is for an API manufacturer, whether in Mumbai, Minneapolis, or Munich, to gain approval for international distribution based on one high standard. This will create efficiencies, improve safety, and reduce costs for American taxpayers.

R Street Institute

1212 New York Ave., NW, Suite 900 Washington, DC 20005
202–525–5717
www.rstreet.org
March 16, 2022

The Honorable Ron Wyden
Chairman
U.S. Senate Committee on Finance
219 Dirksen Senate Office Building
Washington, DC 20510–6200

The Honorable Mike Crapo
Ranking Member
U.S. Senate Committee on Finance
219 Dirksen Senate Office Building
Washington, DC 20510–6200

[164] U.S. Department of Health and Human Services, Food and Drug Administration, Center for Drug Evaluation and Research, and Center for Biologics Evaluation and Research. (2018). Q7 Good Manufacturing Practice Guidance for Active Pharmaceutical Ingredients. Questions and Answers. Guidance for Industry. *FDA.gov*, *https://www.fda.gov/media/112426/download.*

RE: Hearing on "Prescription Drug Price Inflation: An Urgent Need to Lower Drug Prices in Medicare"

Dear Chairman Wyden, Ranking Member Crapo, and Honorable Members of the Committee:

Thank you for the opportunity to submit testimony regarding today's hearing on "Prescription Drug Price Inflation: An Urgent Need to Lower Drug Prices in Medicare." This issue is one of vital importance to millions of Americans, and I applaud the Committee's willingness to address it at such a crucial time.

A recent editorial I authored discusses the topic in detail. I include it below for your consideration.[165]

Thank you again for your leadership on this matter. R Street is happy to advise the Committee in its work or otherwise in any manner that would be helpful.

Respectfully,
Jonathan Bydlak
Director of Governance
Director of the Fiscal and Budget Policy Project

U.S. Edition of the World's Oldest Magazine Policy[166]

"Build Back Better" could limit access to prescription drugs

It's one of the most underreported—and dangerous—consequences of Biden's legislation

December 6, 2021 - 11:05 a.m.
Written by:
Jonathan Bydlak

Much has been written about the expansiveness of the Biden administration's signature priority: the Build Back Better Act (BBB). The legislation is projected by the Congressional Budget Office (CBO) to spend more than $1.6

---

[165] Jonathan Bydlak, "'Build Back Better' could limit access to prescription drugs," The Spectator World, December 6, 2021, https://spectatorworld.com/topic/build-back-better-biden-limit-prescription-drugs.

[166] https://spectatorworld.com/topic-category/policy/.

trillion[167] in its attempts to address countless Democratic priorities ranging from climate change to the expansion of Medicaid.

One aspect of the bill, however, has attracted far less fanfare than it should have: its impact on the cost of prescription drugs.

Provisions in the bill would, among other things, impose rebates[168] on drug manufacturers if prices rise faster than inflation. It's an idea that sounds great in the current moment of creeping inflation, but is ultimately little more than a market distortion likely to produce an array of adverse consequences.

A new University of Chicago study 5 looked at the impact of the bill on "innovation and patient health" and found that BBB would reduce spending on drug research and development by "about 18.5 percent." It concludes that such a reduction might limit research and development, potentially leading to 135 fewer new drugs.

Perhaps most damning, the study also concluded that the corresponding drop in drug production would result in a loss of 331.[169] million life years—a number 31 times larger than the life years lost in the United States as a result of COVID–19. That's presumably not the outcome that Democrats had in mind.

But their proposal doesn't just impact the market for new brand-name drugs. It also would undermine access to affordable generic and biosimilar medicines already approved by the Food and Drug Administration (FDA).

In addition to the inflation rebates, BBB seeks to cap Medicare drug prices by limiting how much the program will pay for prescriptions. While negotiation with manufacturers would result in some savings to the program—$79 billion[170] over 10 years according to the latest CBO estimate—it also would create complications[171] for generics manufacturers, who are critical[172] 8 to keeping prescription costs low in the first place. As another commentator

[167] https://spendingtracker.org/bills/hr5376-117.

[168] https://www.kff.org/health-costs/issue-brief/potential-costs-and-impact-of-health-provisions-in-the-build-back-better-act/.

[169] https://ecchc.economics.uchicago.edu/2021/11/30/issue-brief-the-impact-of-hr-5376-on-biopharmaceutical-innovation-and-patient-health/.

[170] https://pink.pharmaintelligence.informa.com/PS145281/Medicare-Price-Negotiation-Inflation-Rebate-Legislation-Would-Generate-163Bn-CBO-Says.

[171] https://www.statnews.com/2021/11/06/hurried-bills-congress-shouldnt-undermine-vast-savings-generic-biosimilar-drugs/.

[172] https://www.iqvia.com/-/media/iqvia/pdfs/institute-reports/price-declines-after-branded- medicines-lose-exclusivity-in-the-us.pdf.

highlights,[173] "requiring Medicare to negotiate drug prices would upend private-sector negotiations" that are already occurring.

As The Wall Street Journal editorial board recently pointed[174] out, under BBB, "branded drugs will also see less generic competition, which will result in higher prices." They further note that generics on average reduce prices by 30 percent— and once there are four generic entrants in a market, prices drop by nearly 80 percent.

This observation is consistent with past analysis by the FDA, which has broadly found[175] that "greater competition among generic drug makers is associated with lower generic drug prices."

In other words, the more generics manufacturers there are in the marketplace, the more savings for consumers and government alike. Likewise, legislation that threatens such competition ultimately will increase drug prices.

The rise of affordable generics [176] is one of the great healthcare success stories of the last decade. It's a trend that has not only provided quality medication for those who need it, it has also benefited programs like Medicare at a time of otherwise rising healthcare costs.

With inflation[177] and supply chain difficulties [178] continuing to threaten the robustness of the post-pandemic recovery, it's more important than ever that lawmakers pay close attention to the full implications of their policy proposals. Passing along costs and sticking it to drug companies may appeal to populists on both sides, but Americans are unlikely to come out ahead should such misguided policies become law.

Prescription drug reform is one of the few areas where there is genuine bipartisan agreement[179] not only about what policy goals should be, but about the best ways to improve access while keeping costs down.[180] The Biden administration should listen to that consensus and rethink their latest proposal.

---

173 https://www.ntu.org/publications/detail/analyzing-the-new-prescription-drug-pricing-proposal-for-reconciliation.

174 https://www.wsj.com/articles/a-toxic-drug-price-deal-11636415735.

175 *https://www.fda.gov/about-fda/center-drug-evaluation-and-research-cder/generic-competition-and-drug-prices.*

176 https://thehill.com/blogs/pundits-blog/healthcare/343484-one-simple-bipartisan-way-to- help-rein-in-soaring-healthcare/.

177 https://www.washingtonpost.com/business/2021/11/10/cpi-inflation-october/.

178 https://www.cnbc.com/2021/12/01/siemens-chairman-says-supply-chain-chaos-will-last-until-next-summer.html.

179 https://www.grassley.senate.gov/news/news-releases/grassley-leahy-hail-inclusion-creates-act-year-end-spending-agreement.

180 https://www.theamericanconservative.com/the-easiest-way-donald-trump-can-bring-drug-prices-down/.

Jonathan Bydlak is director of the Governance Program at the R Street Institute, a center-right think tank.

Texas Rare Alliance

3575 Far West Blvd., #27892
Austin TX 78731
(512) 688–1914
March 16, 2022

On behalf of nearly 3 million Texans living with a rare disease, approaching 10% of the total rare disease population in the United States, Texas Rare Alliance writes to encourage responsible drug pricing reform that does not negatively impact the continued development of innovative treatments for rare diseases with unmet needs or continued patient access to approved rare disease medications. We ask for the same consideration for patients with common conditions.

Of the more than 8,000 rare diseases, 95% lack an FDA-approved disease-modifying treatment. It is crucial we continue research and development of additional rare disease treatments and that rare disease patients can access disease-modifying treatments upon approval.

We know what price controls have done to patients in other countries—they have resulted in patients, including rare disease patients, having worse access to treatments. They undervalue the lives of people who are chronically ill, disabled, or elderly, and many of these people are rare disease patients.

I. The Unmet Need for Rare Disease Treatments
   A. The Rare Disease Landscape in the United States

The facts are not great. One in 10 Americans, over 32 million, has a rare disease.[181] Half of rare disease patients are children (16 million American children).[182] Rare diseases cause thirty-five percent of the deaths in the first

[181] RARE Facts (n.d.). Global Genes, https://globalgenes.org/rare-disease-facts/.
[182] *Id.*

year of life.[183] Thirty percent of children with a rare disease will not survive until their fifth birthday.[184] There are 7,000 rare diseases.[185]

Ninety-five percent of all rare diseases do not have an FDA-approved disease-modifying treatment.[186] It will take thousands of years to realize treatments for all rare diseases if FDA-approved therapies continue at the current rate.[187]

I am intimately aware of what it means to lack an approved rare disease treatment for your rare disease community. It is devastating. We need more conditions like SMA to cross over from the ninety-five percent of rare diseases that lace an approved SMA treatment to the five percent with an FDA-approved disease-modifying treatment. To achieve this, we must encourage continued research and development of breakthrough therapeutics.

II. Understanding the True Economic Burden of Rare Diseases

The National Economic Burden of Rare Disease Study in the U.S., published by the EveryLife Foundation for Rare Diseases, covered 379 rare diseases affecting 15.5 million people in the U.S. for 2019. The study estimated the overall rare disease economic burden to exceed $966 billion.[188] This included "$418 billion in direct medical cost and $548 billion in indirect and non-medical costs absorbed directly by families living with rare diseases."[189]

Accordingly, in-direct and Non-medical costs (costs absorbed directly by families) in 2019 accounted for nearly 60% of the overall cost.[190] Prescription medications and outpatient prescription administration were only about 10% of the overall economic burden and less than what was spent on inpatient

---

[183] Get the Facts on Rare Diseases (n.d.). Rare Genomics Institute, *https://www.raregenomics.org/rare-disease-facts.*

[184] *Id.*

[185] RARE Facts (n.d.). Global Genes, *https://globalgenes.org/rare-disease-facts/.*

[186] *Id.*

[187] Bock, Eric. (April 17, 2020). Rare Disease Research Progressing, But Could Go Even Faster. NIH Record. 72(8) 1, 8–9, *https://nihrecord.nih.gov/sites/recordNIH/files/pdf/2020/NIH-Record-2020-04-17.pdf.*

[188] EveryLife Foundation for Rare Diseases. (2021). The National Economic Burden of Rare Disease Study, 15, https://everylifefoundation.org/wp-content/uploads/2021/02/The_National_Economic_Burden_of_Rare_Disease_Study_Summary_Report_February_2021.pdf.

[189] *Id.*

[190] *Id.*

care.[191] We can't expect to address affordability if we focus on a small percentage of the problem.

III. Protecting the Pathway to Rare Disease Research

Congress recognized the unmet need for rare disease treatments by passing the Orphan Drug Act (ODA) in 1983.[192] The ODA incentivizes the development of treatments for rare diseases, many of which are life-threatening, and most lack an approved treatment.[193] Congress reaffirmed its commitment to the rare disease community in 2016 by passing the 21st Century Cures Act,[194] a bipartisan effort President Obama signed into law. The Act included many provisions to improve the discovery, development, and delivery of orphan therapies for rare disease patients, together with substantial NIH funding.[195]

IV. The Commitment to Rare Disease Research Is Paying Off

2018 represented a historic year for the rare disease community. For the first time, rare disease approvals exceeded general approvals from the Center for Drug Evaluation and Research (CDER) at the FDA.[196] "In 2018, 34 of CDER's 59 novel drugs (58%) were approved to treat rare or 'orphan' diseases that affect 200,000 or fewer

Americans."[197] Increased approvals of rare disease treatments are a welcome sign for the rare disease community. We must avoid barriers to research and development to ensure the continued development of innovative FDA-approved therapies for rare diseases with unmet needs.

---

[191] *Id.*

[192] Orphan Drug Act of 1983. Pub L. No. 97–414, 96 Stat. 2049.

[193] Rare Diseases at FDA. (February 20, 2020). U.S. Food and Drug Administration, *https://www.fda.gov/patients/rare-diseases-fda.*

[194] Public Law 114–255, 130 Stat. 1033. To Accelerate the Discovery, Development, and Delivery of 21st Century Cures, and for Other Purposes. Enacted: December 13, 2016, *https://www.congress.gov/114/plaws/publ255/PLAW-114publ255.pdf.*

[195] Huron, Jennifer. President Signs 21st Century Cures Medical Innovation Bill Into Law (December 13, 2016). National Organization of Rare Disorders, *https://rarediseases.org/president-signs-21st-century-cures-bill-law/.* Rare Diseases at FDA. (February 20, 2020). U.S. Food and Drug Administration, *https://www.fda.gov/patients/rare-diseases-fda.*

[196] Center for Drug Evaluation and Research. Advancing Health Through Innovation: 2018 New Drug Therapy Approvals, *https://www.fda.gov/files/drugs/published/New-Drug-Therapy-Approvals-2018_3.pdf.*

[197] *Id.*

V. Rare Disease Research Benefits Us All

Research for rare diseases greased the wheels for a COVID–19 vaccine. Before the COVID–19 pandemic, most had not heard of mRNA technologies. This is not true for researchers in the rare disease community. There are more than 145 ongoing mRNA clinical trials for rare diseases, including Cystic Fibrosis.[198] This represents more than 25% of all mRNA clinical trials.[199] Rare disease researchers pivoted to work on developing treatments and vaccines for COVID–19. One of these researchers is Dr. David Fajgenbaum, a clinician and researcher who also happens to be a rare disease patient with Castleman Disease.[200]

Today, mRNA COVID vaccines protect most vaccinated patients in the U.S. As of April 28, 234.6 vaccines have been administered in the U.S. 226.5 million of the vaccines—96.5%—have been the Pfizer and Moderna mRNA vaccines.[201] We need research into breakthrough technologies like mRNA technology to continue and protect all of us.

VI. History Has Taught that Setting Prices Doesn't Work

Being a Texan, it is hard not to see the impact government interference in pricing has had on other sectors. U.S. price controls on oil, gasoline, and petroleum in the 1970s resulted in a sharp decline in domestic oil production, increasing reliance on foreign oil,[202] creating lines for miles and hours along highways as vehicles waited for gas, despite FTC warnings.[203,204] Another example in the U.S. is the Federal Reserve adoption rules imposing fee caps

---

198 CBI Insights. (February 3, 2021). What Are mRNA Therapies, and How Are They Used for Vaccines? Research Briefs, *https://www.cbinsights.com/research/what-are-mrna-therapies/.*

199 *Id.*

200 Moffitt, Debra. (May 27, 2020). Rare Disease Hunter Dr. David Fajgenbaum Takes on COVID–19, *https://www.cslbehring.com/vita/2020/david-fajgenbaum-takes-on-covid19.*

201 Fry, Erika and Rapp, Nicolas. (April 28, 2021). 55% of U.S. Adults Have Gotten a COVID Vaccine. See How Your State Is Doing, Fortune, https://fortune.com/2021/04/28/covid-vaccine-tracker-update-us-state-by-state-pfizer-moderna-johnson-and-johnson-data-coronavirus-vaccines-april-2021/.

202 Rafuse, Jack. (June 7, 2007). History 101: Price Controls Don't Work. *Chicago Tribune, https://www.chicagotribune.com/news/ct-xpm-2007-06-07-0706061080-story.html.*

203 Mitchell, Dan. (April 16, 2020). The Case Against Price Controls. International Liberty, *https://danieljmitchell.wordpress.com/2020/04/16/the-case-against-price-controls/.*

204 *Id.*

for debit card transactions in 2011[205] that decreased access to credit products by consumers and *failed to lower consumer fees or pass on savings*[206],[207]

Innovation and technology have led to an improved quality of life for Americans.

Innovation and technology are the answer and historically have led to an improved quality of life for all Americans.

VII. Price Controls Would be Disastrous for Access to Medications

According to the Galen Institute, 89% of new medicines introduced between 2011 and 2018 are available in the U.S. compared to 62% in Germany, 60% in the U.K., 50% in Japan, and 48% in France.[208] In its analysis of H.R. 3, the CBO estimated that the resulting reduced revenues over a decade between "$.05 trillion to $1 trillion would lead to a reduction of 8 to 15 new drugs coming to market. It is difficult to know in advance the nature of these drugs or to quantify the effect of foregone innovation on health."[209] The CBO estimated the cost of creating and maintaining the system to implement H.R. 3 would increase spending at around $3 billion over a 6-year period.[210]

Comparably, the Build Back Better Act (BBBA) would result in 135 fewer new drugs and a loss of 331.5 million life years in the U.S. by 2039.

We find that H.R. 5376 will reduce revenues by 12.0 percent through 2039, and therefore that the evidence base predicts that R&D spending will fall about 18.5 percent, amounting to $663 billion. We find that this cut in R&D activity leads to 135 fewer new drugs. This drop in new drugs is predicted to generate a loss of 331.5 million life years in the U.S., 31 times as large as the 10.7 million life years lost from COVID–19 in the U.S. to date. These estimated effects on the number of new drugs brought to market are 27 times larger than projected by CBO, which finds only 5 drugs will be lost through 2039, equaling a 0.63 percent reduction.[211]

---

205 *Id.*

206 *Id.*

207 *Id.*

208 The Editorial Board. (October 4, 2019). Pelosi's Expensive Drug Bill. *The Wall Street Journal, https://www.wsj.com/articles/pelosis-expensive-drug-bill-11570228189.*

209 Swagel, Phillip. (October 11, 2019). Effects of Drug Price Negotiation Stemming From Title 1 of H.R. 3, the Lower Drug Costs Now Act of 2019, on Spending and Revenues Related to Part D of Medicare, CBO, *https://www.cbo.gov/system/files/2019-10/hr3ltr.pdf.*

210 *Id.*

211 https://cpb-us-w2.wpmucdn.com/voices.uchicago.edu/dist/d/3128/files/2021/08/Issue-Brief-Drug-Pricing-in-HR-5376-11.30.pdf.

That is a hefty cost for a system that could prove as disastrous as the oil, gasoline, and petroleum controls of the 1970s and the more recent failed debit card transaction fee caps beginning in 2011. It is a cost that will be paid in worsened health outcomes—and deaths—in the rare disease and greater patient communities.

VIII. Inflation Penalties Would Lead to Empty Medicine Cabinets

In February, U.S. inflation reached a 40-year high of 7.9%.[212] However, consumer prices that included gasoline, food outpaced the inflation rate, with gasoline increasing 22% in two weeks.[213] If our government had inflation penalties in place for food and gasoline, retailers could not afford to supply food and gas. Our pantries, refrigerators, and our tanks would be empty.

Similarly, pharmaceutical and biopharmaceutical companies cannot supply medications to patients when circumstances increase their supply costs above inflation. Although our government is not considering inflation penalties on food and gas, it is on our medications. It places U.S. patients in danger of having empty medicine cabinets devoid of their medications.

IX. My Experience with QALY-Based Cost-Effectiveness Analysis

When policymakers talk about coverage and reimbursement strategies for health care treatments based on their value or cost-effectiveness, they rely on a discriminatory metric called the quality-adjusted life year that devalues lives lived with disabilities and chronic conditions—particularly rare diseases. Foreign countries rely on the metric to justify restricting access to care that they do not view as cost- effective. Our 10-year-old son, Hunter, diagnosed with SMA Type I, has a QALY of .2. This means his life is valued at 80% less than our daughters in perfect health who have QALYs of 1. ALS is another example worth noting because it has a QALY of -.05. This tells ALS patients and their loved ones that having ALS is worse than being dead.

We are blessed that Hunter hasn't been directly impacted by the QALY. However, I did move the family back to our St. Louis home at the height of the COVID–19 pandemic following the death of Michael Hickson in Austin

---

[212] https://www.bloomberg.com/news/articles/2022-03-10/u-s-inflation-hits-fresh-40-year-high-of-7-9-before-oil-spike.

[213] *https://apnews.com/article/gas-prices-record-high-russia-ukraine-ac7fcc350ad1f1c71d b4185b99fef112.*

by a doctor who employed a QALY rationale to deny treatment because the doctor didn't perceive Michael as having a quality of life.

It was a sucker punch. I packed up everything and ran away fast and temporarily returned to St. Louis, where I knew St. Louis Children's Hospital saw value in Hunter, worked hard to save him so many times and provided his Spinraza treatments.

I also witnessed Hunter's friend Ben impacted by QALYs. Ben and Hunter started the Spinraza EAP together—with positive health outcomes. After FDA approval, insurers did not view Spinraza as cost-effective for patients like Ben, who depended on a machine to help him breathe. Ben's mom, Melissa, cried. She asked why Ben's life wasn't worth saving too. Eventually, he found coverage from a patient assistance program until being covered under Medicaid. We oppose metrics that devalue our children's lives. We refuse to save our children only to have a health system adopt QALYs that gives upon them.

The Institute for Clinical and Economic Review (ICER) conducts value assessments relying on QALYs for treatments such as Spinraza. I testified that Hunter had not been hospitalized since starting treatment in 2016. The year before, we feared for his life. It is also imperative to commence treatments presymptomatically to afford the patients the best possible health outcomes and quality of life. I testified to ICER about all of the costs of SMA that no one considers, such as the daily respiratory protocol such as albuterol nebulizer treatment, the extensive daily stretching physical therapy to preserve and improve movement, occupational therapy to improve movements related to education, and navigating the world, and speech including oral stimulation to improve both speech and swallow, not to mention nutrition and medical equipment, most of which is not covered by insurance. Yet, their assessment using a QALY measure failed to capture any of the significant economic aspects of that drug for my family. ICER ultimately determined that Spinraza was not cost-effective.

In 2018, when CVS Caremark threatened to use a QALY-based benchmark for what drugs they would cover in a benefit package being marketed to their employer clients, it created a moment of panic for people that rely on these innovations to survive. Thankfully, advocacy worked against CVS Caremark, and they stopped marketing that benefit package. Still, we constantly fear payers using these cost-per-QALY benchmarks to determine what they will or will not cover. I cannot imagine the fate of families like mine if we were to explicitly endorse the use of discriminatory metrics in Medicare and Medicaid. 89% of new medicines introduced between 2011 and 2018 are available in the U.S. compared to 62% in Germany, 60% in the U.K., 50% in Japan, and 48% in France. The Congressional Budget Office, assuming the use of QALYs in its analysis of the impact of legislation to control drug prices in the House of Representatives, H.R. 3, estimated a reduction of 8 to 15 new drugs coming to market and acknowledged difficulty quantifying the effect of foregone innovation on health.

Thankfully, the National Council on Disability, an independent federal agency advising Congress and the administration on disability issues, has recommended that Congress unambiguously bar the use of QALYs. Their research found that QALYs would prioritize providing treatment to a non-disabled population with a longer theoretical life expectancy and otherwise perfect health over a population with a disability or chronic condition.

They also found that simplified value assessments do not account for the complex experience of patients with rare diseases that are not well-represented in the research literature, particularly for communities of color. QALYs do not take into account clinical expertise on rare disorders that may not have extensive research literature available for use in value assessments. QALYs often rely on research that does not adequately account for the ways in which many people—especially, though not exclusively, those with rare conditions—may have medication responses that vary dramatically from the average. For individuals with rare conditions or who come from groups underrepresented in research, like people with disabilities and people of color, the inability of QALYs to account for information that primarily exists within clinical knowledge but has not yet made it into the research literature constitutes a serious problem. Many cancer drugs are not considered valuable enough to cover in the U.K. due to their use of QALYs. Historically, the United Kingdom has used QALYs to justify not covering the limited drugs available for Alzheimer's disease, even when they cost the equivalent of a cup of coffee. The use of a cost-per-QALY analysis in the United Kingdom delayed access to cystic fibrosis treatments in the United Kingdom.

America's sense of morality and ethic of equality makes it a bridge too far to deny or devalue care to those with significant lifetime health needs just because they may never achieve a pre-conceived notion of optimal health. The implications are even more significant for communities of color that are underrepresented in the research literature that informs value assessment. Therefore, we need a consistent national policy that makes it clear that federal programs cannot use discriminatory metrics such as QALYs to drive reimbursement and coverage. While the law bars Medicare from using QALYs, state Medicaid programs have recently started to openly ref- erence

QALYs, and legislation considered by Congress to reduce drug prices opens the door to their use in Medicare decisions.

X. Patients Conflate Rising Out-of-Pocket Insurance Costs with Drug Costs

According to CMS, Out-of-Pocket spending by patients grew 4.6% in 2019 to $406.5 billion, comprising 11% of healthcare spending.[214] Retail prescription prices decreased in 2019 by .4%. Prescription drugs represent 10% of healthcare spending.[215] Growth in retail prescription drug spending increased by 5.7% but was attributed to growth in the use of prescriptions drugs in terms of the number of prescriptions dispensed.[216] Our population is aging, and aging individuals use more prescriptions. Hospital and physician and clinical services increased more dramatically than prescription drugs in 2019 at rates of 6.2% and 4.6%, respectively. This represents a combined 51% of healthcare spending.[217]

XI. Patients Need Responsible Reform that Improves Access to the Medications They Need

A. Medicare Part D Out-of-Pocket (OOP) Limits for Beneficiaries

The BBBA does provide benefits that should be retained for Medicare beneficiaries. Many disabled and elderly Medicare patients are currently forced to choose between paying a mortgage, rent, putting food on the table, or paying for the medications they need. Medicare beneficiaries in that situation lose no matter what choice they make. The OOP limits for beneficiaries would be capped at $2,000 under BBBA. It would also be spread over the year so that beneficiaries wouldn't face paying the entire $2,000 in the first month to access their medications.

B. Pharmacy Benefit Manager (PBM) Oversight and Transparency

Drug pricing increases are traceable to the emergence of PBMs and their practices that benefit PBMs and payors to the detriment of U.S. patients. At

[214] National Health Expenditures 2019 Highlights (2020), CMS, *https://www.cms.gov/files/document/highlights.pdf.*

[215] *Id.*

[216] *Id.*

[217] *Id.*

best, PBMs operate as contractual middlemen to insurers, and at their worst, PBMs are wholly owned by plans. PBMs act as gatekeepers to the formulary, creating a race to the bottom between drug manufacturers to gain a coveted spot on the formulary. The PBMs also demand rebates, concessions, and fees from manufacturers. To pay the demanded rebates, concessions, and fees, manufacturers increase the price that the insurer pays. Then, the PBMs and insurers complain to the press and policymakers that drug prices are rising too fast and too much.

Fortunately, some states have caught on and have enacted legislation that protects patients from some unscrupulous practices such as penalizing patients with higher copays for using a network pharmacy of their choice over a PBM-owned pharmacy, mandating patients use the PBM-owned mail order pharmacy, or from reimbursing PBM-owned pharmacies at higher rates than other pharmacies.

However, to truly understand the practices of PBMs and the impact on the health care ecosystem, we must first know what those practices are, how much the PBMs and insurers make, and what, if any, benefit is passed on to beneficiaries. Consequently, we cannot improve the situation until there is transparency on all sides. California has made strides in this effort, with PBM reform providing oversight and transparency.[218] Several state and federal laws have banned PBM gag clauses that prevent pharmacies from disclosing when the retail price for medication is lower than the co-insurance price. Arkansas legislation even goes as far to penalize and fine PBMs in addition to banning the gag clauses.[219]

C. Innovation and Competition Are the Solutions to Lower Drug Prices

Just as innovation and competition in the oil industry led to the U.S. escaping the clutches of OPEC (not the disastrous pricing mandates that led to rationing, empty gas tanks, and mile-long lines at the gas stations), it will be innovation and competition that reduce drug pricing and result in the proliferation of innovative treatments for rare diseases with unmet needs. Some of the innovations come from surprising sources, such as innovative regulatory reform at the FDA that makes platform clinical trials possible that

---

218 https://leginfo.legislature.ca.gov/faces/billTextClient.xhtml?bill_id=201720180AB315.

219 https://custom.statenet.com/public/resources.cgi?id=ID:bill:AR2018010H1010&ciq=ncsldc3&client_md=9a13edc9b4b75c06b9f201a9884a52cf&mode=current_text.

could create shared clinical trial fees from smaller pharmaceutical and biopharmaceutical companies that would increase the number of clinical trials for rare and orphan conditions with unmet needs.

XII. Conclusion

We can improve the rare disease community by ensuring continued research and development for the 95% of rare diseases without an FDA-approved disease-modifying treatment. We must respect the lives of chronically ill, disabled, and elderly individuals. Their lives matter, and we cannot afford to discount their lives at any cost. With all of us working together to embrace innovation and technology, we can expedite rare disease treatments as we did with COVID–19 vaccines. We witnessed what is possible, and treating rare disease patients is just as crucial as protecting lives from COVID–19. Please consider the negative implications that imposed drug pricing would have on the development of rare disease treatments—as well as common conditions that lack disease-modifying treatments like Alzheimer's and Diabetes— and access to those treatments. Thank you for your consideration. If you have any questions or would like to discuss our statement, please contact me at khrystal@txrare.org or by phone at (512) 688–1914.

With gratitude,
Khrystal K Davis, J.D. Founding President

Taxpayers Protection Alliance

1101 14th St., NW, Suite 1120
Washington, DC 20005

Statement of Daniel Savickas, Government Affairs Manager

I am pleased to be able to submit this statement for the record on behalf of the Taxpayers Protection Alliance (TPA). TPA is a non-profit non-partisan organization dedicated to educating the public through the research, analysis and dissemination of information on the government's effects on the economy. TPA, through its network of taxpayers will hold politicians accountable for the effects of their policies on the size, scope, efficiency and activity of government and offer real solutions to runaway deficits and debt.

TPA has done extensive work to help lower the costs of prescription drugs in the United States. We strive to promote policies that will lower costs for patients and lessen the financial burden on taxpayers across the nation. We also strive to increase competition in the marketplace to achieve those objectives. The following statement was published as an editorial piece in TownHall on November 19, 2021 and is a product of those aforementioned efforts. I thank the committee in advance for its dedication to this issue and consideration of the views expressed below.

Prescription Price Controls Harm Access to Life Saving Medication

As Published in Townhall—November 19, 2021 by Daniel Savickas

It is no secret that the costs of prescription drugs are very high in the United States. Studies from Harvard Medical School indicate that one in four American patients have foregone a prescription because the cost was too high. With the costs of everything else beginning to rise due to the pandemic, inflation, and the global supply chain crisis, it is even more possible that more Americans will have to choose between treating their illnesses and affording basic necessities. This is unacceptable.

Access to medicine and prescriptions is a problem that touches many families in the United States. Naturally, lawmakers are trying to ameliorate this problem through legislation. Unfortunately, the prevailing proposal on Capitol Hill is a set of command-and-control policies slipped into the "Build Back Better" reconciliation spending plan. The plan would implement restrictions and price controls on the market. This would actually harm the companies most likely to offer affordable solutions, generic and biosimilar drug manufacturers.

Generic drugs are manufactured very similarly to brand name products. They have the same active ingredient as their branded competitor and are often very similar in other characteristics, such as safety, strength, and intended use. Biosimilars are manufactured to have the same impacts as the branded drug, but are more complex in their manufacturing to be considered as identical in the way generics are.

Generics and biosimilars come to market to compete with the brand name alternative once the initial patent expires on the brand name product. Generics and biosimilars are most notable because of their prices. According to the

Food and Drug Administration (FDA) data, generics are on average 80 to 85 percent less expensive than branded drugs, and biosimilars are roughly 10 to 37 percent less expensive.

Creating more competition in the market between branded drugs, generics, and biosimilars will be key to any strategy to lower the prices of prescription medicines. During the years-long period where the branded drug has market exclusivity, generic and biosimilar manufacturers need to be able to reliably forecast the market to hit the ground running when market access begins. Price controls and government negotiations that are based on changing benchmarks and arbitrary numbers erode that ability. Generics and biosimilars will be left in the dark in terms of what type of investment is needed to create a successful, widely available product.

Price controls shift demand, drastically alter supply calculations, and obscure the true value of medications already available. Such proposals reflect a fundamental misunderstanding about the nature of prices. Prices are merely a signal of value from consumers and suppliers based on a host of factors. Price controls treat the symptoms of what's wrong with the current system, but not the underlying cause. That would be like shutting off "low battery" notifications on your phone instead of plugging your phone into a charger. If generics and biosimilars can't read the signals that prices send and the market behavior that follows, they will be at a severe disadvantage when it comes time to market their products.

These price controls come in the form of government "negotiations" with drug manufacturers. First, a negotiation is hardly fair or based on actual value when one party is the government, which has a monopoly on force and threatens punitive action should talks fall through. Proponents of the plan tout the fact that negotiation benchmarks will be tied to international market valuations. However, international markets are substantially different from the American one. In the U.S., patients have more access to newer medicines, which is partly responsible for higher prices. This negotiation further obfuscates value and will lead to decreasing availability and investment. Generics will bear this shift heavily.

Another price control in the package is an inflationary penalty. This penalty would implement a steep tax on drug manufacturers who raise the price of their drugs faster than the rate of inflation. First, this will incentivize drug makers to come to market at a higher list price to hedge their bets, in case a price hike might be needed in the future. That is because labor supply, manufacturing costs, and supply chain shortages—like those we're seeing now—can increase costs faster than inflation. This would necessitate a change, but without the ability to make it, prices would have to start astronomically high to protect investment.

Secondly, such a percentage-based benchmark would disproportionately impact generic drug makers, whose prices are already far lower. Because of the discrepancy, a minuscule price hike by a generic would trigger the penalty. This provision is not an incentive to lower prices; instead it's an incentive for brands to start high and a punishment for the manufacturers that are offering affordable medicines.

Competition is the surest way to lower the price of any product on the market, and prescription drugs are no exception. Generic and biosimilar drug manufacturers have been helping offer far more affordable alternatives for years. While lawmakers in Washington think they are going after pharmaceutical companies charging the highest prices, the manufacturers of all life-saving medications will be impacted. The biggest price of all, however, will be paid by the patients and families that rely on them.

Chapter 2

Constitutional Challenges to the Medicare Drug Price Negotiation Program*

Hannah-Alise Rogers

Summary

Congress created the Medicare Drug Pricing Program (the program) through the budget reconciliation measure known as the Inflation Reduction Act (IRA; P.L. 117-169), which became law on August 16, 2022. The program allows Medicare to negotiate the prices of certain Medicare drugs directly with drug manufacturers for the first time. The Centers for Medicare and Medicaid Services (CMS), the division of the U.S. Department of Health and Human Services (HHS) tasked with administering the program, has issued guidance to explain the program's initial implementation. On August 29, 2023, CMS selected the first 10 Medicare Part D drugs that will be subject to negotiated prices in 2026.

In summer 2023, several drug manufacturers and trade associations representing manufacturers challenged the law before federal district courts across the country. The plaintiffs argue that the law is unconstitutional under the First, Fifth, and Eighth Amendments, and they also allege violations of the Nondelegation Doctrine and the Spending Clause. This report explains and contextualizes the plaintiffs' constitutional claims by analyzing relevant U.S. Supreme Court jurisprudence.

The plaintiffs argue that the IRA violates the First Amendment because it forces manufacturers to sign a pricing agreement with the Secretary of HHS that characterizes the negotiated price of the drug as "fair," which

* This is an edited, reformatted and augmented version of Congressional Research Service Publication No. R47682, dated September 6, 2023.

In: Medicare's Prescription Drug Pricing
Editor: Lloyd M. Porter
ISBN: 979-8-89530-728-1

amounts to compelled speech. The plaintiffs also argue that the IRA violates the Fifth Amendment, both the Due Process Clause and the Takings Clause. First, the plaintiffs claim that the IRA violates the Due Process Clause because it lacks the requisite procedural safeguards, including notice, the opportunity to be heard, and the potential for judicial review. Second, the plaintiffs allege that the law constitutes a taking of both tangible (drugs) and intangible (patents) property. Some of the plaintiffs claim that the program amounts to a per se taking, while others argue that it constitutes a regulatory taking.

A few of the plaintiffs argue that the IRA violates the Eighth Amendment Excessive Fines Clause because the excise tax to which manufacturers of selected drugs that do not comply with the statute will be subjected is really a punishment disguised as a tax. The trade association plaintiffs argue that the IRA violates the Nondelegation Doctrine by ceding too much power to the Secretary of HHS to set drug prices. Finally, several plaintiffs argue that the IRA cannot be justified on the basis of Congress's Spending Clause power because the IRA does not condition the receipt of federal funding on a manufacturer's participation in the program. The plaintiffs further allege that even if the IRA could be said to impose such a condition, the statute does not provide adequate notice of the condition, the condition is not related to the purpose of the spending and is unconstitutionally coercive, and compliance with the condition would violate manufacturers' other rights under the Constitution.

The report concludes by identifying relevant considerations for the 118th Congress as the litigation proceeds. At least one drug manufacturer has filed a preliminary injunction, seeking to halt CMS's implementation of the program until the litigation is resolved. Some stakeholders predict that the litigation could reach the U.S. Supreme Court.

Congress created the Medicare Drug Price Negotiation Program (the program), in a budget reconciliation measure known as the Inflation Reduction Act (IRA), which became law on August 16, 2022.[1] Beginning in June 2023, several pharmaceutical manufacturers and tradeassociations filed lawsuits in various federal district courts alleging that the program was unconstitutional. These cases, brought against the U.S. Department of Health and Human Services (HHS) and the Centers for Medicare and Medicaid Services (CMS), were filed in D.C. District Court, the U.S. District Court for the Southern District of Ohio, New Jersey District Court, the U.S. District Court for the Western District of Texas, the U.S. District Court for the Northern District of

[1] Inflation Reduction Act of 2022, P.L. 117-169, 136 Stat 1818. The IRA is codified in multiple titles of the *U.S. Code*. The relevant sections of the Medicare Drug Price Negotiation Program are found at 42 U.S.C. §§ 1320f-1 *et seq*.

Illinois, the U.S. District Court for the District of Connecticut, and the U.S. District Court for the District of Delaware.[2] Taken together, the cases bring a variety of facial constitutional challenges against the IRA, including under the First, Fifth, and Eighth Amendments; the Nondelegation Doctrine; and the Spending Clause.[3] At least two of the plaintiffs also argue that the CMS guidance implementing the program violates the Administrative Procedure Act.[4]

The IRA authorizes the Secretary of HHS, via CMS, to negotiate the prices of certain qualifying, single-source drugs directly with manufacturers for the first time.[5] The program will apply to certain single-source prescription drugs and biological products covered by Medicare Part B (physician-administered drugs) and Medicare Part D (retail prescription drugs).[6] The IRA instructs CMS to implement the first three years of the program (price years 2026-2028) through "program instruction or other forms of program

---

[2] Complaint, Merck & Co. v. Becerra, No. 23-1616 (D.D.C. Jun. 6, 2023), ECF No. 1 [hereinafter Merck Compl.]. Complaint, U.S. Chamber of Commerce, et al. v. Becerra, No. 23-0156 (S.D. Ohio, Jun. 9, 2023) ECF No. 1 [hereinafter Chamber of Com. Compl.]; Complaint, Bristol Myers Squibb Company v. Becerra, No. 23-3335 (D.N.J. Jun. 16, 2023), ECF No. 1 [hereinafter Bristol Myers Compl.]; Complaint, Pharmaceutical Research and Manufacturers of America (PhRMA) et al. v. Becerra, No. 23-0707 (W.D. Tex. Jun. 21, 2023), ECF No. 1 [hereinafter PhRMA Compl.]; Complaint, Janssen Pharmaceuticals Inc. v. Becerra, No 23-3818 (D.N.J. July 18, 2023), ECF No. 1 [hereinafter Janssen Compl.]; Complaint, Astellas Pharma U.S., Inc. v. Becerra, No. 23-4578 (N.D. Ill. July 14, 2023), ECF No. 1 [hereinafter Astellas Compl.]; Complaint, Boehringer Ingelheim Pharmaceuticals, Inc., v. Becerra, No. 23- 01103 (D. Conn. Aug. 18, 2023), ECF No. 1 [hereinafter Boehringer Compl.]; Complaint, AstraZeneca Pharmaceuticals LP v. Becerra, No. 23-0931 (D. Del. Aug. 25, 2023), ECF No. 1 [hereinafter AstraZeneca Compl.].

[3] Complaints *supra* note 2.

[4] AstraZeneca Compl. at 7; Boehringer Compl. at 8. This Report only addresses the plaintiffs' constitutional challenges.

[5] Inflation Reduction Act of 2022, Pub. L. No. 117-169, §§ 11001-02, 136 Stat. 1818 (codified at 42 U.S.C. §§ 1320f-1-1320f-7).

[6] The statute's definition of "qualifying single source drug" distinguishes between drug products and biological products. 42 U.S.C. § 1320f-1(e)(1)(A)-(B). For a drug product to be a qualifying single-source drug, the drug must be a covered Part B or Part D drug and (1) be approved by the U.S. Food and Drug Administration (FDA) and be marketed pursuant to such approval; (2) at least seven years must have passed since the initial approval; and (3) the drug cannot be the listed drug for any approved and marketed generic drug. *Id.* § 1320f-1(e)(1)(A)(i)-(iii). For a biological product to be a qualifying single-source drug, the statute requires the covered Part B or Part D biological product (1) to be licensed under § 351 of the Public Health Service Act (42 U.S.C. §§ 201 et seq.) and be marketed under the license; to have been marketed for at least 11 years from the date of initial licensure; and (3) not to be the reference product for any other licensed and marketed biosimilar. *Id.* § 1320f-1(e)(1)(B)(i)-(iii).

guidance."[7] As described in previous CRS reports, CMS began implementing the Medicare Drug Price Negotiation Program by issuing Initial Guidance on March 15, 2023.[8] CMS subsequently issued Revised Guidance on June 30, 2023, to address stakeholder concerns regarding the selection of negotiation-eligible drugs and the factors to be considered when evaluating maximum fair prices (MFPs).[9] In accordance with the statute, on August 29, 2023, CMS selected the first 10 drugs for price negotiation.[10] The MFP negotiations are to conclude by August 1, 2024, and the MFP is to take effect in 2026.[11]

This report explains and contextualizes the plaintiffs' constitutional claims, relying on relevant Supreme Court jurisprudence.[12]

---

[7] The statute directs CMS to carry out the first three years of the program (price years 2026-2028) "by program instruction or other forms of program guidance." 42 U.S.C. § 1320f note. In its Revised Guidance, CMS states that it "will develop its policies for 2029 and all subsequent initial price applicability years of the Negotiation Program through notice-and-comment rulemaking." CMS REVISED GUIDANCE, *infra* note 8, at 2.

[8] CENTERS FOR MEDICARE AND MEDICAID, MEDICARE DRUG PRICE NEGOTIATION PROGRAM: INITIAL MEMORANDUM, IMPLEMENTATION OF SECTIONS 1191–1198 OF THE SOCIAL SECURITY ACT FOR INITIAL PRICE APPLICABILITY YEAR 2026, AND SOLICITATION OF COMMENTS (Mar. 15, 2023), https://www.cms.gov/files/document/medicare-drug-price-negotiation-program-initial-guidance.pdf [hereinafter CMS INITIAL GUIDANCE]. For a description of the Medicare Drug Price Negotiation Program, the CMS Guidance, and the statute's limitations on judicial review, *see* CRS Report R47555, *Implementation of the Medicare Drug Price Negotiation Program: Centers for Medicare and Medicaid Guidance and Legal Considerations*, by Hannah-Alise Rogers (2023). For a complete summary of the IRA's changes to Medicare, Medicaid, and private insurance, *see* CRS Report R47396, *Health Care Provisions of the Budget Reconciliation Measure P.L. 117-169*, coordinated by Katherine M. Kehres (2022). For a brief overview of the IRA's changes to the Medicare Program, including an overview of the Medicare Prescription Drug Price Negotiation Program and other changes to Medicare Parts B and D, see CRS In Focus IF12203, *Selected Health Provisions of the Inflation Reduction Act*, by Suzanne M. Kirchhoff (2022).

[9] CENTERS FOR MEDICARE AND MEDICAID, MEDICARE DRUG PRICE NEGOTIATION PROGRAM: REVISED GUIDANCE, IMPLEMENTATION OF SECTIONS 1191–98 OF THE SOCIAL SECURITY ACT FOR INITIAL PRICE APPLICABILITY YEAR 2026, (JUN. 30, 2023), https://www.cms.gov/files/document/revised-medicare-drug-price-negotiation-program-guidance-june-2023.pdf [hereinafter CMS REVISED GUIDANCE].

[10] U.S. DEPT. OF HEALTH & HUMAN SERVS., *HHS Selects the First Drugs for Medicare Drug Price Negotiation*, Press Release (August 29, 2023), https://www.hhs.gov/about/news/2023/08/29/hhs-selects-the-first-drugs-for-medicare-drug-price-negotiation.html.

[11] CMS REVISED GUIDANCE at 117; 42 U.S.C. § 1320f(d)(1).

[12] At the time of this writing, HHS has not had the opportunity to address all of the plaintiffs' claims—the report does not address the validity of the claims being made or any arguments or defenses with which the government may respond.

First Amendment Claim

The First Amendment states, in relevant part, that "Congress shall make no law . . . abridging the freedom of speech."[13] Among other free speech protections, the U.S. Supreme Court has recognized that Free Speech Clause concerns arise when a person or entity is compelled to say or otherwise express a viewpoint that the speaker does not agree with or wish to communicate.[14] At least six plaintiffs have claimed that the IRA violates the First Amendment prohibition against compelled speech.[15]

Under the IRA, the manufacturers of selected drugs are required to enter into agreements with HHS to negotiate, and potentially renegotiate, what the statute calls the "maximum fair price" (MFP) of the drug.[16] If the manufacturers of selected drugs fail to sign an agreement with CMS by October 1, 2023, the manufacturers will be subject to an excise tax, which is described in further detail below.[17] One plaintiff claims that signing such agreements amounts to "forced messaging that promotes the (false) impression that manufacturers . . . agree with prices imposed by HHS decree."[18] Similarly, another plaintiff alleges that the IRA compels manufacturers to "become a spokesperson for promoting the Government's value judgments," by requiring manufacturers to "endorse and express the viewpoint that they 'agree' to HHS-dictated prices, and that those prices are fair."[19] The manufacturer claims the government cannot justify this "compelled-speech regime" because it lacks a "legitimate reason" to force manufacturers to convey these "misleading" messages.[20] The plaintiffs further argue that Congress could regulate drug prices "without burdening a speaker with unwanted speech," and that "[p]rice controls do not require speech

---

[13] U.S. CONST. amend. I. *See also* CONG. RESEARCH SERV., Amdt 1.7.1 *Historical Background on Free Speech Clause*, https://constitution.congress.gov/browse/essay/amdt1-7-1/ALDE_00013537/(last accessed Sept. 1, 2023).

[14] *See, e.g.*, 303 Creative LLC v. Elenis, 143 S. Ct. 2298, 2312 (2023); Nat'l Inst. of Family & Life Advocates v. Becerra, 138 S. Ct. 2361, 2371 (2018).

[15] Merck Compl. at 3; Chamber of Com Compl. at 8; Bristol Myers Compl. at 20; Janssen Compl. at 6; Astellas Compl. at 4; Boehringer Compl. at 6.

[16] *See* 42 U.S.C. 1192f-3(c).

[17] For more information about the excise tax and other penalties to which manufacturers will be subject under the IRA, *see infra* p. 9.

[18] Merck Compl at 17; *see also* Astellas Compl. at 32; Janssen Compl. at 6; Boehringer Compl. at 7.

[19] Bristol Myers Compl. at 20.

[20] *Id.*

controls."[21] It further claims that the government lacks a "legitimate reason" to force manufacturers to convey misleading messages.[22]

In evaluating First Amendment challenges, one critical threshold question a court would consider is whether the government is regulating expressive activity, which is protected by the First Amendment, or only nonexpressive conduct, which is not protected. The Supreme Court has observed that "the First Amendment directs that the government may not suppress speech as easily as it may suppress conduct."[23] The Court has also said that the government can prohibit an agreement to engage in unlawful conduct "brought about through speaking or writing" without violating the First Amendment.[24] "[I]t has never been deemed an abridgement of freedom of speech," the Court has stated, "to make a course of conduct illegal merely because the conduct was in part initiated, evidenced, or carried out by a means of language, either spoken, written, or printed."[25]

With respect to pricing regulations specifically, in *Expressions Hair Design v. Schneiderman*, the Court analyzed whether a state law banning surcharges on credit card purchases violated the First Amendment.[26] The Court observed that a "typical price regulation"[27] might not implicate the First Amendment if it would only regulate conduct.[28] However, if a law regulates "the communication of prices rather than prices themselves," it regulates "speech," thus triggering First Amendment scrutiny.[29] The *Expressions* Court reasoned that the state law regulated speech because rather than dictating the price of goods, it instead prohibited the vendors' means of communicating its prices to customers.[30]

---

[21] Chamber of Com. Compl. at 54.

[22] Id.

[23] 44 Liquormart, Inc. v. Rhode Island, 517 U.S. 484, 512 (1996) (plurality opinion).

[24] Giboney v. Empire Storage & Ice Co., 336 U.S. 490, 502; *see also* Brown v. Hartlage, 456 U.S. 45 (1982).

[25] *Id.*

[26] Expressions Hair Design v. Schneiderman, 581 U.S. 37, 42 (2017). The New York law stated that "[n]o seller in any sales transaction may impose a surcharge on a holder who elects to use a credit card in lieu of payment by cash ...." *Id.*

[27] *Id.* at 47. The Court gave an example of a "typical price regulation" as one that would "regulate the amount that a store could collect" from a buyer. In such an example, the Court said, the regulation would regulate the seller's conduct, because by communicating prices to buyers, "the law—by determining the amount charged—would indirectly dictate the content of [the] speech." In that example, the Court said that the law would only "incidental[ly]" affect speech, because its "primary effect" would be on the seller's conduct. *Id.*

[28] *See, e.g.*, 44 Liquormart, Inc. v. Rhodes Island, 517 U.S. 484 (1996) (plurality opinion).

[29] Expressions Hair Design, 581 U.S. at 48.

[30] *Id.*

Determining whether an activity is sufficiently expressive so as to trigger the First Amendment can involve analyzing various factors. For example, in *Rumsfeld v. Forum for Academic and Institutional Rights (FAIR)*, several law schools argued that the Solomon Amendment, which conditioned the receipt of federal funding on the schools' willingness to allow military recruiters equal access to their campuses, violated the First Amendment.[31] The Court found that "accommodating the military's message does not affect the law schools' speech," because the schools were not actually speaking by hosting on-campus interviews.[32] The Court also did not find the law school's conduct of hosting military recruiters "inherently expressive," because giving the recruiters access to its campus did not "interfere with any message of the school."[33] The Court observed that "[t]he expressive component of a law school's actions is not created by the conduct itself but by the speech that accompanies it."[34] Because explanatory speech was necessary to express the conduct, the Court said this was "strong evidence" that the conduct was not so expressive as to warrant First Amendment protection.[35]

Assuming that a regulation interferes with an expressive activity that triggers First Amendment protection, the next threshold inquiry a court would consider is the appropriate level of constitutional scrutiny to be applied. The First Amendment's protections do not apply with uniformity: different types of regulations will trigger different levels of scrutiny, depending on the type of speech being regulated and how the regulation operates.[36] For example, commercial speech—defined as speech that relates "solely to the economic interests of the speaker and its audience"—is typically afforded intermediate scrutiny under the *Central Hudson* test.[37] As the name suggests, "intermediate" scrutiny is a medium level of constitutional scrutiny. The

---

[31] *FAIR*, 547 U.S. at 48. The case arose when a group of law schools restricted campus access to military recruiters because of the military's policy on homosexuals. *Id.* at 51. In response, Congress enacted the Solomon Amendment. *Id.* The law schools sued, arguing that the "forced inclusion and equal treatment of military recruiters violated the law schools' First Amendment freedoms of speech and association. *Id.* at 53.

[32] *FAIR*, 547 U.S. at 64.

[33] *Id.* at 64. The Court observed, "[l]aw schools remain free under the statute to express whatever views they may have on the … policy [with which they disagree] all the while retaining eligibility for federal funds."

[34] *FAIR*, 547 U.S. at 66.

[35] *Id.*; *see also* United States v. O'Brien, 391 U.S. 367, 376 (1968) (finding that even if a law regulating conduct contains a "communicative element," more is needed in order to "bring into play" the First Amendment).

[36] See generally CRS Report R45700, *Assessing Commercial Disclosure Requirements under the First Amendment*, by Valerie C. Brannon (Apr. 23, 2019).

[37] Cent. Hudson Elec. Corp. v. Pub. Serv. Comm'n, 477 U.S. 557, 561 (1980).

Central Hudson test requires the government to show that the regulation relates to a "substantial" governmental interest that is "directly advance[d]" by the law.[38]

Central Hudson, however, is not the only standard that could apply to messaging concerning price regulations. Government actions compelling speech are usually subject to strict scrutiny—a rigorous standard that laws rarely satisfy,[39] but the Supreme Court has sometimes applied a standard of review even less stringent than intermediate scrutiny to commercial disclosure requirements.[40]

Thus, a court analyzing the plaintiffs' First Amendment arguments in the Medicare Drug Price Negotiation Program litigation may have to address several threshold questions, including whether the act of signing a contract that describes a drug price as "fair" is an inherently expressive activity that warrants First Amendment protection, or whether such action is merely nonexpressive conduct. Assuming that a court were to find the signing of the negotiation contract an expressive activity, it would then likely consider which standard of constitutional scrutiny to apply. Determining the level of scrutiny to be applied would likely require a court to determine the type of speech the IRA regulates (e.g., commercial or noncommercial speech) and how the law operates (e.g., whether it burdens or compels speech).

Fifth Amendment Claims

The Fifth Amendment provides, "No person shall be . . . deprived of life, liberty, or property, without due process of law; nor shall private property be taken for public use, without just compensation."[41] The first clause quoted above, known as the Due Process Clause, requires that the government provide sufficient ("due") procedures before it deprives a person of life, liberty, or property.[42] The second clause, known as the Takings Clause, allows the government to seize a person's property for a public use, but only if the

---

[38] *Id.* at 566.
[39] Nat'l Inst. of Family & Life Advocates v. Becerra, 138 S. Ct. 2361, 2371 (2018).
[40] *Id.* at 2372; *e.g.*, Zauderer v. Off. of Disciplinary Couns., 471 U.S. 626, 651 (1985).
[41] U.S. CONST. amend. V.
[42] *See* CONG. RESEARCH SERV., Amdt 5.5.1 *Overview of Due Process*, https://constitution.congress.gov/browse/essay/amdt5-5-1/ALDE_00013721/(last accessed August 23, 2023).

government pays fair compensation for the taking.[43] All of the plaintiffs argue that the IRA violates some provision of the Fifth Amendment, with some claiming Due Process Clause violations,[44] and others claiming Takings Clause violations.[45] Each of these claims is explored in further detail below.

Due Process Clause

The plaintiffs argue that the IRA violates the Fifth Amendment's Due Process Clause by depriving drug manufacturers of their property without the requisite procedural safeguards.[46] The alleged property at issue is drug manufacturers' "investment-backed patent rights and common- law right to sell their products at market prices free from arbitrary and inadequately disclosed governmental constraints."[47] The plaintiffs insist that the IRA does not comply with the core principles of procedural due process—notice and "the opportunity to be heard"[48]—because they were not given sufficient notice of the IRA's "fundamental change[s] to the legal landscape," which affected investments they made before the IRA was passed.[49] They further argue that because some aspects of CMS's guidance implementing the program were finalized without stakeholder input, there is "no guarantee that they will have an opportunity to be heard on the key decisions that HHS will make over the next three years before the first [MFP] takes effect in 2026."[50] The plaintiffs also claim that the law runs afoul of the Due Process Clause because "the IRA expressly deprives manufacturers of any judicial review of HHS's key decisions."[51]

---

[43] *See* CONG. RESEARCH SERV., Amdt 5.9.1 *Overview of Takings Clause*, https://constitution.congress.gov/browse/essay/amdt5-9-6/ALDE_00013285/#ALDF_ 00022171 (last accessed August 23, 2023).

[44] Chamber of Com. Compl. at 40; PhRMA Compl. at 6.

[45] Merck Compl. at 15; Bristol Myers Compl. at 26.

[46] PhRMA Compl. at 43; Chamber of Com. Compl. at 40; AstraZeneca Compl. at 30.

[47] PhRMA Compl. at 43.

[48] *See* Mathews v. Eldridge, 424 U.S. 319, 333 (1976); Armstrong v. Manzo, 380 U.S. 545, 552(1965).

[49] PhRMA Compl. at 47.

[50] Chamber of Com. Compl. at 40; *see also* AstraZeneca Compl. at 30.

[51] *Id.* at 4;1 *see also* PhRMA Compl. at 43; Astellas Compl. at 4. For more information about the Medicare Drug Pricing Program's limitations on judicial review, *see* CRS Report R47555, *Implementation of the Medicare Drug Price Negotiation Program: Centers for Medicare and Medicaid Guidance and Legal Considerations*, by Hannah-Alise Rogers.

The Supreme Court established the basic framework for considering procedural due process claims in *Mathews v. Eldridge*.[52] The *Mathews* factors address the amount of process required before the government may impair a protected property or liberty interest.[53] This fact-dependent analysis weighs (1) the private interest affected by the government's action; (2) the "risk of erroneous deprivation" of an interest given the current procedures and the value of additional "procedural safeguards"; and (3) the government's interest, including the "function involved" and any burden that additional procedures would entail.[54]

For example, in *Mathews*, a plaintiff sued the Social Security Administration (SSA) after termination of his disability benefits, and the Court addressed whether the Fifth Amendment required that he be given a hearing prior to the termination.[55] The Court cautioned that "[d]ue process is flexible and calls for such procedural protections as the particular situation demands."[56] The Court reviewed the "elaborate" procedures for terminating benefits under the Social Security Act, the various safeguards that the SSA put in place to avoid a mistaken deprivation of benefits, and considered how to balance the high cost of additional safeguards with the need to conserve "scarce fiscal and administrative resources."[57] After weighing the three factors, the Court's majority held that an evidentiary hearing was not required prior to the benefit determination, and that the agency's administrative procedures were sufficient to meet the minimum standard required by the Fifth Amendment.[58]

When considering the plaintiffs' Due Process claim in the Medicare Drug Price Negotiation Program litigation, a court could use the *Mathews* factors to weigh the interests of the drug manufacturers against those of the government and could consider the manufacturers' risk of being deprived of their property.

---

52 Chamber of Com. Compl. at 44; *see also* PhRMA Compl. at 50–52; *see also* Mathews v. Eldridge, 424 U.S. 319 (1976).

53 424 U.S. 319, 334–35.

54 *Id.* at 335.

55 *Id.* at 323.

56 *Id.* at 324 (*quoting* Morrisey v. Brewer, 408 U.S. 471, 481 (1972) (internal quotations omitted)).

57 *Id.* at 339, 345.

58 *Id.* at 349. The Court further observed: "The judicial model of an evidentiary hearing is neither a required, or even the most effective, method of decision making in all circumstances. The essence of due process is the requirement that "a person in jeopardy of serious loss be given notice of the case against him and opportunity to meet it." *Id.* at 348 (*quoting* Joint Anti-Fascist Refugee Comm. v. McGrath, 341 U.S. 123, 171–72 (1951) (internal quotations omitted)).

As part of this inquiry, a court could also analyze the language of the IRA to determine whether it contains sufficient procedural safeguards to protect drug manufacturers' property. Such an inquiry might also address whether CMS, in its implementation of the law, provided sufficient procedural safeguards.

Takings Clause

Other plaintiffs have raised distinct Fifth Amendment claims under the Takings Clause, alleging that the implementation of the IRA constitutes a taking of both tangible property (drugs and biological products) and intellectual property (patents) without just compensation.[59] One plaintiff claims that "the singular purpose of this scheme [in the IRA] is for Medicare to obtain prescription drugs without paying fair market value."[60] Another alleges that the program "is akin to the Government taking your car on terms that you would never voluntarily accept and threatening to also take your house if you do not 'agree' that the taking was 'fair.'"[61]

As with the Due Process Clause allegations made by other plaintiffs, the manufacturers argue that their drugs and patents are property, and that the government is "forcing [them] to provide third parties with 'access' to [their] products at steeply discounted prices."[62] The manufacturers state that such a "compelled transfer of title effects a classic, per se taking."[63] The plaintiffs further allege that the program's pricing mechanism is not "just compensation" because it is not sufficiently connected to fair market value, and in fact, the statute requires the price to be set "significantly below the drug's market value."[64]

The Supreme Court has clarified that the Takings Clause "does not prohibit the taking of private property, but instead places a condition on the exercise of that power" by requiring the government to fairly compensate someone whose property rights are taken.[65] To determine whether a taking has

---

59 Merck Compl. at 15; Bristol Myers Compl. at 26; Astellas Compl. at 4; Janssen Compl. at 27; Boehringer Compl. at 34.

60 Merck Compl. at 2.

61 Janssen Compl. at 6.

62 Merck Compl. at 16; *see also* Boehringer Compl. at 35.

63 Merck Compl. at 16; *see also* Boehringer Compl. at 36.

64 Bristol Myers Compl. at 18; Astellas Compl. at 28.

65 Lingle v. Chevron U.S.A. Inc., 544 U.S. 528, 536 (2005) (quoting First English Evangelical Lutheran Church v. Cnty. of L.A., 482, U.S. 304, 314 (1987)); *see also* CONG.

occurred, a party must demonstrate that the claimed property at issue is protected by the Takings Clause, and that it was "taken" by the government.[66] To show that the taking was unconstitutional, the party must prove either that (1) the taking was not for public use,[67] or (2) the party has not received just compensation.[68]

The Takings Clause applies only to "private property" interests protected under the Fifth Amendment.[69] Personal property (such as pills or vials of a drug) is protected,[70] but the Supreme Court has never directly held that patents are property protected by the Takings Clause.[71] Assuming that the property (whether drugs, patents, or both) is protected, a court would next analyze whether it has been "taken" under two doctrinal frameworks: per se takings or regulatory takings.

Historically, the Court has recognized certain physical invasions of property under a per se rule: an appropriation of property, even if minor, is a taking that requires compensation.[72] For example, in *Loretto v. Teleprompter Manhattan CATV Corp.*, the Court held that a law requiring landlords to permit cable companies to install equipment on the exterior of their buildings constituted a per se taking for purposes of the Takings Clause, because the law authorized a permanent, if only minimal, physical occupation of the property.[73] Other instances in which the Court has recognized a per se taking are when the

---

RESEARCH SERV., Amdt 5.9.2 *Public Use and Takings Clause*, https://constitution.congress.gov/browse/essay/amdt5-9-2/ALDE_00013281/ (last accessed July 10, 2023).

[66] *See, e.g.,* Ruckelshaus v. Monsanto Co., 467 U.S. 986, 1000-01 (1984).

[67] Kelo v. New London, 545 U.S. 469, 483 (2005) ("For more than a century, our public use jurisprudence has wisely eschewed rigid formulas and intrusive scrutiny in favor of affording legislatures broad latitude in determining what public needs justify the use of the takings power.")

[68] *Id.*

[69] *See Ruckelshaus*, 467 U.S. at 1001. For more information, *see* CONG. RESEARCH SERV., Amdt 5.9.3 *Property Interests Subject to Takins Clause*, https://constitution.congress.gov/browse/essay/amdt5-9-3/ALDE_00013282/ (last accessed August 17, 2023).

[70] *See* Horne v. Dept. of Agric., 576 U.S. 350 (2015).

[71] In *Horne*, the Court reiterated its previous observation that "[a patent] confers upon the patentee an exclusive property in the patented invention which cannot be appropriated or used by the government itself, without just compensation, any more than it can appropriate or use without compensation land which has been patented to a private purchaser." 576 U.S. 359–60 (alteration in original) (quoting James v. Campbell, 104 U.S. 356, 358 (1882)).

[72] *See, e.g.* Loretto v. Teleprompter Manhattan CATV Corp., 458 U.S. 419, 434–35 (1982) ("In short, when the 'character of the governmental action' is a permanent physical occupation of property, our cases uniformly have found a taking to the extent of the occupation, without regard to whether the action achieves an important public benefit or has only minimal economic impact on the owner." (quoting Penn Cent. Transp. v. City of New York, 438 U.S. 104, 121 (1978)).

[73] Id.

government took title to a share of a farm's agricultural crop,[74] or when an owner was deprived of all his property's economic use or value.[75]

When the per se framework does not apply, the Court has still recognized a "regulatory taking" when a government action significantly affects property rights, holding that if the regulation "goes too far[,] it will be recognized as a taking."[76] Although the Court has avoided a "set formula to determine where regulation ends and a taking begins,"[77] and has stated that regulatory takings cases require "essentially ad hoc, factual inquiries,"[78] the Court has established some general principles for determining when regulatory takings occur.

In *Penn Central Transportation Co. v. City of New York*, the Court analyzed whether a government regulation amounted to a taking. Factors considered by the Court included (1) "the economic impact of the regulation"; (2) whether the regulation interfered with "distinct investment-backed expectations"; and (3) the character of the government's action.[79] Regarding the third factor, the Court explained that a taking "may more readily be found when the interference with property can be characterized as a physical invasion by a government than when interference arises from some public program adjusting the benefits and burdens of economic life to promote the common good."[80]

The Court applied the *Penn Central* framework in *Ruckelshaus v. Monsanto*, which concerned public disclosure of trade secrets that were submitted by a pesticide manufacturer to the Environmental Protection Agency (EPA).[81] The Court acknowledged that the manufacturer held a property interest in the data containing trade secrets, but it held that the EPA regulation requiring disclosure did not constitute a taking when a manufacturer did not have a "reasonable investment- backed expectation" that the data

---

[74] Horne v. Dep't of Agric., 576 U.S. 351, 361 (2015).

[75] *See* Agins v. City of Tiburon, 477 U.S. 255, 260 (1980); Lucas v. S.C. Coastal Council, 505 U.S. 1003 (1992).

[76] Pa. Coal Co. v. Mahon, 260 U.S. 393, 415 (1922). *See also* CONG. RESEARCH SERV., *Early Jurisprudence on Regulatory Takings*, https://constitution.congress.gov/browse/essay/amdt5-9-5/ALDE_00013284/ (last accessed July 10, 2023).

[77] *Penn. Cent. Transp. Co.*, 438 U.S. at 124.

[78] *Id.*

[79] *Id.* at 124. For more information about the *Penn Central* analysis and how it is used to evaluate regulatory takings, *see* CONG. RESEARCH SERV., *Regulatory Takings and Penn Central Framework*, https://constitution.congress.gov/browse/essay/amdt5-9-6/ALDE_00013285/#ALDF_00022171 (last accessed July 13, 2023).

[80] *Id.* (citation omitted).

[81] Ruckelshaus v. Monsanto, 467 U.S. 986, 990 (1983).

would remain confidential.[82] The Court highlighted that manufacturers voluntarily participated in a regulatory scheme that required their products to be registered with the federal government and that such participation allowed them to sell their products in the U.S. market.[83] The Court also found that the disclosure requirement was rationally related to the legitimate government interest of ensuring safety in the sales and use of pesticides.[84] For these reasons, the Court held the manufacturer did not have a "reasonable investment-backed expectation," and that no regulatory taking occurred.[85]

In considering whether the Medicare Drug Price Negotiation Program constitutes an unconstitutional taking for purposes of the Fifth Amendment, a court would likely need to resolve several questions. As a threshold matter, a court would likely need to address whether drug patents are a form of property protected by the Takings Clause. If so, a court could consider whether the patents or drugs themselves were "taken" by the government. Such an inquiry might assess whether the IRA's processes of selecting drugs for negotiation and determining the MFP of those drugs constitutes a per se taking, or a regulation that goes so far that it should be considered a taking under the *Penn Central* framework. It is unclear whether the plaintiffs could demonstrate a per se taking with the present facts. If a court were to use the *Penn Central* framework to evaluate whether a regulatory taking occurred, the court would likely look at the potential economic impact of the IRA on manufacturers, how it is being implemented, and whether the manufacturers had a "reasonable investment-backed expectation" that they would be able to freely market their products without negotiating Medicare prices with the government.

If a court were to find that a taking of drugs occurred, the next question could be whether the taking was for public use and whether the manufacturers received just compensation for their drugs and other property. Such an inquiry might require the court to look more closely at the MFP and how it was calculated by CMS. As this is a fact-specific analysis, it may be difficult for a court to make this evaluation before the actual MFP is established by CMS.

---

[82] *Ruckelshaus*, 467 U.S. at 1005. The Court found a taking of data submitted during some time periods, based primarily on whether the manufacturer had a "'reasonable investment-backed expectation' that EPA would maintain those data in strictest confidence." *Id.* at 1110.

[83] *Id.* The Court observed that "as long as [the manufacturer] is aware of the conditions under which the data are submitted, and the conditions are rationally related to a legitimate Government interest, a voluntary submission of data by an applicant in exchange for the economic advantages of a [product] registration can hardly be called a taking." *Id.* at 1007.

[84] *Id.* at 1005.

[85] *Ruckelshaus*, 467 U.S. at 1006.

Eighth Amendment Claim

The Eighth Amendment provides that "[e]xcessive bail shall not be required, nor excessive fines imposed, nor cruel and unusual punishments inflicted."[86] Some plaintiffs claim that the IRA's excise taxes and penalties are in fact punishments designed to force manufacturers to comply with the statute's price negotiation scheme.[87] The IRA amended the Internal Revenue Code to create an excise tax on the sale of selected drugs if a manufacturer fails to execute a price negotiation agreement with the Secretary; fails to agree to an initial or renegotiated MFP; or does not submit requested information about the drug to the Secretary.[88] The tax is calculated based on a percentage of the sales during the noncompliance period, starting with 65% for the first 90 days of noncompliance, and reaching up to 95% after 270 days.[89] In addition, separate provisions impose civil money penalties on manufacturers that fail to sell their drug at or below the MFP;[90] violate the terms of the pricing agreement;[91] or provide false information to the Secretary.[92]

The plaintiffs are particularly concerned with the impact of the excise tax, which one characterizes as a "massive penalty."[93] Another plaintiff asserts that "Congress well understood that, in practice, the threat of this ruinous excise tax would force manufacturers to accept whatever price HHS demands."[94] The parties point to the Joint Committee on Taxation's estimate of a similar iteration of the excise tax found in previous legislative proposals as raising "no revenue whatsoever," as well as a similar Congressional Budget Office projection.[95] Manufacturers argue that such projections demonstrate that

---

[86] U.S. CONST. amend. VIII.

[87] Chamber of Com. Compl. at 47; PhRMA Compl. at 55; Boehringer Compl. at 39.

[88] Inflation Reduction Act of 2022, Pub. L. No. 117-169, §11003 (codified at 26 U.S.C. § 5000D).

[89] 26 U.S.C. § 5000D(d). For an example of how the excise tax would be calculated, *see* CRS Report R47396, *Health Care Provisions of the Budget Reconciliation Measure P.L. 117-169*, coordinated by Katherine M. Kehres.

[90] 42 U.S.C. § 1320f-6(a). The CMP is calculated by multiplying by 10 the difference between the MFP and the sale price. *Id.* For example, if a manufacturer sold 100 units of a selected drug at $10 per unit, the total sale would be $1,000. But, if the MFP for that selected drug was $5, the manufacturer would be liable for $5,000 (10 times the number of units sold (100) and the difference between the sale price ($10) and the MFP ($5).

[91] The penalty is $1,000,000 for each day of a violation. 42 U.S.C. § 1320f-6(c).

[92] The penalty is $1,000,000 for each item of false information. 42 U.S.C. § 1320f-6(d).

[93] Boehringer Compl. at 39.

[94] PhRMA Compl. at 25.

[95] PhRMA Compl. at 25; Chamber of Com. Compl. at 28; Boehringer Compl. at 40. The estimate is based on H.R. 5376, the Build Back Better Act (117th Cong.), which proposed a similar excise tax.

Congress intended the excise tax as a punishment for noncompliant manufacturers, because noncompliance is so costly that no manufacturer would risk being subject to the tax.[96] Another plaintiff argues that "[r]egardless of its name, the IRA's 'excise tax' is a penalty," and that "no manufacturer could possibly afford to pay" the amounts owed for noncompliance.[97]

The Supreme Court has found that the purpose of the Excessive Fines Clause is "to limit the government's power to punish,"[98] and has applied the clause to situations in which fines are both imposed by and paid to the government.[99] Although historically applied only to criminal cases, the prohibition on excessive fines can also apply in civil cases.[100] The Court has made clear that the threshold question "is not … whether [the action] … is civil or criminal, but rather whether it is punishment."[101] When analyzing whether a fine constitutes punishment, the Court has looked at the history of the action and whether it could be "properly considered punishment today."[102]

---

[96] PhRMA Compl. at 25.

[97] Chamber of Com. Compl. at 48.

[98] *See, e.g.*, Austin v. United States, 509 U.S. 602, 607–09 (1993) ("Some provisions of the Bill of Rights are expressly limited to criminal casesThe text of the Eighth Amendment includes no similar limitation. Nor does the history of the Eighth Amendment require such a limitation.") *Id.* at 607–08. *See also* United States v. Bajakajian, 524 U.S. 321 (1998) (holding that a punitive civil forfeiture violated the Excessive Fines Clause); *but see* Browning-Ferris Indus., 492 U.S. 257 (1989) (holding that the Eighth Amendment's prohibition on excessive fines did not apply to an award of punitive damages in a civil suit between private parties).

[99] *See* Browning-Ferris Indus. v. Kelco Disposal, Inc., 492 U.S. 257, 266–67 (1989).

[100] *See, e.g., Browning-Ferris*, where, in considering the legislative history behind the Excessive Fines Clause, the Court stated, "Congress did not discuss what was meant by the term 'fines,' or whether the prohibition had any application in the civil context." 492 U.S. 257, 264–65. The Court further observed: "Bail, fines, and punishment traditionally have been associated with the criminal process, and by subjecting the three to parallel limitations the text of the Amendment suggests an intention to limit the power of those entrusted with the criminal-law function of government." *Id.* at 263 (quoting Ingraham v. Wright, 430 U.S. 651, 644 (1977)); *but see* Austin, 509 U.S. at 608, (observing that "some provisions of the Bill of Rights are expressly limited to criminal casesThe text of the Eighth Amendment includes no similar limitation. Nor does the history of the Eighth Amendment require such a limitation)." The Supreme Court recently denied a petition for certiorari in a case in which the Fourth Circuit decided that a civil tax penalty imposed by the IRS was not an excessive fine. *See* Toth v. United States, 143 S. Ct. 552 (2023). Justice Gorsuch filed a dissenting opinion in which he noted "taking up this case would have been well worth our time." *Id.* at 553 (Gorsuch, J., dissenting).

[101] *Austin*, 509 U.S. at 610.

[102] *Austin*, 509 U.S. 619. It is unclear whether the Court would consider a civil tax imposed by the Internal Revenue Code to be a "fine" for purposes of applying the Excessive Fines Clause. In 2016, the United States Bankruptcy Court for the Northern District of Texas observed, "The parties have not cited, nor has the Court located through its own research,

If a fine can properly be characterized as punishment so as to fall within the purview of the Excessive Fines Clause, the Court has next analyzed whether the fine is excessive.[103] In 1998, the Court decided *United States v. Bajakajian*, which addressed whether a civil forfeiture of cash constituted a punishment, and whether the punishment was considered "excessive" for purposes of the Eighth Amendment.[104] The case was brought by a family attempting to smuggle cash onto an international flight in violation of federal law; the government sought full forfeiture of the money.[105] Justice Thomas, writing for a five-Justice majority, held that under the Eighth Amendment, a fine is unconstitutional when its amount is grossly disproportionate to the gravity of the conduct it was designed to discourage.[106] Observing that the amendment's text and history provided few insights as to the level of disproportionality required, the Court undertook a fact- specific inquiry to compare the amount of the forfeiture against the gravity of the offense.[107] The majority held that forfeiture of the entire amount would violate the Excessive Fines Clause, reasoning that the harm caused was minimal as the crime underlying the forfeiture was a failure to report the transfer of money, not the transfer itself.[108] Additionally, "the money was the proceeds of legal activity," and the family did not fit the "class of persons for whom the statute was principally designed" (i.e., tax evaders and money launderers).[109]

A court reviewing the plaintiffs' Eighth Amendment claim would likely need to decide whether the IRA's excise tax constitutes a punishment. To do

---

a single case that holds that a tax penalty is a fine under the Excessive Fines Clause, let alone an excessive fine. In sum, those courts that have been faced with the dilemma of how to apply an Excessive Fines Clause analysis to civil tax penalties have all arrived at largely the same answer—i.e., civil tax penalties … are not fines, and therefore the Excessive Fines Clause is not applicable to them." *In re Wyly*, 552 B.R. 338, 613 (Bankr. N.D. Tex. 2016). The Court has not addressed whether the reasoning from *Wyly* would extend to civil tax penalties in the Internal Revenue Code.

[103] Bajakajian, 524 U.S. at 334.

[104] *Id.* at 328, 334.

[105] *Id.* at 325.

[106] *Id.* Justice Kennedy authored a strongly worded dissent that was joined by Chief Justice Roberts, Justice O'Connor, and Justice Scalia. Justice Kennedy argued, "For the first time in its history, the Court strikes down a fine as excessive under the Eighth Amendment. The decision is disturbing both for its specific holding and for the broader upheaval it foreshadows. At issue is a fine Congress fixed in the amount of the currency respondent sought to smuggle without reporting. If a fine calibrated with this accuracy fails the Court's test, its decision portends serious disruption of a vast range of statutory fines." *Id.* at 344 (Kennedy, J., dissenting).

[107] *Id.* at 336–37.

[108] *Id.* at 337, 339.

[109] *Id.* at 338.

this, a court might ask what Congress intended by enacting the tax, and whether the tax was designed to "punish" manufacturers of selected drugs who did not wish to participate in the program, or who did not comply with its requirements. Because the IRA was enacted as a budget reconciliation measure, the bill progressed through Congress outside of the formal committee process, resulting in a more limited legislative history. It is not clear how a court would proceed in light of this limitation.[110]

If a court reviewing the plaintiffs' claims were to find that the excise tax constitutes a punishment for purposes of the Eighth Amendment, it might next assess whether the tax is excessive. If the court were to look to Justice Thomas' decision in Bajakajian, it would ask whether the excise tax is grossly disproportionate to the conduct it was designed to prevent—in other words, whether the IRA's excise tax is disproportionate to drug manufacturers' actions of charging Medicare higher prices. It might be difficult for a court to undertake this balancing test without additional facts, such as the amount of the negotiated MFP.

The Nondelegation Doctrine Claim

Article I, Section I of the Constitution, known as the Vesting Clause, states, "All legislative Powers herein granted shall be vested in a Congress of the United States, which shall consist of a Senate and House of Representatives."[111] In interpreting these words, the Supreme Court has created what is known as the Nondelegation Doctrine, which is the principle that "Congress cannot transfer … powers which are strictly and exclusively legislative" to another branch of government.[112] All delegations to federal

---

[110] In debating legislative language similar to the IRA, Rep. Shalala argued that Americans "pay more for our prescription drugs than any other country on Earth," but that many Americans "can't afford to benefit" from the scientific advances that have led to the development of lifesaving medications. 165 CONG. REC. H10034 (Dec. 11, 2019) (statement of Rep. Donna Shalala). On the other hand, Rep. Burgess argued that the bill "claims to negotiate drug prices, but with a 95 percent excise tax for manufacturers who fail to reach a price agreement with the government, it is more akin to a hostage taking and then shooting the hostage." *Id.* at H10036 (statement of Rep. Michael Burgess). It is unclear whether and to what extent a court might find the legislative history of predecessor bills persuasive in considering whether the excise tax is designed as a punishment.

[111] U.S. CONST. art. I, § 1.

[112] Gundy v. United States, 139 S. Ct. 2116, 2123 (2019). *See also* Mistretta v. United States, 488 U.S. 361, 371 (1989) ("The nondelegation doctrine is rooted in the principle of separation of powers that underlies our tripartite system of government."). For an overview of the

agencies must, therefore, be accompanied by an "intelligible principle" that both constrains and guides the agency in its implementation of the law.[113] The trade association plaintiffs argue that the IRA runs afoul of the Nondelegation Doctrine because "Congress delegated unfettered discretion to HHS to set prices however it wishes."[114] Similarly, a manufacturer argues, "Congress has impermissibly delegated sweeping authority to implement price controls without providing a clear standard to guide the agency's discretion …."[115] The trade association plaintiffs contrast the Medicare Drug Price Negotiation Program with other price-setting programs, such as the regulation of natural gas companies, which the plaintiffs argue are implemented with satisfactory procedural safeguards, including notice-and-comment rulemaking and the opportunity for judicial review.[116]

The plaintiffs specifically argue that the IRA's delegation of authority to the Secretary lacks an intelligible principle.[117] As an example, they point to the factors the Secretary is to consider in developing the MFP, which they purport "provide[] no guidance whatsoever about how the agency should weigh those factors."[118] They argue the program is further unlawful because it establishes only a ceiling price which the MFP cannot exceed, while simultaneously directing HHS to "achieve the lowest [MFP] for each selected drug."[119] The plaintiffs describe the program as "unique and unprecedented,"

Nondelegation Doctrine, *see* CONG. RESEARCH SERV., *Art. I, S.1.5.1 Overview of Nondelegation Doctrine*, Constitution Annotated, available at https://constitution.congress.gov/browse/essay/artI-S1-5-1/ALDE_00000014/#ALDF_00016513 (last accessed July 26, 2023). For more information on the Nondelegation doctrine and its history, *see* CONG. RESEARCH SERV., *Art. I, S.1.5.2 Historical Background on Nondelegation Doctrine*, Constitution Annotated, available at https://constitution.congress.gov/browse/essay/artI-S1-5-2/ALDE_00000009/(last accessed July 26, 2023).

113 *Mistretta,* 488 U.S. at 372 ("Applying this 'intelligible principle' test to congressional delegations, our jurisprudence has been driven by a practical understanding that in our increasingly complex society, replete with ever changing and more technical problems, Congress simply cannot do its job absent an ability to delegate power under broad general directives.") *Id.* In *Mistretta*, the Court further observed that "no statute can be entirely precise," and that as a result, "some judgements involving policy considerations[] must be left to the officers executing the law and to the judges applying it." *Id.* at 415. *See also* J.W. Hampton, Jr., & Co. v. U.S., 276 U.S. 394, 409 (1928) ("If Congress shall lay down by legislative act an intelligible principle to which the person or body authorized [] is directed to conform, such legislative action is not a forbidden delegation of legislative power.").

114 PhRMA Compl. at 31; *see also* Boehringer Compl. at 6.

115 Boehringer Compl. at 6.

116 *Id. referencing* 15 U.S.C. §§ 717c, 717r (regulation of natural gas companies); 16 U.S.C. §§ 824d, 824e (regulation of electric utilities); 39 U.S.C. § 3622 (regulation of mail products).

117 *Id.* at 30.

118 *Id.*

119 Chamber of Com, Compl. at 43.

claiming that "[d]espite the IRA's breathtaking delegation of power to HHS, the statute lacks both the requisite "intelligible principle" and the constitutional safeguards necessary to ensure accountability, rationality, and fairness" in price setting.[120]

Although Congress may not simply give away its legislative powers, the Supreme Court has recognized that Congress needs "flexibility and practicality . . . to perform its functions," and that it "may confer substantial discretion on executive agencies to implement and enforce the laws."[121] As a result, the Court has generally used the rather lenient intelligible principle test to uphold delegations.[122] In fact, the Court has not held a statute unconstitutional on the basis that Congress impermissibly delegated authority to another branch of government since 1935, when it decided *A.L.A. Schechter Poultry Corp. v. U.S.* and *Panama Refining Co. v. Ryan.*[123]

The *Schechter Poultry* and *Panama Refining* cases arose in the context of the Great Depression when Congress delegated authority to the executive branch to regulate various economic activities, including allowing the President to prohibit the interstate transport of excess petroleum.[124] In finding a violation of the Nondelegation Doctrine, the *Panama Refining* Court

---

[120] *Id.* at 36.

[121] Gundy v. United States, 139 S. Ct. 2116, 2123 (2019) (plurality opinion) (Gorsuch, J., dissenting) (cleaned up)).

[122] Although the nondelegation doctrine has generally been used to uphold congressional delegations under the intelligible principle test, Justices Gorsuch, Roberts, and Thomas have indicated that it may be time for the Court to revisit the doctrine. *Gundy* 139 S. Ct. at 2131 (2019). At least when it comes to delegations that allow for a noncongressional entity to directly restrict an individual's liberty, these three Justices seem to call for a new nondelegation doctrine standard. *See Id.* at 2134. Justice Gorsuch remarked, "[I]t's undeniable that the 'intelligible principle' remark [in *J.W. Hampton*] eventually began to take on a life of its own. We sometimes chide people for treating judicial opinions as if they were statutes, divorcing a passing comment from its context, ignoring all that came before and after, and treating an isolated phrase as if it were controlling. But that seems to be exactly what happened here." *Id.* at 2139.

[123] A.L.A. Schechter Poultry Corp. v. United States, 295 U.S. 495 (1935) and Panama Refining Co. v. Ryan, 293 U.S. 388 (1935). For more information about the history of the nondelegation doctrine, *see* CONG. RESEARCH SERV., *Art. I, S.1.5.3 Origin of Intelligible Principle Standard*, Constitution Annotated, available at https://constitution.congress.gov/browse/essay/artI-S1-5-3/ALDE_00001317/ (last accessed July 26, 2023).

[124] *Schechter*, 295 U.S. at 526; *Panama Refining*, 293 U.S. at 433. The Court distinguished *Schechter* from *Panama Refining* by observing that the issue in *Schechter* was whether Congress had given adequate definition to the "codes of fair competition" under the National Industry Recovery Act, such that the President could interpret that term. *Schechter*, 295 U.S. at 530–31. *Panama Refining*, on the other hand, concerned the "range of discretion given to the President" to prohibit the interstate and foreign commerce transportation of petroleum. *Id.* at 530.

observed, "Congress did not declare in what circumstances that transportation [of petroleum] should be forbidden Congress left the matter to the President without standard or rule, to be dealt with as he pleased."[125] For these reasons, the Court said, even though the President was acting on behalf of the public interest in hopes of spurring the economy and easing the impact of the Great Depression, Congress violated the Nondelegation Doctrine by ceding its legislative function to the executive branch without sufficient guidance.[126]

A court evaluating the plaintiffs' Nondelegation Doctrine challenge in the Medicare Drug Price Negotiation Program litigation would likely turn to the intelligible principle test to determine whether Congress provided CMS with enough legislative direction to implement the program in accordance with its vision. In doing so, a court might look at 42 U.S.C. § 1320f-3, the section of the statute outlining the process for CMS to develop an initial offer for the MFP. The statute calls for CMS to "develop and use a consistent methodology and process" for the price negotiation, in order to "achieve the lowest maximum fair prices for each selected drug."[127] It goes on to list various factors that the Secretary "shall consider" when developing an initial offer.[128] The statute does not dictate how much weight the Secretary should give each factor or otherwise rank their importance. A court reviewing the plaintiffs' Nondelegation Doctrine challenge could evaluate whether these provisions contain enough of an intelligible principle with sufficient "standard[s] or rule[s]" to guide CMS through the negotiation process. The plaintiffs would have the burden of showing why the standards in the IRA differ from other delegations previously upheld by the Court.

---

125 *Panama Refining*, 293 U.S. at 419. The Court also observed that "[t]he President was not required to ascertain and proclaim the conditions prevailing in the industry which made the prohibition [on transporting petroleum] necessary." *Id.* at 418.

126 *Id.* at 430. The Court observed: "When, therefore, such an administrative agency is required as a condition precedent to an order, to make a finding of facts, the validity of the order must rest upon the needed finding. If it is lacking, the order is ineffective." *Id.* at 433.

127 42 U.S.C. § 1320f-3(b)(1).

128 42 U.S.C. § 1320f-3(c)-(e). The factors are based both on data submitted by manufacturers—demonstrating facts such as research, development, and production costs, federal financial support the manufacturer received, and patent and regulatory exclusivity information—as well as evidence of alternative treatments, including therapeutic alternatives to the drug, as well as their cost and availability. *Id.* at (e)(1)-(2).

Spending Clause Arguments

Article I, Section 8, Clause 1 of the Constitution, known as the "Spending Clause," provides, "The Congress shall have Power To lay and collect Taxes, Duties, Imposts, and Excises, to pay Debts and provide for the common Defence and general Welfare of the United States."[129] The pharmaceutical manufacturer plaintiffs argue that Congress's power under the Spending Clause cannot justify the IRA's regulatory scheme.[130] First, the plaintiffs assert that the IRA is not a valid spending condition, because it does not condition federal Medicare reimbursement on a manufacturer's compliance with the terms of the statute.[131] Instead, one plaintiff alleges, the IRA "commands manufacturers to comply and levies monetary penalties for failure to do so."[132] Another plaintiff argues that the IRA "unconstitutionally conditions participation in Medicare" on its "relinquishment" of its constitutional rights.[133]

Another manufacturer further argues that even if Congress created a funding condition in the IRA, the statute does not provide "clear notice" of the condition.[134] According to one plaintiff, "there is no offer . . . to accept," and thus the "choice" to comply with the statute and participate in the Medicare program is "illusory," because due to the structure of the tax, manufacturers may gain relief only by completely extricating themselves from Medicare.[135]

---

129 U.S. CONST. art. I, § 8.

130 Bristol Myers Compl. at 24; Merck Compl at 22; Janssen Compl. at 6; Boehringer Compl. at 42.

131 Bristol Myers Compl. at 24–25; Merck Compl. at 21.

132 Bristol Myers Compl. at 24; Merck Compl. at 21. The monetary penalties to which the manufacturers refer are the law's excise tax, which is based on a percentage of the selected drug's total revenue, not just its Medicare revenue. *See* 26 U.S.C. §5000D.

133 Boehringer Compl. at 42.

134 *See* Bristol Myers Compl. at 24 ("Here, the IRA does not set forth conditions on Medicare or Medicaid reimbursement, or provide for exclusion from those benefit programs if a manufacturer does not cooperate. [The IRA's] indirect, convoluted scheme does not "unambiguously" condition a manufacturer's receipt of federal funding on its acceptance of the IRA's mandates.") *Id.*

135 Merck Compl. at 21; *see also* 26 U.S.C. § 5000D(b). The manufacturers point out that in order to withdraw from participation in these programs, federal law requires them to give notice of their decision to terminate, and the IRA "delays [their] ability to terminate … for between 11 and 23 months." Merck Compl. at 24 (citing 42 U.S.C. § 1395w- 114a(b)(4)(B)(ii)) (regarding the allowable duration of Medicare Coverage Gap Discount Program agreements and a manufacturer's right to terminate such an agreement). In effect, the manufacturers argue that they would have had to withdraw from Medicare and Medicaid by January 2022, before the IRA was even enacted, to avoid the excise taxes. Bristol Myers Compl. at 24. As one plaintiff summarizes the issue: "In short, once a manufacturer is sucked into the IRA's vortex of forced below-market sales, it has at its disposal no

Another manufacturer claims the statute is "unconstitutionally coercive because it leverages vast, unrelated benefits to induce distinct transactions that the Government wants."[136] Another manufacturer argues that because manufacturers can only "escape" the program by "withdrawing *all* . . . products from Medicare and Medicaid—not just the drug selected for the Program," this amounts to a "gun to the head."[137]Additionally, the plaintiffs state that the IRA unlawfully conditions receipt of their Medicare reimbursement payments on the "abandonment of their First and Fifth Amendment rights," in violation of the doctrine of unconstitutional conditions.[138]

The Supreme Court has interpreted the Spending Clause to allow Congress "wide latitude" in attaching conditions to federal funding while simultaneously recognizing four main constitutional restrictions on such conditions.[139] First, Congress must articulate clear notice of the funding condition.[140] In *Pennhurst State School and Hospital v. Halderman*, for example, the Court observed, "The legitimacy of Congress' power to legislate under the spending power thus rests on whether the state voluntarily and knowingly accepts the terms of the 'contract.'"[141] The Court held that

---

evidenced means of escape." Merck Compl. at 12. In its Revised Guidance, CMS has attempted to resolve this issue by allowing for an expedited termination of Medicare participation for manufacturers of selected drugs who do not wish to participate in negotiations. *See* CMS REVISED GUIDANCE at 120-21.

[136] Merck Compl. at 23.

[137] Janssen Compl. at 4.

[138] Bristol Myers Compl. at 25; Janssen Compl at 6.

[139] South Dakota v. Dole, 483 U.S. 203, 206 (1987) ("Incident to this [spending] power, Congress may attach conditions on the receipt of federal funds, and has repeatedly employed the power 'to further broad policy objectives by conditioning receipt of federal moneys upon compliance by the recipient with federal statutory and administrative directives.'" (quoting Fullilove v. Klutznick, 448 U.S. 448, 474 (1980)).

[140] *See generally*, CONG. RESEARCH SERVICE, *Art. I S.8.C1.2.1 Overview of Spending Clause*, Constitution Annotated, available at https://constitution.congress.gov/browse/essay/artI-S8-C1-2-1/ALDE_00013356/ (last accessed July 10, 2023); CRS Report R46827, *Funding Conditions: Constitutional Limits on Congress's Spending Power*, by Victoria L. Killion (July 1, 2021).

[141] 451 U.S. 1, 13, 17 (1984). The federal statute at issue created "a federal-state grant program" wherein the federal government provided financial assistance to participating states to create programs to care for the developmentally disabled. *Id.* at 1. States' participation in the program was voluntary; to receive federal funding, states were required to comply with various provisions in the bill. *Id.* A resident of Pennhurst State School and Hospital, a facility that provided care to the developmentally disabled, brought a class action challenging the facility's "inhumane" conditions and asserting patients' rights under the Federal Constitution and the "bill of rights" provisions of the statute authorizing the grant program. *Id.* at 2. Congress created explicit funding conditions in other sections of the statute, which outlined "procedures and sanctions to ensure state compliance with its

Congress must impose funding conditions "unambiguously," so that States could "exercise their choice knowingly, cognizant of the consequences of their participation," and that there could be "no knowing acceptance if a State is unaware of the conditions."[142]

Other limitations that the Court has placed on Congress's power under the Spending Clause include whether the condition is related to the underlying purpose of the spending; whether the condition is unconstitutionally coercive; and whether the condition can be characterized as an "unconstitutional condition."[143] In *South Dakota v. Dole*, the Court observed that "conditions on federal grants might be illegitimate if they are unrelated to the federal interest in particular … programs."[144] In *Dole*, for example, the Court found that conditioning the receipt of federal highway funds on states adopting a minimum drinking age was sufficiently related to the federal interest in "safe interstate travel."[145]

Although Congress may condition federal funding, "in some circumstances the financial inducement offered by Congress might be so coercive as to pass the point at which 'pressure turns into compulsion,'" in violation of federalism principles.[146] In *NFIB v. Sebelius*, the Court invalidated a section of the Patient Protection and Affordable Care Act (ACA) that withheld all federal Medicaid funding from states that did not expand their Medicaid programs in accordance with the law on the basis that such changes violated the anticoercion principle described in *Dole*.[147] The Court characterized the ACA's changes to the Medicaid program as "dramatic[],"

---

requirements." *Id.* at 12. In determining whether the Bill of Rights provisions constituted a condition, the Court likened the funding conditions to a contract, wherein the federal government is offering federal funds in exchange for the state's compliance with a condition on how the funds can be used or on the state's adoption of a particular policy. *Id.* at 17. Although *Pennhurst* addresses funding conditions in the context of states, its reasoning has been applied to funding conditions that Congress places on private entities receiving federal funding as well. *See, e.g.*, Gonzaga Univ. v. Doe, 536 U.S. 273 (2002).

142 *Pennhurst*, 451 U.S. at 17.

143 South Dakota v. Dole, 483 U.S. 203, 207–08 (1987). For more detailed information about the restrictions the Court has placed on Congress's ability to place conditions on the receipt of federal funding, *see* CONG. RESEARCH SERVICE, *Art. I S.8.C1.2.1 Overview of Spending Clause*, Constitution Annotated, available at https://constitution.congress.gov/browse/essay/artI-S8-C1-2-1/ALDE_00013356/ (last accessed July 10, 2023); and CRS Report R46827, *Funding Conditions: Constitutional Limits on Congress's Spending Power*, by Victoria L. Killion (July 1, 2021).

144 *Dole*, 483 U.S. 203, 207 (1987).

145 *Id.* at 208. ("Indeed, the condition imposed by Congress is directly related to one of the main purposes for which highway funds are expended–safe interstate travel.") *Id.*

146 *Id.* at 211 (*quoting* Steward Machine Co. v. Davis, 310 U.S. 548, 590 (1937)).

147 National Federation of Independent Business (NFIB) v. Sebelius, 567 U.S. 519 (2012).

because if a state opted not to comply with the statute, it would "lose not merely 'a relatively small percentage' of its existing Medicaid funding, but *all* of it."[148] The Court reasoned that the Medicaid expansion essentially created a "new program," and that "Congress is not free to … penalize States that choose not to participate in that new program by taking away their existing Medicaid funding."[149]

Finally, the Court has held that Congress may not use its Spending Clause power to "induce the States to engage in activities that would themselves be unconstitutional."[150] Under this "independent constitutional bar" principle, for example, a condition that would require states to violate the First Amendment rights of their citizens would be an unconstitutional spending condition.[151]

Congress may condition funds to both governmental (e.g., states or federal agencies) and nongovernmental (e.g., private businesses) recipients.[152] Whether each of the Spending Clause limits discussed above applies to conditions on private entities, however, is unsettled. Although the Supreme Court has applied the clear notice principle in a case involving a private funding recipient,[153] it has not ruled on whether the relatedness or anticoercion limitations—which are rooted in federalism concerns—also apply to conditions on funding to private entities, such as drug manufacturers.[154]

In the Medicare Drug Price Negotiation Program litigation, a court analyzing whether Congress exceeded its power under the Spending Clause would likely need to address the threshold question of whether Congress

---

[148] *Id.* at 575, 581.

[149] *Id.* at 587.

[150] *Dole*, 483 U.S. 210. This principle has come to be known as the "unconstitutional conditions" doctrine. The Fifth Circuit has described the doctrine as examining "the extent to which government benefits may be conditioned or distributed in ways that burden constitutional rights or principles." Pace v. Bagalusa City Sch. Bd., 403 F.3d 286 (5th Cir. 2005) (en banc).

[151] *See* discussion of First Amendment Claims, *supra* p. 2.

[152] *See, e.g. Dole*, 482 U.S. 203; Gonzaga Univ. v. Doe, 536 U.S. 273 (2002). The plaintiffs' complaints do not address whether the Court's limitations on constitutional conditions apply equally to private entities and the states.

[153] *Gonzaga Univ.*, 536 U.S. 273.

[154] *See* Northport Health Servs. v. HHS, 438 F. Supp. 3d 956, 970–71 (W.D. Ark. 2020) ("No part of the Court's decision in *NFIB* touched on the government's power to place conditions on private entities. In fact, Courts of Appeals have held time and time again that the participation of private entities in Medicare and Medicaid is always voluntary, and providers can avoid regulations to which they object by choosing not to participate in Medicare or Medicaid."), *aff'd on other grounds*, 14 F.4th 856 (8th Cir. 2021). For more information on the distinctions between private and governmental entities with respect to the constitutional limitations on Congress's power under the Spending Clause, *see* CRS Report R46827, *Funding Conditions: Constitutional Limits on Congress's Spending Power*, by Victoria L. Killion (July 1, 2021).

actually conditioned Medicare reimbursement on the manufacturer of a selected drug's participation in the program. In so doing, a court might look at whether the IRA creates an "unambiguous" condition on Medicare spending, and if drug manufacturers could be said to "voluntarily and knowingly" accept the terms of the IRA when choosing to participate in Medicare. If a court were to find that Congress conditioned Medicare reimbursement on participation in the program, it could look at whether the condition was related to the purpose of the reimbursement for the manufacturer's products and whether the manufacturers are being coerced into participation as a result of the IRA's excise tax and other noncompliance penalties. However, it is unclear whether a court would find all of these factors applicable to a drug manufacturer, which is a private entity, as much of the Spending Clause doctrine has been built around the relationship between Congress and the states.

Concluding Considerations

A number of studies have shown that the United States spends more per capita on retail prescription drugs than other developed countries. For example, using 2019 data, the Organization for Economic Cooperation and Development (OECD) found that the average prescription drug spending per capita in the United States was more than double the average across other OECD countries.[155] The Congressional Budget Office (CBO) estimated that the Medicare Drug Price Negotiation Program would lower the federal budget deficit by $25 billion and that by 2031, Part D prices would be 8% lower, and Part B prices 9% lower, as a result of the negotiations.[156]

Although the program may result in a deficit reduction, some stakeholders have contended that the IRA will negatively affect future drug research and development by stifling innovation.[157] Some manufacturers have claimed that

---

155 Pharmaceutical Expenditure, ORGANISATION FOR ECONOMIC COOPERATION AND DEVELOPMENT, https://www.oecd-ilibrary.org/sites/2493ee95-en/index.html?itemId=/content/component/2493ee95-en#indicator-d1e13542 (last accessed Sept. 5, 2023). The OECD data are for retail prescription drugs and over-the-counter products. *Id.*

156 How CBO Estimated the Budgetary Impact of Key Prescription Drug Provisions in the 2022 Reconciliation Act at 5, 19, CONGRESSIONAL BUDGET OFFICE (Feb. 2023), https://www.cbo.gov/system/files/2023-02/58850-IRA-Drug- Provs.pdf. *See also* Michael Erman et al., *Bristol Myers, Pfizer, AbbVie Drugs Likely to Face U.S. Price Negotiation*, REUTERS (Mar. 13, 2023), https://www.reuters.com/business/healthcare-pharmaceuticals/bristol-myers-pfizer-abbvie- drugs-likely-face-us-price-negotiation-2023-03-13/.

157 Daniel Gilbert, *As Drugmakers Slam Medicare Price Controls, Wall Street Shrugs*, WASH. POST (Aug. 29, 2023) https://www.washingtonpost.com/business/2023/08/29/medicare-

it will incentivize pharmaceutical companies to delay research for drugs used to treat smaller patient populations.[158] In a September 2022 cost estimate for the IRA, the CBO estimated that "the number of drugs that would be introduced to the U.S. market would be reduced by about [one] over the next 2023-2032 period," and "about [five] over the subsequent decade, and about [seven] over the decade after that."[159] It may take years for the U.S. drug market to realize the full effects of the legislation, as more and more drugs will be subject to negotiation in the future. For example, 10 drugs were selected for negotiation in price year 2026, 15 drugs will be selected for each of price years 2027 and 2028, and 20 drugs will be selected in 2029 and every year thereafter.[160] Additionally, for the first two years of the program, CMS will only select Part D drugs; Part B drugs will not become eligible for negotiation until price year 2028.[161]

Litigation over the program is ongoing, and additional cases with similar or new allegations may follow. Some stakeholders have characterized the lawsuits as a "legal crusade" that is being "strategically designed to reach the U.S. Supreme Court," while some legal scholars have characterized the litigation as an "uphill climb[]."[162] At the time of this writing, several plaintiffs and the government have filed or expressed their intention to file motions for summary judgment, which could speed up judicial consideration.[163] Additionally, at least one plaintiff has filed a motion for a preliminary injunction, seeking to immediately halt CMS's implementation of the program altogether on the basis that the program violates due process under long-standing Sixth Circuit precedent.[164]

---

drug-price-pharma-companies-stock/?utm_campaign=wp_the7&utm_medium=email&utm_source=newsletter&wpisrc=nl_the7.

158 Rachel Cohrs, *Genentech Weighs Slow-Walking Ovarian Cancer Therapy to Make More Money Under Drug Price Reform*, STAT+ (Aug. 10, 2023), https://www.statnews.com/2023/08/10/genentech-drug-price-cancer/.

159 Summary Estimated Budgetary Effects of Public Law 117-169 at 15, CONGRESSIONAL BUDGET OFFICE (Sept. 7, 2022), https://www.cbo.gov/system/files/2022-09/PL117-169_9-7-22.pdf. CBO stated that "[t]he amounts in this estimate are in the middle of the distribution of possible outcomes, by CBO's assessment, and they are subject to uncertainty." *Id.*

160 42 U.S.C. § 1320f-1(a)(1)-(4).

161 42 U.S.C. § 1320f-1(d)(1)(A).

162 Ian Lopez, *Drugmakers Prep Medicare Pricing Suits for March to High Court*, BLOOMBERG LAW (Aug. 17, 2023).

163 *See, e.g.*, Order, Merck & Co. v. Becerra, No. 23-1616 (D.D.C. Jun. 28, 2023), ECF No. 14.

164 Memorandum in Support of Motion for Preliminary Injunction, U.S. Chamber of Commerce, et al. v. Becerra, No. 23-0156 (S.D. Ohio, Jun. 9, 2023) ECF No. 29.

While the litigation proceeds, CMS's Revised Guidance attempts to address several stakeholder concerns, some of which could affect the litigation.[165] For example, the guidance attempts to clarify CMS's consideration of the negotiation factors for the establishment of the MFP, which drug manufacturers and others have claimed are overly broad and do not specify the weight the Secretary will assign to each factor.[166] The agency's Revised Guidance also responded to the more than 7,500 comments it received after the release of the Initial Guidance in March 2023.[167] Through the Revised Guidance, CMS also advises that it intends to create additional "patient-focused listening sessions" to enable both the public as well as drug companies "to engage with CMS during the negotiation process."[168]

The fate of the program may depend in part on how courts resolve the various claims made by the parties. Courts could decide to uphold the entire statute, uphold parts of it while striking down others, or declare the entire statute unconstitutional. Absent additional action from Congress, the outcome of the litigation may have a substantial impact on how effectively CMS will be able to carry out the program and uphold its stated goals of lowering prescription drug prices for Medicare beneficiaries.

---

165 *See generally*, CMS REVISED GUIDANCE, *supra* note 8.

166 *Id.* at 46–50; *see also* Chamber of Com. Compl. at 37.

167 CMS Released Revised Guidance for Historic Medicare Drug Price Negotiation Program (Jun. 30, 2023), https://www.cms.gov/newsroom/press-releases/cms-releases-revised-guidance-historic-medicare-drug-price- negotiation-program.

168 *Id.*

Chapter 3

Administrative Procedure Act Challenges to CMS's Implementation of the Medicare Drug Price Negotiation Program*

Hannah-Alise Rogers

Congress created the Medicare Drug Price Negotiation Program (the program) in 2022 through a budget reconciliation measure known as the Inflation Reduction Act (IRA). The IRA authorizes the Secretary of the Department of Health and Human Services (HHS) to negotiate the prices of certain single-source drugs and biological products under Medicare Part B (physician administered drugs) and Medicare Part D (retail prescription drugs). The IRA directed the HHS Centers for Medicare and Medicaid Services (CMS) to implement the first three years of the program (known as price years 2026-2028) through "program instruction or other forms of program guidance." For the initial price years 2026 and 2027, only Medicare Part D drugs are eligible for selection; Part B drugs become eligible for selection in price year 2028.

The IRA requires HHS to publish a list of selected drugs, enter into agreements with manufacturers of the drugs selected for negotiation, negotiate a maximum fair price (MFP) for those drugs with manufacturers, and monitor manufacturer compliance with program requirements. CMS began implementing the program by issuing Initial Guidance in March 2023, which was subsequently updated in Revised Guidance in June 2023. In accordance with the statute, CMS selected the first 10 drugs for price negotiation on August 29, 2023, including AstraZeneca's drug Farxiga and Novo Nordisk's Fiasp and NovoLog products.

---

* This is an edited, reformatted and augmented version of Congressional Research Service Publication No. LSB11112, dated January 31, 2024.

In: Medicare's Prescription Drug Pricing
Editor: Lloyd M. Porter
ISBN: 979-8-89530-728-1

Beginning in June 2023, several pharmaceutical manufacturers, including AstraZeneca and Novo Nordisk, as well as pharmaceutical trade associations, sued CMS in various federal district courts across the country. At least nine lawsuits have challenged the constitutionality of the program on various grounds, including under the First, Fifth, and Eighth Amendments. In addition to these and other constitutional arguments, AstraZeneca and Novo Nordisk also claim that CMS's implementation of the program violates the Administrative Procedure Act (APA).

This Sidebar explains the APA arguments made in AstraZeneca and Novo Nordisk's cases. (For more information on the constitutional claims, see CRS Report R47682, Constitutional Challenges to the Medicare Drug Price Negotiation Program.) In both cases, the pharmaceutical companies and the government have filed cross motions for summary judgment. In AstraZeneca's case, the Delaware district court heard oral argument on the parties' cross motions for summary judgment on January 31, 2024, but has not yet issued a decision. In Novo Nordisk's case, the parties are scheduled to file briefs for their motions for summary judgment through the end of March 2024.

Legal Background

The APA is a federal statute that permits judicial review of "agency action[s] made reviewable by statute," as well as "final agency action for which there is no other adequate remedy in a court." The APA directs reviewing courts to "hold unlawful and set aside agency action, findings, and conclusions," when they are "arbitrary, capricious, an abuse of discretion, or otherwise not in accordance with law." Additionally, agency actions that are characterized as "ultra vires" may also be reviewed under the APA. In an ultra vires action, even a statute that precludes judicial review of an agency's determinations may be reviewed by a court if the agency's action can be characterized as violating an unambiguous statutory mandate.

Defining a Qualifying Single Source Drug

Before selecting the first 10 drugs for negotiation, the Secretary of HHS identified the pool of "qualifying single source drugs" (QSSD) in accordance with the statute. For price year 2026, for a small molecule drug to be a QSSD, it had to be a Medicare Part D drug that (1) was approved by the U.S. Food and Drug Administration (FDA) and marketed pursuant to such approval, (2) had been FDA-approved for at least seven years, and (3) did not have an approved and marketed generic version. For a biologic to be a QSSD, the product had to be a Medicare Part D drug that (1) was licensed under the Public Health Service Act (PHSA) and was marketed under the license, (2) had been licensed for at least 11 years, and (3) did not have a licensed and marketed biosimilar.

After CMS identified the QSSDs, it calculated the Medicare program's total Part D expenditures for each QSSD by looking at Part D prescription drug cost and payment (PDE) data between June 1, 2022, and May 31, 2023. The 50 drugs with the highest expenditures were considered "negotiation-eligible drugs."

In determining if a QSSD meets the definition of a negotiation-eligible drug, the IRA directed CMS to "use data that is aggregated across dosage forms and strengths of the drug, including new formulations of the drug . . . and not based on the specific formulation or package size of the drug." After applying any relevant statutory exceptions, CMS then selected the top 10 highest-spend Medicare drugs for negotiation. (For more specific information on how drugs are selected, see CRS Report R47555, *Implementation of the Medicare Drug Price Negotiation Program: Centers for Medicare and Medicaid Guidance and Legal Considerations*.)

In its Initial Guidance, CMS stated it would apply the data aggregation provision discussed above to the definition of what it considered a single QSSD. CMS stated that "all dosage forms and strengths of the drug with the same active moiety and the same holder of a New Drug Application (NDA)," even if the products are marketed under different NDAs, would be treated as one drug for QSSD determinations.

Similarly, CMS said that all dosage forms and strengths of a biologic "with the same active ingredient and the same holder of a Biologics License Application (BLA)," even if the products are marketed under different BLAs, would be considered the same QSSD. CMS received a variety of stakeholder comments in response to this Initial Guidance, which it addressed in the Revised Guidance. In that guidance, CMS defended its decision to define QSSD so that multiple products with the same active ingredient could be selected as a single QSSD, stating that "the aggregation rules under [the IRA] are clear." While some stakeholders suggested that a QSSD should be defined based on each distinct NDA or BLA, CMS responded that such an approach would be "inconsistent" with the statute.

Bona Fide Marketing of a Product

As described above, the IRA's definition of QSSD is limited to small molecule drugs and biologics with no generic or biosimilar versions on the market. Thus, if a product has approved and marketed generic or biosimilar competition, it will not qualify as a QSSD for purposes of selection for price negotiation. In its Initial Guidance, CMS stated that it will consider a competing generic drug or biosimilar to be marketed "when the[] data reveal that the manufacturer . . . has engaged in bona fide marketing of that drug or product." CMS advised that the agency "intends to monitor whether robust and meaningful competition exists in the market." In responding to stakeholder comments about the "bona fide marketing" requirement, CMS noted in its Revised Guidance that "Congress contemplated that a generic or biosimilar must have a continuing presence on the market in order to affect CMS's determination whether a drug should be selected" as a QSSD.

Drug Manufacturers' Motions for Summary Judgment

AstraZeneca's Arguments

Both AstraZeneca and Novo Nordisk have challenged CMS's definition of QSSD and the bona fide marketing requirement under the APA. In its motion for summary judgment, AstraZeneca argues that CMS's QSSD definition and the bona fide marketing requirement violate the plain language of the IRA and are arbitrary and capricious under the APA. The drugmaker claims that multiple drug products can be the same QSSD "*only* where the . . . products were approved by the FDA under the same NDA or BLA," and that CMS "lacks the authority to aggregate different drug products approved under different NDAs or BLAs" as the same QSSD. AstraZeneca argues that QSSDs should be based on an NDA or BLA, not on active ingredients, because the IRA definition of QSSD references the definition of a "covered Part D drug" in the Medicare statute, which, in turn, references the definition of "covered outpatient drug" in the Medicaid statute, which is tied to a drug product's distinct NDA or BLA. The company further alleges that the effects of CMS's QSSD policy "will be felt across AstraZeneca's product portfolio," because the existing definition could subject a new Farxiga product to immediate price negotiation, if the product contains the same active ingredient as the original product. AstraZeneca also says that the QSSD definition is arbitrary and capricious because it "discourages" manufacturers from improving their existing products.

With respect to the bona fide marketing requirement, AstraZeneca claims that CMS's interpretation is contrary to the plain language of the IRA as well as arbitrary and capricious. The manufacturer argues that "[n]owhere in the law did Congress include qualifying language that might narrow or otherwise change the ordinary meaning of the word 'marketed.'" AstraZeneca describes the IRA's marketing requirement as a "check-the-box inquiry," and points to an existing Medicaid Drug Rebate Program policy that defines "marketed" by reference to when a product is available for sale. The company also argues that in *Asgrow Seed Co. v. Winterboer*, the Supreme Court found that the term marketing "ordinarily refers to the act of holding forth property for sale." AstraZeneca claims that CMS's "holistic" and "totality of the circumstances" inquiry is too subjective and as a result of CMS's bona fide marketing requirement, a product's price could be subject to negotiation while also being subject to generic competition.

Novo Nordisk's Arguments

Novo Nordisk takes a slightly different approach in its summary judgment motion, claiming that CMS exceeded its statutory authority in several ways, including by selecting more than 10 drugs for negotiation and by selecting QSSDs that have generic or biosimilar competition. The drug maker argues that by selecting six of its NovoLog and Fiasp products as a single QSSD, CMS violated the IRA's requirement that CMS select no more than 10 drugs for price year 2026. Similar to AstraZeneca, Novo Nordisk says that QSSDs should be based on each NDA or BLA, because FDA approvals and exclusivities are product specific, noting that the IRA "says nothing about active moieties or active ingredients."

The company also argues that CMS's focus on the active moiety, rather than a specific product, has led to the selection of both Part B and Part D drugs, in violation of the IRA, which provides that only Part D drugs may be selected for negotiation in 2026. The manufacturer points out that some of its Fiasp products are covered primarily under Part D, while others are covered primarily under Part B, but that CMS has included both types of products on the list of selected drugs. Novo also argues that the IRA's provision limiting administrative and judicial review should not apply, alleging that CMS's action is ultra vires under the APA (i.e., beyond its legal authority).

Government's Cross Motions for Summary Judgment

The government opposed the drug manufacturers' motions and filed cross motions for summary judgment in both cases, making both procedural and substantive arguments. The government first asserts that AstraZeneca lacks standing to bring the APA challenges, because the company did not demonstrate that the QSSD definition impacted Farxiga's selection. According to the government, Farxiga is manufactured under a single NDA and has one dosage form, two strengths, and no currently approved, generic competitors. Thus, the government says, AstraZeneca was not actually harmed by CMS's interpretation of the QSSD definition and lacks standing to challenge it.

The government next argues that the plain text of the IRA precludes judicial review of both AstraZeneca and Novo Nordisk's claims, including their ultra vires challenges. The government relies on several D.C. Circuit cases upholding provisions limiting judicial review in other parts of the Medicare statute, arguing that Congress's express preclusion of judicial review in the IRA makes the QSSD definition and the selection of drugs unreviewable. The government points to DCH Regional Medical Center v. Azar, where a hospital challenged a Medicare payment amount, but where the Medicare Act limited judicial review of "any estimate" the Secretary used to calculate the payment. The D.C. Circuit upheld a district court's dismissal of the case, finding that judicial review was precluded because the methodology HHS used to calculate the payment amount was "inextricably intwined" with the estimate itself. Even though the hospital argued that the action was reviewable under the APA as ultra vires, the court disagreed, finding that CMS's payment methodology was not an "obvious violation of a clear statutory command." The government makes similar arguments in its summary judgment motions against AstraZeneca and Novo Nordisk, arguing that because the statute precludes judicial review of the selection of drugs, the manufacturers' challenges to CMS's authority to "prescribe methodologies" for purposes of selection are "inextricably intwined" with the selection itself and thus should fail.

On the merits, the government argues in both cases that using active moieties and ingredients in the QSSD definition does not violate the IRA. In the government's view, a drug's particular NDA is irrelevant because the statute clearly states that CMS should use "aggregated data across multiple dosage forms and strengths," and directs CMS to apply the negotiated price across different forms and strengths of the drug. The government characterizes the manufacturers' interpretation of the data-aggregation provision as "nonsensical" and asserts that the Revised Guidance is not arbitrary or capricious because CMS reasonably explained its approach to the QSSD definition. The government claims that an NDA-based approach would violate the statute, because different dosage forms and strengths of a drug can be approved under multiple NDAs, depending on how the manufacturer applies for FDA approval. The government points to the statute's "repeated references to the possibility that a single negotiation-eligible drug would comprise multiple dosage forms, strengths, and formulations—and have multiple FDA approvals," and argues that these references "would make no sense if Congress had intended CMS to follow FDA's product-specific approach." The government further reasons that the QSSD definition ensures that drug manufacturers will not engage in "product hopping" as a way of avoiding negotiation, and that there is nothing arbitrary about a newly marketed product being subject to price negotiation.

With respect to Novo Nordisk's argument that the QSSD conflates Part B and Part D drugs in violation of the statute, the government says the statute "directs CMS to select drugs based on relative spending—and makes only Medicare Part D spending a relevant ranking criterion for price applicability years 2026 and 2027." In other words, the government says it is "immaterial" that the manufacturer's insulin drugs are reimbursed under both Parts B and D, because the "practical effect" of the statute is that Part B drugs are not selected for negotiation in price year 2026 unless they also have the highest Part D expenditures. The government argues NovoLog meets both criteria and thus that the drug is not exempted from selection simply because it also receives reimbursement under Part B.

Lastly, the government argues that CMS's bona fide marketing standard is consistent with the IRA. The government explains that the standard is needed to ensure that manufacturers cannot avoid the Negotiation Program by contracting with a generic competitor to launch a de minimus amount of a generic drug or biosimilar, thereby exempting it from the QSSD definition. The government also argues that the specific language of the IRA indicates that Congress intended for CMS to "exercise some judgment in applying the standard," and that the manufacturers' interpretation of the IRA would render the marketing requirement "meaningless." The government also disputes the relevance of other CMS interpretations of 'marketing' that the manufacturers assert lack a bona fide requirement, arguing that in those instances de minimis marketing was not a concern.

Considerations for Congress

As litigation over the Medicare Drug Price Negotiation continues to unfold, many observers are keeping a close eye on both the constitutional and APA arguments being made in the cases. Several of the manufacturers' arguments challenging CMS's guidance seem to raise larger questions, including how much leeway an agency should have to interpret a statute and how specific Congress needs to be when limiting judicial review or directing an agency to issue guidance. A variety of stakeholders and a few Members of Congress have expressed direct interest in the legal developments or have requested leave to file amicus briefs. Absent additional action from Congress, the outcome of the litigation may have a substantial impact on how effectively CMS will be able to carry out the program and uphold its stated goals of lowering drug prices for Medicare beneficiaries.

Chapter 4

Affordable Prescriptions Now: Examining Legislation to Lower Costs for Seniors*

Special Committee on Aging

Friday, July 1, 2022
Fayetteville, GA

The committee met, pursuant to notice, at 10:13 a.m., at Fayette Senior Services, 4 Center Drive, Fayetteville, Georgia, Hon. Raph- ael Warnock, Member of the Committee, presiding.

Present: Senator Warnock

Opening Statement of Senator Raphael Warnock, Member of the Committee

Senator WARNOCK. Good morning to everybody. Thank you so very much for being here. This U.S. Senate Special Committee on Aging field hearing here in the State of Georgia will come to order. The purpose of this hearing titled, Affordable Prescriptions Now, Examining Legislation To Lower Costs For Seniors, is to examine the urgent importance of lowering prescription drug costs for hard- working Georgia families, especially our senior citizens, and so I am glad to be here in Fayetteville today.

---

* This is an edited, reformatted and augmented version of Hearing Before the Special Committee on Aging, United States Senate, Serial No. 117–19, dated July 1, 2022.

In: Medicare's Prescription Drug Pricing
Editor: Lloyd M. Porter
ISBN: 979-8-89530-728-1

I want to acknowledge the presence of the Mayor. Mayor Johnson, thank you so very much for being here. Other officers and elected officials, thank you for hosting us for this important hearing. I want to thank the Fayette County Senior Services Center for hosting this important field hearing at their facility today, and I also want to thank the folks who are able to join us here in person and for the many folks who are watching us online.

As I travel around the State and as I talk to Georgians, one thing is clear, Georgians are doing our best to navigate a changing economy but are being crushed by the rising cost of prescription drugs. As a voice of Georgia in the U.S. Senate, I have been focused on pushing through legislation to lower costs on everything, from prescription drugs, to gas, to groceries, and seniors shouldn't have to choose between buying groceries and buying the drugs that they need, and so we are focused on this. We are also focused on holding corporations accountable for making record profits, record profits, right now, in the middle of the pandemic, record profits on the back of Georgians who have been paying record prices, the pain you feel and the profits that they are enjoying are connected, and you can't talk about one without the other, and so something I hear consistently from Georgians, especially seniors, is about how they are being squeezed by the high cost of prescription drugs and the burden it puts on their health and on their wallets. During a recent call with the Georgia AARP members, I heard from J.C. Irons, a senior citizen from Cherokee County, whose out-of-pocket costs for prescription drugs ranges from $4,000 to $7,500 per year.

He shared that since he is on a fixed income, he is often not able to buy all of the drugs prescribed to him. If you cannot afford your medication, then you don't have affordable health care now. Plain and simple, but this isn't just a Georgia problem, this is an issue that touches seniors all across our country.

The AARP says that the average older American takes 4.7 prescription drugs per month, typically on a chronic basis, and more than four in five seniors say drug costs are unreasonable. Additionally, nearly 25 percent of older Americans who take prescription drugs say it is difficult for them to afford their prescription drugs, including about one in ten who say it is, ''very difficult,'' very difficult in the evening of their lives and struggling with the costs of something that is very basic, so vital, and necessary, so this issue is personal for me. This is about something much bigger than politics. It is about my mother. You know, my mom is 84 years old, and I think about her, and people like her, and I think about the parishioners in my own church that I have counseled over the years who have had to deal with the consequences of rationing lifesaving medication like insulin because they couldn't afford it.

One of my seniors, who is in her 90's, a classmate and schoolmate of her childhood buddy M.L., they called him Martin Luther King Jr., texting me this morning. She texts in her 90's. Talking about the challenges of managing her health care, and so I am focused on fighting the good fight for her and for my mother and so many others. Focused on lowering prescription drug costs in the Senate, and so I am a proud member of the Aging committee.

I am glad to be chairing a field hearing in Georgia today, a first for our State, so it is a historic hearing we are having to explore this issue that I know is top of mind for many Georgians. This hearing will unpack the current challenges our seniors are facing brought on by high drug costs, and it will highlight benefits of lowering prescription drugs for all Georgians, but especially for seniors.

One of the major reasons we are here is that Georgia seniors can't keep waiting for Washington to take action. That is the message I took away from my visit to East Point's Oak Street Health Clinic back in May, where seniors told me about the stress that is being caused by high prescription drug costs.

I am looking forward to hearing from our witnesses today who will underscore why it is so very important that Congress take urgent action now to tackle this issue and lower prescription drug costs. I am also looking forward to exploring in this hearing what Washington can do in the short term and in the long term to lower drug costs for our seniors.

For my part, I am proud to be leading the charge with several legislative proposals to fix this critical issue, including some policies that we will discuss today, like capping out-of-pocket costs and allowing Medicare to negotiate drug prices. While the Affordable Care Act set an annual limit on out-of-pocket costs for people with private insurance, Medicare beneficiaries, which includes many, if not most of our seniors Georgians, currently lack that basic protection, can't negotiate the price.

What kind of capitalism is that, where you don't get to negotiate the price of something you are buying? According to the Kaiser Family Foundation, 1.2 million seniors face out-of-pocket drug costs of more than $2,000 in 2019. No senior citizens should have to choose between buying groceries and taking necessary medication, but today and as these statistics demonstrate, far too many seniors face an impossible choice.

That is why I support allowing Medicare to negotiate and bring down the cost of prescription drugs, and I am pushing my colleagues in Congress to make this happen. It is also why I introduced the Cap and Drug Cost for Seniors Act legislation to cap annual cost of—annual out-of-pocket costs for seniors at $2,000 for the entire year, and you may have heard I am also championing the Affordable Insulin Now Act that would cap the cost of insulin for seniors on Medicare, as well as individuals on private plans at $35 per month. That in a State where 12 percent of the adults have diabetes and $1 in $4 in our health care system is spent on people with diabetes, and so I am so glad to be holding this hearing today because we are closer than ever to getting critical legislation to lower drug costs across the finish line and I won't stop pushing until we get it done. I plan to use today's discussion to help move our efforts in Washington forward by underlining the importance of Congress taking urgent action right now on this issue in the very next work period when we return from the 4th of July.

That will be a good time to declare seniors' independence from incredibly high prescription drug costs. I look forward to hearing more from our witnesses on this very topic, and I thank you again for being here, Mayor and so many others, to share your experience and your expertise.

Before we begin, I want to remind the witnesses to please keep their remarks and questions to 5 minutes, something that the Senator did not manage to do——

The privilege of the chair. I am going to ask you to keep your remarks and your questions of 5 minutes, and I will turn to an introduction of our witnesses. I am pleased to introduce, first of all, Mr. Lee Baker, who served as the President of AARP, Georgia. I have a fine feeling for AARP.

A couple of years ago, my daughter, who is a toddler, she got an invitation to join a preschool. They, you know, they saw that it was her birthday, and they said, dear Chloe, we would like to invite you to our preschool, and I was turning 50, and in that same batch of mail, I got my invitation to join AARP—preschool AARP.

Mr. Baker is a graduate of Georgia Tech. He has been a tireless advocate for the aging population for over a decade. He has years of experience in financial resiliency and understands just how important it is for seniors to be able to afford their prescription drugs. Thank you, Mr. Baker. Thank you all for being here.

Thank you for your expertise. Our next witness is Ms. Elizabeth Ernst, State Director of Protect Our Care, Georgia. Protect Our Care is a national health organization that works to find ways to make health care more affordable and accessible.

Ms. Ernst has been working as an advocate for various patient, consumer rights, and environmental protection issues important to Americans for 15 years and has been a strong voice for improving access to health care in our

State. Thank you so very much, Ms. Ernst, for being here. Next—well, here is the test, Dr. Keerthi Gogineni. Okay?

Dr. GOGINENI. Yes, I recognize that name.

Senator WARNOCK. A dual provider in both oncology and hem tology. She works with patients at Grady, a safety net hospital in Atlanta, and thank God for Grady, and Emory University Hospital as well. Dr. Gogineni has firsthand experience in seeing how exorbitant prescription drug costs lead to difficult choices for patients and compromises their ability to get treatment.

As a breast oncologist, she has guided patients through a complex maze of treatment options, and as an associate professor, she has taught residents and fellows about health policy issues affecting oncology. Thank you so very much, Dr. Gogineni, for being with us today and sharing your expertise with the committee, and then finally, last but not least, our next witness is Ms. Gretchen Spring from Marietta.

Ms. Spring spent the last 6 years as a caregiver for her late husband, Peter, who lost his battle with Alzheimer's disease earlier this year. Prayers and strength to you.

Ms. SPRING. Yes. Thank you.

Senator WARNOCK. She will share the stress and the burden that she and Peter faced just to purchase the prescription drugs they needed. Ms. Spring and Peter had to max out their credit cards and take out personal loans for food so they could afford their medications, but I will allow her to tell her own story. We now turn to our witnesses for their statements, and we will begin with Mr. Baker.

Statement of Lee Baker, CFP, Past President, AARP Georgia, Atlanta, Georgia

Mr. BAKER. Thank you, Senator. AARP, on behalf of our 38 million members across the country, including over 1 million members right here in Georgia, and all older Americans nationwide, appreciates the opportunity to submit testimony on this important hearing and historic hearing of the Senate Aging committee.

High prescription drug prices hit older Americans particularly hard. On average, Medicare Part D enrollees take between four and five prescriptions per month, often for chronic conditions that will require treatment for the rest of their lives. At the same time, Medicare beneficiaries have a median annual income of just under $30,000. One-quarter have less than $8,500 in savings.

Here in Georgia, the average annual cost of prescription drug treatment increased 26.3 percent between 2015 and 2019, while the annual income of Georgia residents only increased by about 18 percent. This population simply does not have the resources to absorb rapidly escalating prescription drug prices, and many are facing the reality of having to choose between their medications and rising prices for other basic needs, like food and housing.

In the case of one of our other members here in Georgia, Eleanor, someone in her late 60's, she spends about $200 each time she refills her glaucoma eyedrops. She is able to get by for now, but she wonders what is going to happen if she needs any other prescription medications in the future. Unfortunately, Eleanor isn't alone. We know that the No. 1 reason someone does not fill their prescription is the cost.

For years, prescription drug prices—increases have dwarfed even the highest rates of general inflation. If consumer prices had risen as fast as drug prices over the last 15 years, gas would actually be about $12 a gallon. Milk would be $13 a gallon. Just in January, the drug industry raised prices on over 800 prescription medications, just as they have increased prices for decades, including three-fourths of the top 100 drugs with the highest spending in Medicare Part D.

AARP is mindful that high and growing prescription drug prices are affecting all Americans in some way. Their high cost is passed along to everyone with health coverage through increased health care premiums, higher deductibles, and other forms of cost sharing. We have also seen massive increases in prescription drug spending under public programs like Medicare and Medicaid.

These escalating costs will eventually affect all of us in one form or another through higher health care costs, higher taxes, cuts to Medicare or Medicaid, or some combination of all of the above. In other words, every single American taxpayer is paying for higher prescription drug prices regardless of whether or not you are taking medicine yourself. Fortunately, there is action that the Senate can take right now, and we hope they do when they get back from the 4th of July break.

There is long, longstanding and overwhelming bipartisan support among voters for allowing Medicare to negotiate with drug companies for lower prices. The policies before the Senate, that Senator Warnock is leading on, including Medicare negotiation, as he mentioned, capping out-of-pocket costs on the Medicare Part D, and for insulin, and penalizing drug companies that increase their prices faster than the general rate of inflation will provide long overdue relief to older Americans across the country.

These policies, taken together, will help reduce drug prices and out-of-pocket costs. This is important because real relief for seniors and all Americans must include policies that get to the root of the problem, the high prices set by drug companies. America's seniors aren't the only ones who stand to benefit.

Lowering prescription drug prices will also save the Medicare program and taxpayers hundreds of billions of dollars every year. Medicare spends more than $135 billion on prescription drugs. Nationally, we have survey data that shows that the vast majority of older adults support each proposed measure being discussed in Congress to reduce drug prices.

The most favored initiative was allowing Medicare to negotiate for drug prices, winning over 87 percent of older adults. Seventy- eight percent support putting a cap on out-of-pocket costs that older adults pay for their prescription drugs under Medicare Part D. Clearly, Americans are fed up with paying three times what people in other countries pay for the same drugs.

More than 4 million people across the country, including over 92,000 here in Georgia, signed a petition to demand lower prices for prescription drugs. There will never be a better time than now, this historic opportunity in front of Congress. Now is the time to get it done.

Senator WARNOCK. Thank you so very much for your testimony, Mr. Baker. Ms. Ernst, you may begin.

Statement of Elizabeth Ernst, State Director, Protect Our Care Georgia, Atlanta, Georgia

Ms. ERNST. Thank you so much, Senator Warnock, and thank you for your leadership and for inviting Protect Our Care to submit testimony on the importance of lowering prescription drug costs for our seniors. Seniors are at the center of America's drug pricing crisis. As many as one in four seniors nationwide struggle to afford prescription drugs, with higher rates among more vulnerable groups, including low income, people of color, and those in poor health.

Yolanda H. is a 70 year old diabetic living in Albany. As she is in the Medicare donut hole, she is charged $300 for each of her three diabetes medications. That is $900 a month for a senior who lives solely on her Social

Security income. She rations her life saving medicines so she can eat or pay other living expenses, and as a result, she has experienced vision loss, kidney compromise, and painful neuropathy, and unfortunately, Yolanda isn't alone. In 2017, 32 percent of Georgia residents reported they stopped taking medications as prescribed due to cost, and every day, drugmakers exploit our broken health care system by hiking the prices of lifesaving medications in order to make record breaking profits.

Between 2019 and 2020, half of all drugs covered by Medicare Part D had price increases equal to or greater than the rate of inflation, and a 2020 congressional report traced the steep price hikes of the cancer drug Revlimid to the desire of executives to meet company revenue goals and shareholder earning targets.

In Georgia, this drug price rose 44 percent from 2015 to 2020. This extraordinary corporate greed has serious consequences on our public—our nation's public health. A recent study found that increasing out-of-pocket drug costs by only $10 created a 33 percent increase in mortality due to a decrease in medicine accessibility.

This is a distressing choice that Eustacia from Marietta is all too familiar with. She is a 64 year old Air Force—retired Air Force veteran who struggles not only with her high prescription drug costs not covered by her VA plan, but also for her 80 year old mother who was on Medicare. When her mother drug prices increased, Eustacia and her sisters pooled their money together to pay for her drugs.

She worries about what will happen as her and her mother's drug costs continue to rise when they are both on fixed incomes. It is really a cruel game Georgia's seniors and their families are forced to play all as a result of corporate greed, and yet research shows that drug companies could lose $1 trillion in sales and still be the most profitable industry. Skyrocketing prescription drug prices are affecting all Georgians, not just seniors.

In recent years, Georgia residents and their insurers have spent more on prescription drugs and for out of pocket medicines than most States in the U.S. We have also seen massive increases in prescription drug spending under Medicare and Medicaid. Not only are Georgia taxpayers bearing these price hikes, these high costs are also passed along to everyone with health insurance through increased premiums, increased deductibles, and the like, and simply put, every single Georgia—Georgian is paying for high prescription drug costs regardless of who is taking the medications, and that is a hard pill to swallow. The problem is only going to get worse without intervention. The policies

Senator Warnock has championed will provide immediate relief to all Americans.

Under his Affordable Insulin Now Act, which caps patients out of cost insulin—out of pocket insulin cost at $35 a month under Medicare and private plans, seniors like Yolanda will be able to afford her life saving medications without compromising a basic quality of life, and by reducing out-of-pocket costs under Medicaid Part D through Senator Warnock's Capping Drug Costs for Seniors Act families like you Eustacia's will not have to face the possibility of making the choice of which family members stay healthy and which can't.

Coupled with his Medicaid Save Lives Act and the Medicare drug pricing negotiation proposals before the Senate, these critical bills attack the high prices set by the pharmaceutical industry. Americans are sick and tired of paying these high, exorbitant drug prices, and as the country continues to recover from the economic and health crisis brought upon by the pandemic, American families can no longer afford to wait.

We ask that Congress seize this opportunity to lower prescription drug prices through these popular policies. The time for fair, affordable drug pricing is now. Thank you.

Senator WARNOCK. Thank you so very much, Ms. Ernst. Dr. Gogineni?

Statement of Keerthi Gogineni, MD, MSHP, Associate Professor Hematology-Oncology, Emory University School of Medicine, Atlanta, Georgia

Dr. GOGINENI. Thank you. Hello, everyone. Thank you, Senator Warnock, for inviting me to speak today about the importance of lowering prescription drug costs for our Nation's seniors. I am an Associate Professor of Hematology and Medical Oncology at Emory University School of Medicine.

I began taking care of patients with cancer 15 years ago, and now specialize in the care of patients with breast cancer at Grady Memorial Hospital and Emory Winship Cancer Institute. As a general disclaimer, please understand that these views I am about to share are my own opinions and not that of my employer. There has been thrilling progress in the field of oncology.

New drugs offer greater chances of cure and enable us to tell a patient with incurable cancer that they can live for years despite a metastatic diagnosis. Increasingly, the latest targeted agents are pills, which is a huge advance for patients' quality of life. To not be hooked up to IV chemotherapy multiple times a month is game changing, but the optimism afforded by new oral drugs has been countered by the astounding price tags that accompany these medications, and that is why passing legislation like your Capping Prescription Costs Act is so important for everyday Americans seeking quality care. The patients I take care of come from many different walks of life, but no matter their socioeconomic background, the strain a cancer diagnosis places on a patient and their household is profound. In addition to the physical and emotional toll, at least half struggle with the financial toxicity of the diagnosis.

The impact on patients living in rural areas, and on black and Hispanic patients is even greater. According to the CDC, one in three Americans experiences financial burdens due to necessary medical care. This burden is even more striking for cancer patients who have greater out-of-pocket costs for lifesaving care. Half of Medicare beneficiaries with cancer spend at least a 10th of their income toward out-of-pocket treatment costs, including prescription drugs. Keep in mind, the average age of a patient diagnosed with cancer is 66.

Many, therefore, will be on Medicare. There is a spiral that begins with diagnosis. Treatment often means patients have to work less, which means less income and depletion of savings, which in turn affects their ability to afford treatment. The monthly costs of these drugs force patients to make impossible decisions between being able to get their medication versus paying for rent versus paying their electric bills.

High out-of-pocket costs associated with novel anti-cancer drugs prolong the time it takes to start therapy and compromise the ability to stay on therapy, and ultimately staying on a drug affects whether a patient's cancer stabilizes or progresses. People who get diagnosed with cancer are 2.65 times more likely to declare personal bankruptcy.

Horrifyingly, patients who declared bankruptcy had a 79 percent greater risk of dying compared to the cancer patients who did not have to declare bankruptcy. Mrs. X was first diagnosed with breast cancer in 2012 and thought she was cured. Unfortunately, her cancer came back 10 years later.

When she came to see me in February, her metastatic breast cancer was getting worse on her current treatment. Although she had stage four disease, Mrs. X still had options that could prolong her life by years with hopefully minimal side effects. I prescribed two oral drugs called Exemestane and a drug called Afinitor or Everolimus. When she followed up in March, a month later, she shared that she would not been able to start the Afinator because it was too expensive.

Without insurance, this drug would have cost $6,000 a month. Now, Mrs. X had insurance. In fact, she would been employed by the Federal Government. Her insurance required her use of the generic version of the drug. However, the monthly co-pay would still amount to $1,450, absolutely unaffordable, especially for seniors who are typically on a fixed income.

We tried to get her access to a manufacturers assistance program, but to qualify, she had to be prescribed the branded drug. Her insurance repeatedly denied permission to do so, despite us explaining in a series of appeals that the generic drug was still unaffordable and that the branded drug would enable access to copay assistance. Her social worker applied for support from three different foundations, but funds had dried up.

Finally, we were able to get a patient assistance program to supply her drug through this December. It took 4 months of effort, from the patient to a dedicated pharmacist, and social worker to get a patient with health insurance onto a standard of care regimen for her metastatic breast cancer.

This is one patient's story. Multiply this by the nearly 1.9 million Americans diagnosed with cancer each year. Many of our patients with cancer are seniors. Given the soaring costs of oral anti-cancer therapy, lowering prescription drug costs is literally lifesaving. It is difficult enough for a person to receive a cancer diagnosis, but to then realize promising treatments are out of reach because they are unaffordable, is devastating.

This is why Senator Warnock's Capping Drug Costs for Seniors Act is so critical. On behalf of our patients and my colleagues, I thank you for your time and help.

Senator WARNOCK. Thank you so much for your expertise and care of so many patients and for your statement this morning, and now, Ms. Spring, you may begin.

Statement of Gretchen Spring, Caregiver, Marietta, Georgia

Ms. SPRING. Senator Warnock, thank you for having me here today to speak about my experience with expensive prescription drugs. My experience is, unfortunately — [technical problems.] My name is Gretchen Spring, and I am a proud resident of Marietta, Georgia. I am a widow and a retired caregiver. In 2016, my husband Peter was diagnosed with Alzheimer's by a neuropsychiatrist. During my 6 years of being the caregiver, I had to keep as active as possible, or my husband would have passed away 1 year or 2 years prior than he did. On April 7th of this year, after almost 17 years—thank you—

of marriage, the love of my life passed away. Yesterday would have been our 17th anniversary. His condition had required him to use many different medications, 11 total. He was on Eliquis for heart condition and Namenda to slow down the process of Alzheimer's.

We were paying an arm and a leg for Eliquis and Namenda. Spending $250 to $300 a month per medication and that was with insurance. I was even on a first name basis with everybody at the pharmacy. We were in our golden years, but the only people that were seeing gold were the pharmaceutical companies, and this is in addition to the costs of my own prescriptions.

The cost was overwhelming. Peter and I had Part D coverage through Medicare Advantage plans, but my husband's medication broke the bank. We are talking about $800 to $1,000 out of pocket every month. With 15 prescriptions between the two of us, we would easily spend at least $12,000 a year. I loved Peter dearly and I did everything I could to keep him healthy.

When he was diagnosed with Alzheimer's, he had to leave the workforce and I started my fourth career as caregiver, which played havoc on our finances, but at the same time, it was also important to me to listen to our doctors about our health. That meant putting the costs of our medications on credit cards, sometimes maxing our limits, and the last thing a senior citizen wants is — on a fixed income, is using a credit card with 21 to 28 percent interest.

Due to my husband's expensive prescription drugs, we also had to delay making needed updates to make our home more comfortable, and sometimes we had to make difficult decisions about purchasing basic essentials like groceries. At one point, we even reached out to family members about setting up a Go Fund Me page because of the strain on our finances.

It was only because of the generosity—of friends' generosity and our pension funds that we didn't go into debt. We went through $60,000 of pension money. Addressing the high costs of prescriptions is an issue that is personal to me. My husband has passed, but there are many, so many seniors and families in our State who are struggling to afford lifesaving medications. Let me be clear, we don't have a choice when it comes to prescriptions.

It is simply wrong and unethical that seniors are faced with these decisions. Senator Warnock, your leadership on this issue means a lot for you Capping Drug Costs for Seniors Act, which would cap out of pocket cost of $2,000 per year for people on Medicare—would have made all the difference for my husband and I.

I am a proud 74, and it is with your continued support on lowering costs, that I am looking forward to 75 with more reasonable prescription costs. In closing, it is past time Congress addresses high prescription drug costs, and I am just one of many with the story about struggling with the affordable medications.

Thank you again for the opportunity to speak with you today. I look forward to addressing any questions you may have.

Senator WARNOCK. Thank you so very much of Ms. Spring, and again, prayers and strength to you. Thank you for your statement and thanks to all of our witnesses. I want to begin now a round of questions, and I am going to ask everyone to just take a second and check and make sure your phone is on silent as we proceed with the questions.

There are over 1 million AARP members in the State of Georgia, and many of these members are struggling to afford their prescription drug costs. Even with Medicare Part D, seniors face high out- of-pocket costs, and that is unacceptable. Mr. Baker, can you talk about the difficulties that AARP members right here in Georgia experience when trying to afford their medications?

Mr. BAKER. Yes, it is one of those things that candidly is heart wrenching. We would get calls, and with technology, some of those calls that would go into our State office would funnel to my laptop or my cell phone, and I hear calls from seniors saying we simply need help.

As Senator Warnock mentioned the last 10 to 12 years doing this work with AARP at that same time as trustee, chair of our church, and Senator Warnock, very familiar with the situation where members come to a place where they feel they can get help, and so frequently, Sunday afternoons after service, we are back in the finance room trying to figure out how we can help somebody that is now in a situation where they can't help themselves. It is an incredible strain, particularly on the seniors here in Georgia. It is a strain on their families, you know, caregivers.

We are sitting here now with two people that are or have recently been caregivers on this panel this morning. It is a strain. The strain of being a caregiver leaks over into other aspects of your life. They are stressed, and so they begin taking medication, so it is a bit of a domino effect.

As I mentioned earlier in the testimony, you may not be taking medication, but you are affected. Right now, I don't take any medications right now, other people in my home do, and we have had those stories. One of my children is allergic to fish, and getting an EpiPen is not an enjoyable experience, and sometimes it is challenging to even get it, and so the ability to navigate the system, particularly for our seniors, when you don't have the support system in place to help you argue, if you will, at the pharmacy, to navigate, if I use this program, can I use that program, it is incredibly difficult, and some people simply throw up their hands and they shouldn't have to do that.

Senator WARNOCK. What are some things that Congress could do that would directly help your members, AARP?

Mr. BAKER. One of the biggest things—and I am happy that we heard a little bit of news yesterday, as I understand it, that through the reconciliation process, it appears that perhaps we are going to get some movement on allowing Medicare to negotiate prescription drug prices.

Again, as you mentioned early on—you know, in my day job, I am a financial advisor. I help people grow and keep their wealth, so I have no problems with a capitalist society, but as you said, what kind of capitalism is it that does not allow me to negotiate the price and that is a problem, so if there is any one big thing at AARP that we support to help this, that could bring about relief literally in the span of, I guess, the next 18 months, is allowing Medicare to negotiate prices, and so again, we fully support that, and I would say immediately and really big impact, that is the one.

Senator WARNOCK. I agree with that, which is why I am pushing to get us to be able to negotiate the costs or Medicare to be able to negotiate the cost of prescription drugs, as the VA currently does. In addition to that, capping the cost of insulin and capping the cost of prescription drugs.

In all of your testimony today, all of you have made clear that our health care system is failing patients, and even for those with insurance, like Medicare Part D, as you point out Dr. Gogineni, prescription drugs can be out of reach due to the high out-of-pocket costs, so Dr. Gogineni, could you share with us what you experienced as a provider when your patients cannot afford their medication and how that can literally affect their health outcomes? Can you say more about that?

Dr. GOGINENI. Sure. Thank you for the question. You feel like you are failing—sure—I, you know, I pride myself on being able to talk to a patient about their diagnosis and options for treatment with compassion, and I really want to be able to inject hope into that process, and I want to be able to tell folks that we are going to be able to give you the most effective drug we can for what you are going through.

I don't want to have to tell people I can't get you that drug because it is simply not affordable even though you have insurance, and so it is devastating. I mean, people are already under a great deal of strain from the diagnosis and then trying to cope around coming up with a plan for how they are going to manage this and then to have to spend the energy and the time, and it is a full time job trying to get access to some of these medications, and without a doubt, you know, your ability to start something on time and how that stabilizes a cancer, and if you can't get the drug, you can't— you can't control that cancer, and people suffer from the side effects of what that cancer is causing and the strain of knowing that they are waiting to get started.

You know, people are very motivated to get treated and invested in getting better, and to not be able to empower them to actually do that is not what I set out to do.

Senator WARNOCK. Sure. Sure, and in your testimony, you spoke about how it took 4 months for a patient with metastatic breast cancer—?

Dr. GOGINENI. Yes.

Senator WARNOCK To get the care that she needed, and it was only through your persistence and other colleagues that you were finally able to get medication. Meanwhile, the disease is not waiting, right, so can you talk about some of the other hoops that you as a provider have had to jump through just to give financial assistance to your patients?

Dr. GOGINENI. Yes. I think we were educated in school about how to make a diagnosis and how to treat people. We were not educated to navigate the maze of the financial system around treatment. I am really lucky that I have staff that work with me, like the pharmacists and like the social workers, to try to do everything we can to get access for affordable medication, but it does not mean that happens overnight. Frequently, there are processes where we are trying to secure less costly drug assistance programs, foundations, and you can't necessarily do those things in parallel. You have to sort of get denied by one and then you go on to the next one, so this process, in terms of the time it takes, accumulates and all the while this person is sitting there untreated, and it is not often that medications in cancer are interchangeable. There is a hierarchy of what works best and what works less well, so the idea of substituting for something that's less effective is just—you know, when someone has a limited amount of time, and you are trying to make the most of that time, it is you really want to give them the best shot possible without having to compromise.

Senator WARNOCK. Thank you so much for your answer. Health care access and affordability, as you point out, go hand in hand. If you can't afford it, you can't access it, and it doesn't matter if they are some of the best and most effective medications on the market if patients are not able to afford them.

One drug that treats cancer costs over $1,000 per day, according to the AARP. Ms. Ernst, how bad are the health care access and affordability challenges facing Georgia families and seniors? How bad is it out there?

Ms. ERNST. Thank you for that question, and it is pretty bad. I mean, I think that we have heard a lot of stories, and these are just a few that we can all share about how difficult it is, and I think we know from research that patients with high out-of-pocket drug costs often are more likely to avoid treatment, abandoned treatment, or interrupt treatment, and this leads to worse health care outcomes.

I spoke about Yolanda in my opening remarks, and where she has rationing her diabetes medication, which she needs to stay alive, and as a result, she was experiencing vision loss and kidney compromise, but one part of that story that I didn't share is that, as a result of the worry and the stress of struggling to stay alive, and either through getting her medications or being able to eat or house herself, she developed terrible depression and anxiety as a result, and from that, you know, to get treatment, the mental health treatment she needs costs more money, so it is just, the cycle—the cycle of violence continues, all because she could not get her insulin and her diabetes medication, and it is—so it is a domino effect that we are seeing, and as you share, it is personal. With Gretchen, it is personal. I think everyone in this room has a story about a family member or a community member or a neighbor about how high drug costs are affecting our health outcomes. We see people in pain. We see people forgoing treatment.

Doctors are put in a terrible position of either having to prescribe a different form of a medication that might not be as effective, but it is cost effective for the patient, so the patient just continues with like, you know—not as an effective form of treatment. That has happened to a gentleman, Alex, where he couldn't afford his asthma medication and ends up losing his voice and having major lung complications, so you know, it affects us all and it is something that we can do something about. Everyone is eager to make this happen, and we appreciate, from Protect Our Care, your willingness to take this issue head on, and——

Senator WARNOCK. How would a provision like capping the costs of seniors to no more than $2,000 per year impact the folks that you are seeing on the ground here in Georgia?

Ms. ERNST. Well, I think Yolanda would be able to survive and not have painful nerve damage, and she wouldn't develop depression and anxiety, so she could take care of her grandchildren.

She could be an active member of the community. Also, too, it saves taxpayers a tremendous amount of money. One thing that we haven't talked about is how a lot of times patients don't know the cost of those drugs until it is time to fill them. Pharmacies fill them. They don't pay for them. They go unclaimed, and then that just gets absorbed by the entire health care system, and then everyone in this room is paying for those high prescription drug costs in our premiums and our deductibles, so that is—those are just a couple of examples.

Senator WARNOCK. So all of us have a stake in lowering the cost of prescription drugs?

Ms. ERNST. Absolutely. Absolutely.

Senator WARNOCK. I am always deeply appreciative when folks can share their personal stories in a forum like this, and that is why I am so glad that Gretchen Spring is here, that we can hear directly from you and your voices in the conversation.

Can you say a little bit more? You talked about the care you had to provide to your husband, Peter, and your marriage of nearly 17 years, but I do think it is important sometimes to put a human face on the public policy we would make or fail to make. Can you say just a little bit more about Peter?

Ms. SPRING. Wow. You got a couple days?

Senator WARNOCK. No, but we have a couple of minutes though.

Ms. SPRING. Okay——

Senator WARNOCK. Tell me—and tell me about some of the challenges he faced. You know, what were some of the medical and health challenges he faced that required prescription drugs as you were navigating your way—?

Ms. SPRING. Okay. I am sorry to say, Senator Warnock, I cannot do that. I never knew I could live with somebody 24/7 and enjoy their company as much as I did it, and it ended up being a godsend for me. Peter was a very affectionate person. He was a very humorous person. His humor put a smile on my face every day.

The trauma for me came in the last year because all of a sudden he became more of a child, and the stressful part was the fact that he couldn't take care of himself—of going to the bathroom. He was on depends. I was having to change the beds every day, and that, you know—and there is nothing, there are no prescriptions to stop that at all, and you just have to write it out. The reason he ended up in the condition is because of affordability. He stopped taking his drugs because he couldn't afford them, and it wasn't until I stepped in and started taking over all the finances that I understood more of what was going on with prescription drugs.

Senator WARNOCK. In addition to the stresses of care, you had the stress of the cost of care?

Ms. SPRING. Yes—I mean, I was taking care of an adult child, and that adult child was not going to grow up. End of story, and that is the reality of it. I even—and. I hate to admit this, but I smoke because that was my tranquilizer, because I knew if I took tranquilizers, they would put me to sleep because I am very susceptible to that medication. I was on antidepressants.

You know, I did request our primary care doctor. Fortunately for me, we had a primary care doctor that we were seeing every 3 months that was making sure that the medications we were on were right. She was working hand in hand with the cardiologist. The cardiologist, primary care doctor were working hand in hand with the pharmacist. I mean, yes——

Senator WARNOCK. So you are managing all of these things and costs at the same time and—thank you so much for sharing your deeply personal story and helping to put a human face on this issue.

It is clear from the testimony today that lowering prescription drug costs for seniors will have an immediate and a lasting impact on the lives of everyday people, and I am glad that there is clear bipartisan movement right now to addressing this issue, and I will keep fighting until we get something done. That said, we also need to make it clear that this is an urgent matter that needs to be addressed expeditiously.

As we close, I would like to ask each of you to take this opportunity, each of our witnesses, to speak more broadly about the importance of lowering prescription drug prices right now, even here in Fayetteville, Georgia. We are on the official record. This is a congressional hearing, and in just a couple of minutes, would you tell us what you would like to say to Congress about the importance of addressing this issue of the cost of prescription drugs for seniors? We will start again with Mr. Baker.

Mr. BAKER. Senator Warnock, and everyone here, particularly you, Senator Warnock, I hope you will forgive me or allow me a little bit of poetic license and say to yourself and other Members of Congress why we can't wait. We can't wait because we are in the midst of a longevity revolution.

People are going to live longer and longer, and in most instances, be taking medication for an extended period of time. The reason we can't wait is because we have got a whole lot of things coming at us. We have got inflation. We are paying more at the pump. We are paying more at the grocery store and having to make those choices, and there is no other relief in sight. We can't wait, frankly, because it is unjust to have to hear Gretchen's story. That is it.

Senator WARNOCK. Thank you. Thank you so much. Ms. Ernst. Ms. ERNST. Thank you for that question, and I think it is something that we on this panel too say time and time again, day in and day out, we cannot wait because people are dying. People are getting sicker.

We are disrupting families and costing everyone more for lower quality of care, all because of prescription drug costs. It is just been unregulated—or not negotiated, and the time is now. We see the need. The benefit is great, and the proposals on the table are solid and popular and the time is now, and let's not wait any longer.

Senator WARNOCK. Thank you so much. Dr. Gogineni.

Dr. GOGINENI. Yes. Thank you. No one plans to get cancer, and we have had this revolution in new drugs and novel treatments, but it is meaningless if people can't access this. The strain of a diagnosis and treatment is tough enough without then having to navigate trying to actually be able to afford drugs that are life-saving.

This is why it is absolutely critical that Medicare be able to negotiate for drug prices. It is critical for patients to be able to have a cap on those annual drug costs, and we are asking for people to have access to available treatment, and I think that—I mean, this is fundamentally a human right, and I think we need to catch up on the legislative side.

Senator WARNOCK. Thank you so much. Finally, Ms. Spring.

Ms. SPRING. I personally feel like we are in the dark ages when it comes to our prescription drugs because they are so expensive. They don't need to be that way. They really don't, you know. No one, you know—I mean, at one point I was going to set up a Go Fund Me just to pay for our prescriptions, and it is like, that is not fair to me and that is not fair to anybody else, you know. It is like you said, we—like all of you said, we should be able to live a healthy life and it be—not be so outrageously expensive.

Senator WARNOCK. Thank you. I want to thank all of our witnesses today for contributing your time, your expertise, and also your deep experience with this issue. It is unacceptable that in our country, one of the richest in the world, seniors are making impossible decisions about whether or not to pay for lifesaving medication or other basic essentials.

No one should be forced to choose between affording their medication and putting food on the table, but these decisions are all too real for Georgia seniors. Their testimony from—the testimony from our witnesses today has shown how important it is that Congress acts, and acts on this issue right now.

I am glad that we could bring together voices from our great State on this issue, from Dr. Gogineni, a provider at a safety net hospital, Grady in Atlanta, to Mr. Baker, a leader with the AARP, to Ms. Ernst, a strong advocate for improving access to affordable health care, to Gretchen Spring, and whose testimony was especially powerful, thank you. I will keep your words, especially with me, as we continue this fight in the Senate. No one should be forced with the decisions that Ms. Spring and her husband faced, but unfortunately, that will continue to be the reality of our country if we do not do something about it, and that is what I am pushing us to do in the Senate. We don't have time to wait. We can't wait.

To our witnesses, thank you so very much for your advocacy. Thank you so very much for your stories. Stories I will keep in mind as I work to lower the cost of prescription drugs, and thank all of you for participating today.

I see that there are members of our General Assembly who are here, other elected officials, and those who serve in law enforcement, and just concerned citizens. It is great to be in Fayetteville for this important hearing.

Thanks, everybody. This concludes the hearing. [Whereupon, at 11:15 a.m., the hearing was adjourned.]

Appendix: Prepared Witness Statements

AARP Statement for the Record for the United States Senate Special Committee on Aging Field Hearing on Affordable Prescriptions Now: Examining Legislation to Lower Costs for Seniors July 1, 2022 Fayetteville, Georgia[#]

Lee Baker
Past President, AARP Georgia

AARP, on behalf of our 38 million members, including over one million members in Georgia, and all older Americans nationwide, appreciates the opportunity to submit testimony on this important hearing of the Senate Aging Committee.

High prescription drug prices hit older Americans particularly hard. On average, Medicare Part D enrollees take between four and five prescriptions per month, often for chronic conditions that will require treatment for the rest of their lives. At the same time, Medicare beneficiaries have a median annual

[#] For further information contact: Glen W. Fewkes Health Care Access and Affordability Government Affairs gfewkes@aarp.org.

income of just under $30,000. One-quarter have less than $8,500 in savings. In Georgia, the average annual cost of prescription drug treatment increased 26.3% between 2015 and 2019, while the annual income for Georgia residents only increased 18.8%. This population simply does not have the resources to absorb rapidly escalating prescription drug prices and many are facing the reality of having to choose between their medications and rising prices for other basic needs such as food or housing.

In the case of one of our members here in Georgia, Eleanor B (late 60s) spends about $200 each time she refills her glaucoma eye drop prescription (Travatan Z). She is able to get by for now, but she wonders what will happen if she needs any other prescription medications in the future. Unfortunately, Eleanor isn't alone. We know the number one reason someone does not fill a prescription is because of the cost.

For years, prescription drug price increases have dwarfed even the highest rates of general inflation. If consumer prices had risen as fast as drug prices over the last 15 years, gas would now cost $12.20 a gallon, and milk would be $13 a gallon. Just in January, the drug industry raised prices on over 800 prescription medications—just as they have increased prices for decades—including three-quarters of the top 100 drugs with the highest spending in Medicare Part D.

AARP is mindful that high and growing prescription drug prices are affecting all Americans in some way. Their high cost is passed along to everyone with health coverage through increased health care premiums, deductibles, and other forms of cost-sharing. We have also seen massive increases in prescription drug spending under public programs like Medicare and Medicaid.

These escalating costs will eventually affect all of us in the form of higher health care costs, higher taxes, cuts to Medicare or Medicaid, or all of the above.

In other words: every single American taxpayer is paying for high prescription drug prices, regardless of whether you are taking medicine yourself.

Fortunately, there is action the Senate can take right now. There is long-standing and overwhelming bipartisan support among voters for allowing Medicare to negotiate with drug companies for lower prices. The policies before the Senate that Senator Warnock is leading on – including Medicare negotiation, capping out of pocket costs under Medicare Part D and for insulin, and penalizing drug companies that increase their prices faster than inflation – will provide long-overdue relief to older Americans across the country.

These policies, taken together, will help reduce drug prices and out-of-pocket costs. This is important because real relief for seniors and all Americans must include policies that get to the root of the problem: the high prices set by drug companies.

America's seniors aren't the only ones who stand to benefit. Lowering prescription drug prices will also save the Medicare program and taxpayers hundreds of billions of dollars. Every year, Medicare spends more than $135 billion on prescription drugs.

In December 2020, a survey commissioned by AARP Georgia and conducted by the bipartisan team of Fabrizio Ward and Hart Research Associates showed Georgians across the aisle agree on the need for affordable medication and action by their members of Congress. An overwhelming majority of Georgians over age 50 – regardless of party – agree: they are more likely to support a Senate candidate who advocates to allow Medicare to negotiate with drug companies (Republicans 93%, Democrats 94%).

Nationally, our survey data also show that vast majorities of older adults support each proposed measure being discussed in Congress to reduce drug prices. The most favored initiative was allowing Medicare to negotiate for the price of drugs, winning over 87% of older adults; 78% support putting a cap on out-of-pocket costs that older adults pay for their prescription drugs under Medicare Part D; and 71% support penalizing drug companies that raise their prices faster than inflation. Furthermore, 80% of older Americans surveyed believe that drug prices can be lowered without affecting innovation.

Clearly, Americans are fed up with paying three times what people in other countries pay for the same drugs. More than four million people across the country, including over 92,000 here in Georgia, signed a petition to demand lower prices for prescription drugs. There will never be a better time to lower drug prices than the historic opportunity in front of Congress. Now it's time to get it done! Thank you again to the Special Aging Committee for holding this hearing in Georgia, and to Senator Warnock for inviting us here to raise awareness about this critical issue.

Testimony to the Senate Special Committee on Aging Hearing: Affordable Prescriptions Now: Examining Legislation to Lower Costs for Seniors Statement of Liz Ernst, State Director, Protect Our Care Georgia

Senator Warnock, thank you for your leadership and for inviting Protect Our Care to submit testimony on the importance of lowering prescription drug costs for our seniors.

Seniors are at the center of America's drug pricing crisis. As many as one in four seniors nationwide struggle to afford prescription drugs, with higher rates among more vulnerable groups, including low-income, people of color, and those in poor health.[1]

Yolande H. is a 70 year old diabetic living in Albany, Georgia. As she is in the Medicare "donut hole", she is charged $300 for each of her three diabetes medications —that's $900 a month for a senior who lives solely on her Social Security income. She rations her life-saving medicines so she can eat or pay other living expenses. As a result, she's experienced vision loss, kidney compromise, and painful neuropathy.

Unfortunately, Yolande isn't alone. In 2017, 32 percent of Georgia residents reported that they stopped taking medication as prescribed due to cost.[2]

Every day, drugmakers exploit our broken health care system by hiking the prices of life saving medicines in order to make record breaking profits. Between 2019 and 2020, half of all drugs covered by Medicare Part D had price increases equal to or greater than the rate of inflation.[3] A 2020 congressional report traced the steep price hikes of the cancer drug Revlimid to the desire of executives to "meet company revenue targets and shareholder

---

[1] Ashley Kirzinger, Tricia Neuman, Juliette Cubanski, Mollyann Brodie, "Data Note: Prescription Drugs and Older Adults," KFF (August 9, 2019), accessed on June 28, 2022, https://www.kff.org/health-reform/issue-brief/data-note-prescription-drugs-and-older-adults/.

[2] "How Georgia Residents Are Impacted By High Rx Costs," AARP (2021), accessed on June 28, 2022, https://www.aarp.org/content/dam/aarp/politics/advocacy/2019/09/rx-state-info graphic-three-issues- georgia.pdf.

[3] Juliette Cubanski, Tricia Neuman, "Prices Increased Faster Than Inflation for Half of All Drugs Covered by Medicare in 2020," KFF (February 25, 2022), accessed on June 28, 2022, https://www.kff.org/medicare/issue-brief/price-increases-continue-to-outpace-inflation-for-many-medicare- part-d-drugs/.

earnings goals."[4] In Georgia, Revlimid's price rose 44 percent from 2015 to 2020.[5]

This extraordinary corporate greed has serious consequences for our nation's public health. A recent study found that increasing out-of-pocket drug costs by only $10 dollars created a 33 percent increase in mortality, due to a decrease in medication accessibility.[6]

his is the distressing choice Eustacia M. from Marietta, Georgia is all too familiar with. Eustacia is a 64 year old, retired Air Force veteran, who struggles not only with her own high prescription drug costs not covered by her VA plan but also for her 80 year old mother, who is on Medicare. When her mother's drug costs increase, Eustacia and her sisters pool their money to pay for them. She worries about what will happen as both her and her mother's drug costs continue to rise when they are both on fixed incomes.

It's a cruel game Georgia seniors and their families are forced to play — all as a result of corporate greed. Yet, research shows that drug companies could lose $1 trillion in sales and still be the most profitable industry.[7]

Sky rocketing prescription drug prices are affecting all Georgians, not just seniors. In recent years, Georgia residents and their insurers have spent more on prescription drugs and for out- of-pocket medicines than most states in the U.S.[8] We have also seen massive increases in prescription drug spending under Medicare and Medicaid.[9] Not only are Georgia taxpayers bearing these price hikes, these high costs are also passed along to everyone with health insurance through increased premiums, deductibles and the like. Simply put, every single Georgian is paying for high prescription drug prices, regardless of who is taking the medications.

---

[4] U.S. Congress, House, Committee on Oversight and Reform, *Drug Pricing Investigation, Celgene and Bristol Myers Squibb-Revlimid.* 116th Cong. H.R. rpt. No.116-122, at i (2020) (staff report), accessed June 28, 2022, https://oversight.house.gov/sites/democrats.oversight.house.gov/files/Celgene%20BMS%20Staff%20Rep ort%2009-30-2020.pdf.

[5] Leigh Purvis,Stephen W. Schondelmeyer, "Rx PriceWatch Reports," AARP Public Policy Institute, accessed June 28, 2022, https://doi.org/10.26419/ppi.00073.000.

[6] Amitabh Chandra, Evan Flack, and Ziad Obermeyer, "The Health Costs of Cost-Sharing," National Bureau of Economic Research (February 2021), accessed June 28, 2022, https://doi.org/10.3386/w28439.

[7] Jeromie Ballreich, Sean Dickson, "How Much Can Pharma Lose?:A Comparison of Returns Between Pharmaceutical and Other Industries", West Health Policy Center (2019), 10, accessed June 28, 2022, https://s8637.pcdn.co/wp-content/uploads/2019/11/WHPC_White-Paper_How-Much-Can-Pharma- Lose_FINAL-November-2019.pdf.

[8] Beau Evans, The Staggering Cost of Prescription Drugs in Georgia," *State Affairs,* August 24, 2021, accessed June 28, 2022, https://stateaffairs.com/GA/44-the-staggering-cost-of-prescription-drugs-in- georgia.

[9] Ibid.

The problem is only going to get worse without intervention. The policies Senator Warnock is championing will provide immediate relief to all Americans. Under his Affordable Insulin Now Act, which caps patients' out-of-pocket insulin costs at $35 a month under Medicare and private plans, seniors like Yolande would be able to afford her life saving medications without compromising a basic quality of life. By reducing out-of-pocket costs under Medicare Part D through Senator Warnock's Capping Drug Costs for Seniors Act, families like Eustacia's would not have to face the possibility of making the choice of which family members can remain healthy and which ones can't. Coupled with his Medicaid Saves Lives Act and the Medicare drug pricing negotiation proposals before the Senate, these critical bills attack the root of the problem: the high prices set by the pharmaceutical industry.

Americans are sick and tired of paying three times the amount that people in other countries pay for the same drugs. As the country recovers from the economic and health crisis brought about by the COVID-19 pandemic, American families can no longer afford to wait. We ask that Congress seize the opportunity to lower prescription drug prices through these popular policies. The time for fair, affordable drug prices is now.

Keerthi Gogineni, MD, MSHP, Associate Professor Hematology-Oncology, Emory University School of Medicine Testimony to the Senate Special Committee on Aging Hearing: Affordable Prescriptions Now: Examining Legislation to Lower Costs for Seniors

Hello everyone,

Thank you Senator Warnock for inviting me to speak today about the importance of lowering prescription drug costs for our nation's seniors. I'm an Associate Professor of Hematology and Medical Oncology at Emory University's School of Medicine. I began taking care of patients with cancer fifteen years ago and now specialize in the care of patients with breast cancer at Grady Memorial Hospital and the Emory Winship Cancer Institute.

As a general disclaimer, please understand that these views I'm about to share are my own opinions and not that of my employer.

There's been thrilling progress in the field of oncology. New drugs offer greater chances of cure and enable us to tell a patient with incurable cancer they can live for years, despite a metastatic diagnosis. Increasingly, the latest targeted agents are pills- which is a huge advance for patients' quality of life. To not be hooked up to IV chemotherapy multiple times a month is game changing. But the optimism afforded by new oral drugs has been countered by the astounding price tags that accompany these medications. That's why passing legislation like Senator Warnock's Capping Prescription Costs Act is so important for everyday Americans seeking quality care.

The patients I take care of come from many different walks of life.

But no matter their socioeconomic background, the strain a cancer diagnosis places on a patient and their household is profound. In addition to the physical and emotional toll, at least half struggle with the financial toxicity of the diagnosis. The impact on patients living in rural areas, and our Black and Hispanic patients is even greater.

According to the CDC, one in three Americans experiences financial burdens due to necessary medical care. This burden's even more striking for cancer patients, who have greater out of pocket costs for life-saving care. Half of Medicare beneficiaries with cancer spend at least a 10th of their income towards out-of-pocket treatment costs, including prescription drugs. Keep in mind, the average age of a patient diagnosed with cancer is 66. Many will therefore, be on Medicare.

There's a spiral that begins with diagnosis. Treatment often means patients have to work less, which means less income and depletion of savings, which in turn affects their ability to afford treatment. The monthly costs of these drugs force patients to make impossible decisions between being able to get their medication vs paying for rent vs paying their electric bills. High out-of-pocket costs associated with novel anticancer drugs prolong the time it takes to start therapy and compromise the ability to stay on therapy. Ultimately, staying on drug affects whether a patient's cancer stabilizes or progresses.

People who get diagnosed with cancer are 2.65 times more likely to declare personal bankruptcy. Horrifyingly, patients who declared bankruptcy had a 79% greater risk of dying compared to cancer patients who did not have to declare bankruptcy.

Mrs. X was first diagnosed with breast cancer in 2012 and thought she was cured. Unfortunately, her cancer came back 10 years later. When she came to see me in February, her metastatic breast cancer was getting worse on her current treatment. Although she had Stage IV disease, Mrs. X still had options that could prolong her life by years with hopefully minimal side effects. I prescribed two oral drugs - Exemestane and a drug called Afinitor or

Everolimus. When she followed-up in March, she shared that she'd not been able to start the Afinitor because it was too expensive.

Without insurance, the drug would have cost $6000 a month. Now, Mrs. X had insurance. In fact, she'd been employed by the federal government. Her insurance required use of the generic version of the drug. However, the monthly copay would still amount to $1450- absolutely unaffordable, especially for seniors who are typically on a fixed income.

We tried to get her access to a manufacturer's assistance program, but to qualify, she had to be prescribed the branded drug. Her insurance repeatedly denied permission to do so, despite us explaining in a series of appeals that the generic drug was still unaffordable and that the branded drug would enable access to copay assistance. Our social worker applied for support from three different foundations, but funds had dried up. Finally, we were finally able to get a patient assistance program to supply her drug through December. It took four months of effort from the patient, a dedicated pharmacist and social worker to get a patient with health insurance onto a standard of care regimen for her metastatic breast cancer.

This is one patient's story. Multiply this by the nearly 1.9 million Americans diagnosed with cancer each year.

Many of our patients with cancer are seniors. Given the soaring costs of oral anti-cancer therapy, lowering prescription drug costs is literally life-saving. It's difficult enough for a person to receive a cancer diagnosis. But to then realize promising treatments are out of reach because they're unaffordable is devastating. That's why Senator Warnock's Capping Drug Costs for Seniors Act is so critical. On behalf of our patients and my colleagues, I thank you for your time and help.

Testimony of Gretchen Spring Senate Committee on Aging Affordable Prescriptions Now: Examining Legislation to Lower Costs for Seniors July 1, 2022

Senator Warnock, thank you for having me here today to speak about my experience with expensive prescription drugs. My experience is unfortunately all too common.

My name is Gretchen Spring. I am a proud 74 years old and I'm a resident of Marietta, GA. Presently, I am a widow and retired caregiver. In 2016 my husband, Peter, was diagnosed with Alzheimer's disease by a neuropsychiatrist. During my 6 years of being a caregiver, I had to keep us as active as possible or my husband, my best friend, would have passed away a year or two sooner.

On April 7 of this year, after almost 17 years of marriage, the love of my life passed after reaching Stage 7 of Alzheimer's disease. In fact, yesterday would have marked our 17th anniversary.

His condition had required him to use many different medications – 11 total. He was on Eliquis for a heart condition and Namenda, a medication to slow down the process of Alzheimer's disease. We were paying an arm and a leg for Eliquis and Namenda, spending $250 to $300 a month per medication— and that was with insurance. I was even on a first name basis with everyone at the Pharmacy due to my weekly visits. We were in our Golden Years but the only people that were seeing gold were the pharmaceutical companies.

And this was in addition to the costs for my own prescription drugs. I take four different prescriptions, and in addition to my husband's 11 medications—the cost was overwhelming.

Peter and I had Part D coverage through a Medicare Advantage plan, but my husband's medications broke the bank. We're talking about $800 to $1,000 out of pocket every month. With 15 prescriptions between the two of us, we would easily spend at least $12,000 in a year on medication alone.

I loved Peter dearly and I did what I could to keep him healthy. When he was diagnosed with Alzheimer's, he had to leave the work force and I started my fourth career as caregiver, which played havoc in our finances. But at the same time, it was also important to me to listen to our doctors about our health. That meant putting the cost of our medications on our credit cards, sometimes maxing out our limits. And the last thing a senior citizen with a fixed income wants is to use the credit cards with 21-28 percent interest rates.

Due to my husband's expensive prescription drugs, we also had to delay making needed updates to make our home more comfortable to live in, and sometimes had to make difficult decisions about purchasing basic essentials, like groceries. At one point, we even reached out to family members about setting up a GoFundMe page because of the strain on our finances. It was only because of a friend's generosity and our pension funds that we didn't go into debt - and we went through $60,000 of pension money.

As my testimony today demonstrates, addressing the high cost of prescription drugs is an issue that is personal to me. My husband has passed, but there are so many seniors and families in our state who are struggling to afford life-saving medications. Let me be clear – we don't have a choice when it comes to prescription drugs. It is simply wrong and unethical that seniors are faced with these decisions.

Senator Warnock, your leadership on this issue means a lot. Your Capping Drug Costs for Seniors Act, which would cap out-of-pocket costs at $2,000 per year for people on Medicare, would have made all the difference for my husband and me. I am a proud 74 year old and it's with your continued support on lowering costs that I'm looking forward to 75 with more reasonable prescriptions costs.

In closing, it is past time that Congress addresses high prescription drug costs, and I am just one of many with a story about struggling to afford medications. Thank you again for the opportunity to speak with you today. I look forward to answering any questions you may have.

Index

Q

R

S

T

U

V

W

Y